Foundations of
Language Development
A Multidisciplinary Approach
Volume 2

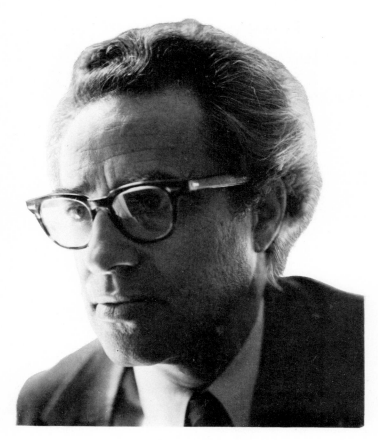

Eric Lenneberg: 1921–1975

Foundations of Language Development

A Multidisciplinary Approach

Volume 2

Edited by

Eric H. Lenneberg

Elizabeth Lenneberg

Department of Psychology
and Department of
Neurobiology and Behavior
Cornell University
Ithaca, New York

ACADEMIC PRESS   New York San Francisco London   1975
A Subsidiary of Harcourt Brace Jovanovich, Publishers

THE UNESCO PRESS   Paris

First published 1975 by THE UNESCO PRESS,
7 Place de Fontenoy, 75700 Paris, France and
ACADEMIC PRESS INC., 111 Fifth Avenue, New York, NY 10003

United Kingdom Edition published by
ACADEMIC PRESS, INC. (LONDON) LTD.
24/28 Oval Road, London NW1

Library of Congress Cataloging in Publication Data
Main entry under title:

Foundations of language development.

   (Unesco symposium)
   Result of the 1968 Symposium on Brain Research and
Human Behaviour, held in Paris.
   Includes bibliographies and index.
   1.   Children—Language—Addresses, essays, lectures.
2.   Languages—Psychology—Addresses, essays, lectures.
3.   Speech, Disorders of—Addresses, essays, lectures.
4.   Writing—Addresses, essays, lectures.
I.   Lenneberg, Eric H.   II.   Lenneberg, Elizabeth.
III.   Symposium on Brain Research and Human Behaviour,
Paris, 1968.   IV.   Title.   V.   Series: United Nations
Educational, Scientific and Cultural Organization.
Unesco symposium.   [DNLM: 1.   Language development—
Congresses.   2.   Language disorders—Congresses.   LB11
LB1139.L3 S989f 1968]
P118.F6   401'.9   74-27784
ISBN 0—12—443702—8 (v. 2) (Academic Press, Inc.)
ISBN 92—3—101313—0 (v. 2) (The Unesco Press)

Eric H. Lenneberg

While these volumes were in the final stages of preparation, Eric Lenneberg died suddenly in White Plains, N.Y., on May 31, 1975. He was a man of boundless intellectual curiosity whose theoretical and integrative skills were without parallel in the study of language, brain, and behavior. Although he is most widely known for his pioneering work on the biological foundations of human language, his ultimate concern was the study of the mind and brain, the problem he was working on just prior to his death. He was the first to propose, in the late fifties, that the human capacity for language can be explained only on the basis of biological properties of man's brain and vocal tract, a point of view that has since been widely accepted and elaborated upon. His experiments and views were summarized in the groundbreaking book, *Biological Foundations of Language*, published in 1967.

Eric Lenneberg was born in Germany on September 19, 1921 and lived there for the first twelve years of his life. In 1933 he emigrated with his parents to Brazil. Seeking broader educational experience, he came to the United States in 1945. After one year's service in the United States Army he entered the University of Chicago in 1947, receiving a B.A. in 1949 and an M.A. degree in linguistics in 1951. He obtained his Ph.D. from Harvard University in 1955 in both psychology and linguistics, and subsequently accepted a post-doctoral fellowship in medical sciences at Harvard Medical School with further specialization in neurology and children's developmental disorders.

From 1959 to 1967 he held faculty positions at Harvard and Massachusetts Institute of Technology while conducting basic research on language development in defective children at the Children's Hospital Medical Center in Boston. From 1967 to 1968 he was Professor of Psychology at the University of Michigan, and in 1968 he accepted an appointment as Professor of Psychology and Neurobiology at Cornell University, which he held to his death. He was the recipient of numerous scholarships, fellowships, and academic honors, including Russell Sage and Guggenheim fellowships and a National Institute of Health Career Award. He was married twice and had two children by his first wife.

Eric Lenneberg, because of his meticulous preparation in several disciplines, was able to bring to the study of language development a new perspective. He brought together the necessary developmental biological evidence in support of his hypothesis that language is a central, maturationally defined mental function which is relatively independent of learning, that "language is the manifestation of species-specific cognitive propensities." This has never been a particularly popular thesis for an empirical psychology, and the recent growth of interest in the language potential of other primates is a typical example of the conflict his theory was to encounter. Nonetheless, research in a wide range of areas related to language pathology, including speech defects, mental retardation, dyslexia, aphasia, and most importantly, deafness, demonstrates the indirect but lasting influence of his work. His application of the biological concept of critical or sensitive periods to the study of language remains a unique and powerful contribution to developmental psycholinguistics.

More fundamentally, Eric Lenneberg's conception of human behavior was different from that held by most research psychologists. Though sometimes called a "nativist," he believed the continuing debate over innate versus environmental factors in human behavior was irrelevant. Behavior for him was "but the outward manifestation of physiological and anatomical interactions under the impact of environmental stimulation." This is a point of view more congenial to biology than psychology, but one certainly destined to become increasingly important in the study of human behavior. His conception of the brain was that of a highly integrated organ constantly changing over time according to certain epigenetic trajectories. Therefore, information-processing or man-machine models of cognitive functioning were of limited value to him because they ignored the fourth dimension of time. He believed that man's functional activity cannot be separated from structural changes in the human brain.

For those of us who knew him, his unique preparation and the creative nature of his intellect made him an extraordinary colleague and teacher. We all gained immeasurably from contact with this courageous and profound thinker. It is to his memory that this volume is dedicated.

Eric R. Brown
New York University

Contents

III. Language in the Clinic

13. Speech Disorders in Childhood

T. T. S. Ingram

14. Language Development in the Absence of Expressive Speech

A. J. Fourcin
With an Introduction By Richard Boydell

15. Mental Subnormality and Language Development

Joanna Ryan

16. Language Development in Malnourished Children

Antonio B. Lefèvre

List of Contributors

Numbers in parentheses indicate the pages on which the authors' contributions begin.

Evelyn Abberton (157), Department of Phonetics and Linguistics, University College London, London, England

Edna Adelson (177), Child Development Project and Department of Psychiatry, University of Michigan Medical Center, Ann Arbor, Michigan

J. de Ajuriaguerra (311), Psychiatric Clinic, University of Geneva, Geneva, Switzerland

M. Auzias (311), National Institute of Health and Medical Research, Paris, France

E. Bay (21), Department of Neurology, University of Düsseldorf, Düsseldorf, Germany

Macdonald Critchley (361), Institute of Neurology, London, England

A. J. Fourcin (157, 263), Department of Phonetics and Linguistics, University College London, London, England

Selma Fraiberg (177), Child Development Project and Department of Psychiatry, University of Michigan Medical Center, Ann Arbor, Michigan

D. B. Fry (137), Department of Phonetics and Linguistics, University College London, London, England

Hans Furth (167), Center for Research in Thinking and Language, Catholic University of America, Washington, D. C.

Henry Hécaen (117), École Pratique des Hautes Études, Paris, France

T. T. S. Ingram (195), Department of Child Life and Health, University of Edinburgh, Edinburgh, Scotland

Marcel Kinsbourne (107), Department of Pediatrics, The Hospital for Sick Children, Toronto, and Department of Psychology, University of Waterloo, Waterloo, Ontario, Canada

Antonio B. Lefèvre (279), Department of Neuro-Psychiatry, School of Medicine, University of São Paulo, São Paulo, Brasil

Eric H. Lenneberg (17), Department of Psychology and Department of Neuro-biology and Behavior, Cornell University, Ithaca, New York

A. R. Luria (49), Department of Psychology, University of Moscow, Moscow, USSR

Susan U. Philips (367), Department of Anthropology, The University of Arizona, Tucson, Arizona

J. B. de Quirós (297), Faculty of Sciences of Human Recuperation. U.M.S.A., and Medical Center of Phoniatric and Audiological Research, Buenos Aires, Argentina

Charles Read (329), Department of English, University of Wisconsin, Madison, Wisconsin

André Roch Lecours (75), Faculty of Medicine, University of Montreal, Montreal, Canada and Faculty of Medicine, University of Paris, Paris, France.

Joanna Ryan (269), Unit for Research on Medical Applications of Psychology, University of Cambridge, Cambridge, England

Orlando L. Schrager (297), Medical Center of Phoniatric and Audiological Research, Buenos Aires, Argentina

Frank Smith (347), Ontario Institute for Studies in Education, Toronto, Ontario, Canada

L. S. Tsvetkova (31), Department of Psychology, University of Moscow, Moscow, USSR

E. Weigl (383), Berlin, Germany, DDR.

James Youniss (167), Center for Research in Thinking and Language, Catholic University of America, Washington, D. C.

O. L. Zangwill (95), The Psychological Laboratory, University of Cambridge, Cambridge, England

Foreword

Foundations of Language Development is a specialized two-volume publication resulting from the 1968 Symposium on Brain Research and Human Behaviour convened by UNESCO in cooperation with the International Brain Research Organization (IBRO) in order to focus attention on the growing importance of brain research in modern society and to demonstrate the relationship between brain research and education, social sciences, and communication. Ambassador Carlos Chagas, the Brazilian Permanent Delegate to UNESCO, chaired the international organizing committee for the symposium, and his leadership extended to most of the ensuing activities, including the preparation of these two volumes. This work attempts to bring together the results of different kinds of studies relevant to the application of brain research to problems in education and more particularly to the problem of language learning in both normal children and handicapped and socioculturally deprived children.

The UNESCO Secretariat was fortunate in securing as editor the late Professor Eric H. Lenneberg of Cornell University, U.S.A., who, with the untiring cooperation of his wife, arranged for the contributions of many eminent specialists in the various research areas. Further, since the problems involved affect a great many people having no specialized background, a version for the layman is being prepared by Dr. Charles P. Bouton of Simon Frazer University, Canada. This will provide facts and advice that parents, medical practitioners, and educators should find of great practical value in attempting to solve problems concerning remedial training in language acquisition in individual cases.

Both publications represent a major contribution to the Anthropology and Language Science in Educational Development (ALSED) programs which UNESCO launched in 1973 with the publication of a collection of papers "Anthropology and language science in educational development" (*Educational Studies and Documents Series No. 11*, Paris, UNESCO, 1973).

UNESCO wishes to express its thanks to the editors, advisors, and contributors to these two volumes on behalf of all those involved in the practical problems of remedial training in language acquisition.

The opinions expressed do not necessarily reflect the views of UNESCO.

Preface

The intention of these two volumes is to bring current viewpoints to the fore and to give an idea of the latest thinking in various areas; it is not an attempt to survey fields, and was not to be used by the contributing authors as a forum to argue any particular case. The book provides many a summary statement on the most recent, important discoveries and issues in the area of language development. Thus it is clear that these volumes will be useful particularly to those who are faced with practical decisions concerning language, including national language policy, language in the classroom, and language rehabilitation.

It is also important to point out that this book is a cooperative and international effort, in keeping with the UNESCO mandate. In these circumstances, the functions of the editors are different from those of an editor of an anthology or of conference proceedings. Particularly, the editors must insure proper representation rather than exercise selectivity according to their own convictions.

We should like to take this opportunity to express our thanks to Albert Legrand, who has helped us with many an editorial and translation problem, to Anton Burgers, whose frequent aid in administrative matters has been invaluable, to Adriano Buzzati-Traverso for his wise guidance and continuing interest in the project, to the advisory and editorial committees for help with the initial planning, and lastly, but most importantly, to Carlos Chagas, who conceived of the original plan for this book, who actively promoted the first stages of the drafting of its contents, and who has since then been our steadfast sponsor, adviser, and friend.

Eric and Elizabeth Lenneberg

Contents of Volume 1

I. Aphasiology

The neurological clinic provides an important source of information on the biological nature of language. Brain disease constitutes nature's own experiments on function. It is often said that psychologists ought to try first to understand normal function before they try to explain what happens to a patient with an illness. This is a shortsighted view. Before we can explain anything, we must know what it is that we wish to explain. The chapters in this section have been included not to describe or explain disease per se, but to highlight the dimensions of the neurological correlates of language. All of the contributors to this section are united by a common article of faith. Disease does not elaborate on normal patterns—does not add complexity—but can only empoverish the normal state of affairs, that is, strip a system of some of its fine detail or disturb a subtle balance. Thus disease "employs a method" of eliminating one or more factors from a well-integrated totality. The outcome is not necessarily a set of undisturbed factors minus one; the elimination may bring about distortions of the system as a whole (or in some instances even leave the system surprisingly undisturbed). But even so, a systematic study of the consequences of disease enables us to piece together a set of connections that would not even have been guessed at had our observations been confined entirely to behavior of the intact organism. It is well to keep in mind that the aphasia-producing condition plays a role similar to the experimentally placed lesion in the brain of an animal.

The chapters of this section are relevant to aphasiology, but must not be regarded as a coherent treatment of the subject. Each author chose a particular topic that he deemed relevant to our more general topic of language development. In some instances, the connection may be more obvious than in others. However, in all cases, the material presented and the theoretical discussions are also interesting in their own right.

1

1. In Search of a Dynamic Theory of Aphasia[1]

Eric H. Lenneberg

The main issues of controversy in aphasiology are briefly analyzed; they are attributed to the difficulties of objective psychological examination of the aphasic patient and to controversies in the ancillary fields of neurology, psychology, and linguistics. Symptoms are sketched out, and the nature of aphasiological evidence is reviewed critically. Special emphasis is placed on the importance of age of the patient at time of lesioning and on the rate of development of the lesion; "neurolinguistic" theories must be able to account not only for the deficits encountered in adult patients with stroke or trauma, but also (a) for the sparing of language functions in certain critical lesions, (b) for the difference in prognosis between juvenile and adult patients, and (c) for the differences in symptomatology among embryological deficits, slowly developing lesions, and fast developing lesions. It is suggested that more satisfactory language theories may emerge from the study of recent formal models in nonequilibrium thermodynamics.

Aphasiology

If one reads the current publications on aphasia from both sides of the Atlantic, one quickly discovers that there are major disagreements with respect to both facts and interpretation. This is true of descriptions of the function and structure of the brain, of physiological facts, of language itself; it is true even of the claims

---

[1] This chapter is a slightly revised version of a paper that appeared in *Daedalus* (1973, *102* [No. 3]) entitled "Comments on the neurology of language."

as to what older authors are supposed to have said or believed. Take, for example, basic views on the general nature of brain function. In this country, there is a tendency to take the computer analogy very literally, engendering a picture of the brain as a collection of more or less independent apparatus interconnected by cables. Personally, I find it hard to reconcile myself with the view that the sensory projection areas in the cerebral cortex should be the localities where "percepts are received;" that cortical association areas should be the "workshops in which percepts are glued together;" that Broca's area (left frontal cortex) should be the "machine that is responsible for the spoken word;" and that Wernicke's area (left temporal cortex) should "convert the raw sounds into perceived speech." There are neurologists whose discussions sound as if cortical loci were "offices" in which decisions are made about specific behavior and where that behavior is programmed and executed. If the communication lines between the "offices" are disrupted, the respective types of behavior are thought to run off independently from one another but are postulated to be otherwise undisturbed. In formulations of this sort, the layman has a hard time separating anatomical facts from highly speculative and sometimes wholly uncorroborated assumptions.

It is true that the brain shows a high degree of anatomical topographical differentiation and specialization that is unparalleled by any other organ. Most of the anatomical facts are beyond dispute today; but not so the "meaning" and function of the structural detail that we can discriminate in the gross or under the microscope. The best example of this is the cerebellum, whose anatomy has been fully worked out but whose function still presents more unsolved than solved problems. When it comes to the cerebral fiber tracts, especially the transcortical ones, there is still disagreement on many basic questions such as, in certain cases, even the direction of flow of impulses. It is very far from clear whether the principal interaction between cortical areas proceeds horizontally across the cortex, or vertically through subcortical relays. At present there is evidence for both, and we must remember that one possibility does not exclude the other. The diagrams that some "neurolinguists" draw, showing cortical centers for various types of language behavior interconnected by directional arrows, are fairly speculative. Moreover, there are logical difficulties in postulating brain centers that are exclusively in charge of specific types of behavior and that operate more or less independently as suborgans. No brain centers comparable in independence to those postulated for language in man have ever been demonstrated in other mammalian cortex. Functional autonomy of brain centers is also unlikely because all nervous tissue is forever active, and the anatomical connectivity of the cortex and the brain as a whole is such that a change in activity in one part of the brain is likely to influence activity in all those parts of the brain to which it is connected. This consideration, which has been particularly stressed by clinical neurologists in Europe (Conrad, 1954; von Monakow, 1914, von Weizsäcker, 1950), leads, however, to explanations of brain function that are quite different from the "behavioral-centers-and-connections" model. Instead of hypothesizing that a lesion has the effect of simply knocking out a particular neuronal component and its correlated specific function, leaving other components and their functions intact, this point of view would put it that a lesion deforms the normal pattern of interaction of a whole network of activities; it therefore does not merely eliminate one capacity from a roster of capacities, but deforms or alters physiological function on a broader base. This would be reflected in behavioral disturbances that could not be pinpointed or characterized in terms of the traditionally accepted psychological processes (arithmetic ability, writing, speaking, pattern perception, etc.), but would be likely to cause aberrations in the performance of a whole variety of tasks, usually affecting some a bit more than others, depending on the location and nature of the lesion.

It would seem that this sort of controversy might easily be settled by empirical investigation of what *actually* happens to patients with brain lesions. Unfortunately, this is not so; in fact, we find neurologists of equal standing and with the same kind of practical experience reporting almost shockingly different findings, including conflicting clinicopathological correlations. In the United States, Geschwind (1965) has argued most persuasively that the lesioned patient's behavior is quite predictable and that it is therefore possible to construct a detailed typology of aphasic symptoms. He has stressed that it is at least theoretically possible to account for every aspect of behavioral deficit by the specific location of one or more lesions. To emphasize the importance of postulated centers and their anatomical connections, he speaks of the resulting constellations of symptoms as disconnection syndromes. It is, however, important to realize that the elicitation of clinical symptoms and their theoretical interpretation is beset with practical problems. What types of tests are to be used? Do patients form sufficiently homogeneous populations to allow test results to be evaluated by sample statistics? Can test results be expressed as numbers and then be used for arithmetic operations? Are naturalistic observations preferable to formal testing, or should one use a combination of these techniques? There is controversy over every one of these questions and many more. It is therefore not so surprising that we often find neurologists unwilling to accept typologies proposed by others. For example, Bay (1967), an aphasiologist of the highest repute in Europe, has argued just as persuasively as Geschwind that any kind of subclassification of the aphasic syndrome is dangerous, and that the fine detail of a particular patient's disabilities, though of theoretical interest, is of no localizing value in the clinic. A position somewhere between those of Geschwind and Bay is that of Luria (1966), who has probably studied more patients with traumatic aphasia than anyone else in the world.

If there are differences in the fields of neurophysiology and neuroanatomy relevant to language, there are even more pronounced disagreements with respect to the psychological interpretation of normal and abnormal language behavior. Here we are faced with the Pavlovians, whose basic behavioral unit is the reflex; the American behaviorists, who postulate associative bonds; the Freudians, with their depth-psychological interpretation; and the Gestaltists, who are concerned with overall patterns. This does not exhaust the possibilities, but will suffice to show

how basic convictions, articles of faith, and often even the investigator's emotions are likely to affect theorizing in this troubled field.

The early aphasiologists did not bother much about the science of linguistics. The medical men simply assumed that the nature of language was something intuitively obvious, and the symptoms they described reflected their naive approach to language. They thought they could discern productive or receptive interference with speech sounds, with words (sometimes subclassified by the traditional parts of speech), with intonation patterns, and with sentences. Some neurologists attributed each of these symptoms to lesions in specific loci (almost as if nature had studied Latin grammar before designing man's brain). Gradually, modern linguistics has begun to exert an influence upon aphasiology, so that now symptoms are often interpreted in terms of particular schools of thought in modern linguistics. But the field of linguistics itself has many divergent points of view, so the increase in sophistication in the analysis of language aberration has brought along a further source of differences in opinion and interpretation of facts. Modern grammarians, particularly those of the Chomsky school, have brought to light a great number of regularities in the way sentences are normally understood and constructed, most of which had not been described before and of which no native speaker had been aware. Students of aphasia have been rightly fascinated by these endeavors, but they have frequently failed to see that only certain aspects of grammatical theory are relevant to aphasia or to the study of the brain mechanisms of language. Generative grammar proposes, for example, certain orders in the application of specified rules of grammar. It might be tempting to see whether these orders correspond to any psychobiological order. Do they reflect physiological events that occur in the course of sentence production or sentence interpretation? Or do they reflect psychological levels of complexity? Unfortunately, from a biological or even a psychological point of view, the linguists' conceptual armamentarium is a somewhat mixed collection. Take, for instance, the rules discussed by Chomsky (1965).[2] These were not intended as physiological or even psychological rules; yet some of them may, perhaps, suggest the existence of some biological process, whereas others are biologically entirely uninterpretable. Branching rules, for example, and their order of application could not conceivably have any physiological correlate whatever. On the other hand, there is, perhaps, some plausibility to the suggestion that transformations that map deep structure onto surface structure have at least a very rough psychological counterpart, namely the changes that take place when an idea or a sentiment is crystallized into a verbal utterance. But even here, we are actually distorting the exact meaning of the grammatical theoretical constructs, and reference to syntactic transformation in the context of psychology or physiology is justifiable only as metaphor.

Apart from the various factions of transformational grammarians, there are

---

[2] Categorial rules, context-free and context-sensitive rewriting rules, branching rules, projection rules, phonological and syntactic redundancy rules, selectional rules, context-free and context-sensitive subcategorization rules, transformational rules, rules of agreement, and others.

several other types of linguistic theory, each one likely to suggest different kinds of observations and tests on the patient. As long as there is such an appalling lack of agreement on theories that relate language to brain function and anatomy, the diversification of linguistic inquiries is likely to prove an *embarras de choix* to aphasiology, rather than an aid.

We have said enough to indicate the many sources of divergent points of view, biases, and articles of faith that turn aphasiology into the confusing and often contradictory field that it is.

SYMPTOMATOLOGY

The traditional source material for aphasiology has been the symptomatology of neocortical lesions in adult patients. Other types of evidence have become available during the last 30 years and will be discussed in the next section. Since it is not my purpose here to evaluate the many different classificatory schemes and their respective theoretical positions, I shall confine myself to a brief discussion of three major types of interference with language performance that are beyond controversy (leaving out the disturbances of articulation and many minor clinical syndromes). The three types may be called (1) *interference with production*, (2) *interference with language knowledge*, and (3) *interference with word finding*.

1. The only interference with production to be discussed here is called Broca's aphasia. The patient can usually read, can often write, using the left (unparalyzed) hand, and can answer questions appropriately by nodding his head or by giving short answers to questions. He gives every evidence that he understands language well and that he knows what he wants to say, but he has great difficulty controlling the motor coordination of the speech muscles (although they are not paralyzed; he can eat and drink without difficulty). The production of every word seems to require inordinate concentration and effort. There are long pauses between words, and every sound comes out slowly and laboriously. Apparently, the strain of speaking is so great that the patient confines himself to the barest minimum of words, resulting in a so-called telegraphic style. Some patients learn to say some few words with relatively greater ease, and make no attempts (or seem unable) to enlarge their oral vocabulary. Those who manage to write seem to have no unusual difficulty remembering words. This clinical picture is associated with a high degree of probability of a left-sided frontal lobe lesion usually involving Broca's area.

2. Interference with language knowledge is more difficult to characterize, since its manifestations are much more varied. I am using the term (it is not part of the standard aphasiological terminology) to cover a multiplicity of symptoms and combinations of symptoms that may either constitute variations on a fairly unified theme, or represent varying degrees of severity of one (or a few) disease processes, or, in fact, be quite independent syndromes. The important point is that, in all cases, some cognitive aspect of language capacity is affected and that this kind of trouble can occur in complete dissociation from the control of oral speech

production. In other words, a patient is sometimes unable to comprehend what is said to him (although his hearing is unimpaired) or to read or write, although he has no difficulty in the motor coordination of the muscles involved in speaking. In fact, some patients become markedly voluble, sometimes to the point of producing an incessant and uninterruptable flow of talk. When this occurs, the utterances are usually filled with neologisms, the phonology may undergo some remarkably consistent alterations, the grammatical structure becomes less varied, and phrases and sentences appear to be constructed in strange ways. Usually, one can only guess at what the patient is trying to say, and in severe cases, it is not even certain that the patient is using his verbal output to communicate anything whatever. When the disorder is less extensive, the patient may answer a question by responding to or even repeating some of the words contained in the question, but he will at once go off on a tangent, so that his answer turns into discourse of an inappropriate and at least partially illogical nature. Most of his words and phrases are quite intelligible, and only occasionally some jargon or paraphasic composition may occur. When asked to give the name of an object—a table, for example—he may start with a well-pronounced neologism such as *blago*; this may sound strange to the patient himself, and he may try again, saying *blagel,* and then, through a number of further approximations, finally reach the correct phoneme pattern. It is noteworthy that a large percentage of patients with abnormally functioning language knowledge seem to be quite unaware of their own difficulties. Some of them are cheerful and always ready to engage in conversation, and if they complain about the communicative process at all, they blame their interlocutor for the breakdown. This condition is called *anosognosia* and is a clear indication that aspects of cognition other than language are often affected by the disease. This complex of symptoms is associated with left-sided parietotemporal lesions.

3. A rather common interference with language is a pronounced difficulty in finding words. This is a vastly exaggerated "tip-of-the-tongue" phenomenon that may become so severe that the patient's speech is completely impaired. One can easily demonstrate that he understands everything that is said to him by phrasing questions in such a way that he can nod yes or no and by giving commands that he can follow. He has no difficulty with motor coordination, because he can repeat words fluently and easily, and one can show that he differs from both the first and second types of patients previously described by asking him a question that calls for words, phrases, or sentences in response. If he is blocked in his answer and one suggests a number of possible answers to him, he will readily choose the correct one and repeat it accurately and naturally. This phenomenon, called *anomia,* may appear with any left-sided cortical lesion, as long as the destruction does not impinge on any of the primary projection areas. If the lesion is focal, it is small; disseminated loss of cells throughout the cortex, however, may produce a similar effect, as, for instance, in the early stages of the presenile dementias (de Ajuriaguerra & Tissot, 1968, and Chapter 19, this volume; Sinclair, Boehme, Tissot, & de Ajuriaguerra, 1966).

This description is sufficient to rough out the general dimensions of aphasic symptomatology. It certainly does not do justice, however, to the many variations and oddities that may be seen in the clinic (for details see Bay, 1969; Geschwind, 1965; Goldstein, 1948; Head, 1926; Luria, 1958, 1970; Pick & Thiele, 1931; de Reuck & O'Connor, 1964).

Cerebral Localization of Functions

The controversy over the problem of cerebral localization is frequently misrepresented or misunderstood. Every serious student of the brain is impressed, even overawed, by the anatomy of the brain, and it is the firm credo of virtually every neurobiologist that tissue differentiation of this degree must have correlates in the realm of physiological function. Consequently, it is a sound and practically universal assumption that localized tissue destruction must, without exception, have a specific effect upon the normal pattern of *physiological* activities. There are, however, serious problems in the way of our ability to identify these effects, and there is outright disagreement over whether such effects are necessarily demonstrable in purely *behavioral* studies. (There is evidence that the organism is capable of internal physiological compensations and readjustments that make detection of behavioral deficits very difficult. There is also a problem of what to look for when we search for behavioral alterations.) As far back as 1909, K. Brodmann (1909), the eminent neuroanatomist who is responsible for the histological maps of the human cortex that are still in use today, wrote:

> *Just as untenable as is the notion of an . . . "association layer" is the assumption of special "psychic center of higher order." Especially recently, we had only too many theories which just like phrenology wanted to localize in certain circumscribed parts of the cortex such complicated mental activities as memory, volition, fantasy, intelligence, or spatial qualities such as a sense for shapes or space. . . .*
>
> *These mental capacities are notions which connote extremely complicated complexes of elementary functions. What has been said above of the presentations for which such physiological cortical processes lie at the bottom of these complex functions is still more valid of such universal "capacities." One cannot think of them arising in any other way as through an infinitely manifold and complex working together of numerous elementary processes, in other words simultaneous functions of numerous cortical parts, probably the whole cortex, perhaps even including subcortical parts* [von Bonin, 1960, p. 215].

A. R. Luria, the Dean of clinical neuropsychology, has repeatedly emphasized the dangers of regarding specific areas in the cortex as the places in which specific psychological processes, including perception, take place (Luria, 1966):

> From the standpoint of modern psychology, the localization of such processes as visual or auditory perception in circumscribed sensory areas of the cerebral cortex, like the localization of voluntary movement and activity in circumscribed areas of the motor cortex, appears . . . more improbable than the localization of respiration or of the patellar reflex in a single, isolated area of the brain [p. 32].

Again, there is no controversy whatever that *some* correlation exists between site and nature of lesion and type of language interference. The disagreements concern the degree of localizability of *specific* language and cognitive disabilities. Further, there is rather sharp disagreement over interpretation of facts. It is because of this that neurologists often find it difficult to persuade their dissenting colleagues simply by exhibiting a deceased patient's lesioned brain, together with an account of his behavioral failures. The temporal correlation between the period of tissue destruction and the periods of observed deficits presents certain problems, as does the *extent* to which the patient was examined and observed. Even the exact determination of the lesion in the specimen presents problems. Usually the brain is simply cut into slices by hand, each slice about one inch in thickness, and an attempt is made to reconstruct the lesion, along with its pathophysiology. Often small blocks of tissue are then prepared for microscopic examination. Under the circumstances, it is possible to miss lesions elsewhere in the brain, and there is always a considerable margin for doubt concerning the secondary or tertiary physiological consequences of destroyed tissues.

The acute clinical syndromes are not the only source of data for theories on brain mechanisms of language. Let us try to place these observations in a more general context.

Evidence for Brain Correlates of Language

TISSUE DESTRUCTION

The most common conditions producing the types of aphasia that are discussed in the literature are stroke, trauma, and surgical lesions. All three circumstances have a very important common denominator: the sudden and catastrophic incapacitation of a large amount of brain tissue that always includes (1) the cerebral cortex (whose thickness is but a few millimeters!), (2) the vascular bed (which extends its arterial tree into regions that go far beyond a circumscribed traumatic or surgical lesion), and (3) the subcortical fiber system (which also affects brain structures and nuclei at considerable distances from the actual site of lesion). Secondary alterations due to sudden lesions include metabolic changes and cellular degeneration; they affect protein synthesis and, in the case of immature brains, the potential for neurogenesis and growth. However, these more far-reaching consequences of sudden tissue destruction are never discussed in the aphasic literature. It is true that we do not know the full range of their effect on behavior, but their very existence should cloud the strict localizationist's crystal ball. There are many insults other than stroke, trauma, and surgical lesions that destroy or alter man's neuroanatomy and neurophysiological processes. Whether these do or do not affect language capacities does not depend merely on the location of the primary lesion, but also on the mode of onset of the disease, on the co-occurrence of other cerebral lesions (a second lesion may under certain circumstances relieve the symptoms caused by the first), and on various other histopathological, metabolic, and biochemical conditions.

Another most important source of data on language function is *abnormal development*, due either to naturally occurring diseases or to man-inflicted deprivations, both environmental and nutritional. The aphasiologists' almost exclusive concentration on a highly selected group of pathologies—pathologies that in one respect are totally different from all others, namely in their mode of onset—has engendered a fairly lopsided view of how the brain controls language. Lesions and pathological conditions that *fail* to interfere with language should play as important a part in our theory construction as do lesions that *do* cause interference. Further, it is difficult to make generalizations about the effect of lesions upon a subject's ability to learn (and to form associations). Usually, tasks become more difficult for the subject, and more training is required to establish learning. But it is at least very rare that simple disconnecting cuts through fiber tracts (excepting the commissures) abolish once and for all the capacity for associative learning. Although an aphasia (say of the second type described) may remain entirely stationary for many years, a patient may nevertheless learn to recognize new faces and to associate names with faces. The age of the patients is of paramount importance here. The young war veteran will have little difficulty in this respect, whereas a patient of sixty or more may be totally unable to learn a single new word or name, even if his general health is fairly good and he continues to live for ten or more years.

ELECTROPHYSIOLOGY

Electrophysiological data are beginning to play an increasing role in aphasiology. They fall into two major categories: extracranial recordings and electrical stimulation of live nervous tissue *in situ* in conscious patients undergoing certain types of neurosurgery. In both categories, one can make observations on the physiology of reception and on the physiology of production of behavior (movements). As far as language is concerned, the extracranial recording techniques have not yet added much to our earlier conceptions of brain mechanisms. The perceptual studies, however, have given us further details of the functional asymmetries between the two hemispheres (Buchsbaum & Fedio, 1969; Kimura, 1964, 1967; Morrell & Salamy, 1971; Wood, Goff, & Day, 1971).

As far as speech production is concerned, EEG data (including averaged potentials) have been disappointing. Ertl and Schafer (1967) reported studies on cortical electrical activities linked to verbal behavior, but in a subsequent article (Ertl &

Schafer, 1969), they questioned their own earlier interpretations. McAdam and Whitaker (1971a) reported observing electrical activity over Broca's area that preceded speech acts and that differed from the activity of the homologous area on the right, but their reports have been severely criticized by Morrell and Huntington (1971), whose own experiments along similar lines failed to lend support to the McAdam and Whitaker findings (see, however, McAdam & Whitaker, 1971b).

The electrical stimulation of brain tissues has resulted in some rather startling observations relevant to both the anatomy and the physiology of language mechanisms. At the same time, it is necessary to stress that these data raise new problems and that there is no intuitively *obvious* way to interpret them. In the first place, there is a curious discrepancy between the behavioral consequences of a lesion and the behavioral consequences of electrical stimulation in the same place when the tissue is healthy. The evidence is primarily taken from animal experiments, but there are analogous data for man. One would expect that behavior produced by stimulation of a given spot could be abolished by the destruction of that spot. But this is not so. There is not much symmetry between destruction and stimulation. A given type of behavior may be elicited from a wide variety of different loci (and histologically different tissues), but lesions in these areas may affect that behavior only negligibly or not at all. On the other hand, the same behavior may be altered by placing lesions in areas where electrical stimulation has no effect. Precisely this condition obtains in man with respect to language. No direct cortical stimulation has ever produced more than vowel-like, drawn-out sounds; and it is rare that patients report hearing articulate utterances when stimulated on the cortical convexity. But cortical destruction can interfere dramatically with language. On the other hand, Schaltenbrand (1965; Schaltenbrand, Spuler, Wahren, & Rümmler, 1971) and others have reported observing patients uttering words and whole phrases upon thalamic stimulation, whereas lesions in the same areas do not produce the types of aphasia described earlier. (In about 10% of thalamotomized patients certain speech disorders do ensue; these defects, however, are usually of a dysarthric or dysrhythmic nature.) In this connection, it may be well to remember that electrical stimulation is always a rather crude interference with ongoing activity, with many uncontrolled variables. Von Holst and von Saint Paul (1963) have shown that in the brains of chickens, at least, the place of electrical stimulation is no more important than the characteristics of the electrical stimulus and the psychophysiological state of the animal at the time of stimulation. They were able to elicit specific sorts of behavior from randomly reached loci by controlling only the nature and moment of the stimulus.

The apparent paradox caused by the incongruity between the consequences of stimulation, on the one hand, and lesioning, on the other, can be resolved if we abandon the simple-minded switchboard model of the brain. The notion of fixed and narrowly located brain centers for specific behavior must also go. Instead, the circuitry appears to have much more widely distributed networks, with rather richly redundant connectivity; experiments such as those initiated by von Holst and von Saint Paul suggest that the *nature of the activity* that goes on in these networks must also be reckoned with in our attempts at model building.

AGE AS A FACTOR IN CORTICAL LOCALIZATION

It is generally known, and is beyond dispute, that focal lesions in young children carry a prognosis different from that of similar lesions in adults. Pathology confined to the left hemisphere (including dysgenesis or surgical removal) and incurred before the end of the second year of life does not block language development, which may even occur at the normal age. If the insult occurs after the onset of language development, but before the end of the child's first decade, a transient aphasia may ensue, but, if the disease is arrested, language is fully recovered within a year or so, even though the left hemisphere may have a fixed and irreversible lesion (Lenneberg, 1967; Wanderley & Lefèvre, 1969). From such evidence we must conclude that the physiological processes of language are not irrevocably destined, from the earliest stage of postnatal brain development, to be located in the left hemisphere. Instead, lateralization is apparently a gradual process of differentiation (functional specialization) concomitant with brain maturation (which in man is much protracted beyond lower primates' maturational histories). At first, both hemispheres can and apparently do partake in the activity patterns that constitute learning and knowing language. As the growing child becomes capable of finer and finer intellectual operations (Inhelder & Piaget, 1964), both structural and functional specializations occur in the neural substrate that polarize activity patterns, displacing those instrumental for language to the left and others, such as those involved in nonverbal processes, to the right. In support of this view, we can cite the effects of sectioning the corpus callosum in adult life, as compared with the effects in adult patients of embryological agenesis of the corpus callosum. If we allow the brain to come to full maturity with the corpus callosum intact, functional asymmetry can develop. If the corpus callosum is severed after formation of this asymmetry, language is strongly localized to the left, many other functions to the right, and the sectioning produces an isolation of language from other aspects of cognition. However, if there has never been a corpus callosum to begin with, so that the hemispheres with their respective cortices have developed without cross-communication, each hemisphere runs its own differentiation history and never loses its capacity for language activities (Sperry, 1968; Gazzaniga, 1970). Thus, the fiber tracts and especially the commissures play a role in the maturational history and may well have embryological functions that deserve to be studied further. A failure of the language functions to lateralize is not an uncommon event; lifelong seizure-proneness in the left hemisphere, for example, seems to interfere with lateralization (Smith, 1966; Ueki, 1966). [For relevant experimental work on animals demonstrating age-correlated functional differentiation of the cerebral cortex, see Bowden, Goldman, Rosvold, and Greenstreet (1971);

Goldman (1971); Goldman, Rosvold, and Mishkin (1970); and Kling and Tucker (1968). For general comments on critical age in man, see Lenneberg (1968).]

In view of these facts, the electrographic evidence of neurophysiological lateralization, cited earlier, should be expanded. Currently, Helen Neville, a graduate student at Cornell University, is attempting to collect similar data in a developmental perspective, in order to obtain a picture of the natural history of the electrical asymmetries. It will be particularly interesting to see whether such a history is changed in children with abnormal language development.

RATE OF LESIONING AND ITS EFFECT ON LANGUAGE INTERFERENCE

A very important but widely ignored fact of neuropathology is the trade-off between rate of growth and size of a lesion. For instance, a tumor that takes many years to grow may assume rather formidable proportions before any symptoms whatever begin to show. When symptoms do develop, they are frequently of the kind that have little localizing value clinically (seizures, headache, vomiting). Even a faster growing, more malignant tumor that destroys tissues in the classical cortical speech and language areas may manifest itself rather differently from sudden destruction of the same tissue by stroke, trauma, or surgery. The classical types of aphasia are by no means obligatory when the lesion is neoplastic. Even the postoperative prognosis does not depend simply on the location and size of the surgical lesion; it depends also on the pathology and morbid history that have led to surgery. Thus the usual ablation studies on animals differ in a fundamental way from surgical procedures on man. The former are done on healthy brains; the latter are not. Notice, however, that it is possible to simulate a condition in experimental animal surgery that approximates a slowly growing lesion in man, with its subsequent surgical treatment. If ablation on animals is carried out in multiple stages, so that only small parts of tissue are removed at a time, and the total ablation is protracted over a period of months or years, then the animal's behavior is no longer irreversibly interfered with and functions may recover (Rosen, Stein, & Butter, 1971; Stein, Rosen, Graziadei, Mishkin, & Brink, 1969). Once more we see that the activity patterns that correspond to behavioral capacities may be only slightly displaced if the insults expand very gradually.

Undoubtedly there are definite limits to this sort of "plasticity." For example, there are many brain structures whose removal is clearly incompatible with the continuance of given functions, no matter how gradually the destruction takes place. But we are talking primarily of a single and specific type of tissue: the cerebral cortex, where it seems that functional localization enjoys a certain degree of freedom under the specific circumstances mentioned (insults during immaturity, or very slow impingement). Even here the functions in the area striata are more fixed than those of Heschl's gyrus, and both these cortical fields are more indispensable than the so-called association cortex.

Preliminaries to Theories on Brain Mechanisms of Language

The neurophysiology of behavior comprises three realms of mechanisms: those concerned with input, those with central integration, and those with output. The first realm includes reception, transduction, and transformation of exogenous stimuli; the third deals with control, regulation, and coordination of muscular activity. The nature of the second realm can be inferred only from the imperfect correlation that exists between input and output. There are many types of input that produce no overt motor output, and many an output (verbal or motor) does not seem to be correlated with any specific environmental input. Registration in our minds of some event need not lead to any immediate or even future predictable motor act. On the other hand, a motor act or an utterance such as "A black scorpion is not dropping on my plate" (which B. F. Skinner told his students was said to him by A. N. Whitehead during a discussion of verbal behavior) need not be evoked by any closely related physical event in the environment.

Up to the present, experimental neurophysiological research and the interpretation of the respective data have been almost exclusively focused on the first and, to a lesser extent, on the third realms. On the other hand, the biology of *knowing language* is essentially a problem of the second realm. Knowing a language means relating, computing, operating on specific aspects of the environment. Learning language means doing these things in very specific ways. Theorizing about brain mechanisms of language is made extremely difficult by our nearly complete ignorance of how any of the processes of the second realm function. The difficulty is not merely the absence of specific facts that may shortly become available. The difficulty is the present lack of even a general or abstract *theoretical model* of how this second realm might work—how behavior and cognition might be related to brain function. The theoretical models that enjoy greatest popularity among neurophysiologists today try to explain how physical patterns (such as the configuration of a chair) might be transformed into "the language of the brain," but they do not face the problem of what happens to the transformed data—what goes on in the second realm. The map-making aphasiologists endeavor to tell us where the neurally encoded speech signal first arrives in the cortex, where it is shunted next, and where it "exists" to produce speech acts. Quite apart from the innumerable questions that surround such functional maps, they would not actually explain what the physiology of language knowledge is even were the anatomical locations by now firmly established. A nervous system is not like a trumpet upon which "the environment" plays a tune by blowing into it. Brains are not passive conveyors of information; they are very active objects, and their activity states are highly unstable, easily perturbed, and subject to modulation from the outside. That is why treating the brain as a communication channel or viewing behavior simply as a function of the input to the system is misleading. It tends to ignore the fact that behavior is in many ways autonomous activity, in the sense that it derives its energy *not* from the stimuli that are behaviorally significant, but from energy stores that are supplied through the body's metabolic activities. Psychologically important stimuli trigger and shape behavior, but the stimuli are not the architects of the principles by which behavior operates; nor is behavior a transform of the input. The relevance of these observations to language is obvious (for elaboration, see Lenneberg, 1967).

The acquisition and maintenance of the language function is a particular example of the general biological problem of how patterns come about and are maintained. It is a special problem within the general problem of biological specificity. We are faced with quite similar problems in the contexts of both evolution and ontogeny. And the problem extends to the field of structure as well as to the field of function (as well as to that of behavior). Thus, our ability to "explain" language biologically is inextricably tied up with our ability to explain the organism's ontogenesis.

The clinical data especially, the relationship between lesioning and age, and the importance of the rate at which cortex is destroyed emphasize the role of morphogenetic processes during the establishment of language capacities. It is only by bringing the notions of embryological regulation, differentiation, and determination to bear upon the functional organization of the human brain during the critical years of language development that we can hope to understand the occurrence and nonoccurrence of language disturbances. Piaget and his colleagues are the only psychologists who have clearly seen the intimate relationship between embryological processes and the unfolding of cognition (Piaget, 1971). Nothing could illustrate better the direct connections between developmental biology and developmental psychology than the neurology of language. As the behavioral capacities become differentiated during growth (Brown, 1974; Sinclair, 1967), the human brain is undergoing its final structural and functional differentiation as well (Jacobson, Chapter 6, this volume; Lenneberg, 1967). It is especially the functional differentiation that should be of interest to the student of behavior and language. Functions do not suddenly start when the "machine has been assembled," as in a computer that is suddenly ready to be used. Cognitive functions and the capacity for language knowledge have an epigenetic history; they are the transforms of earlier, less specialized functions and their correlated physiological processes. The cerebral activity patterns that constitute the use and knowledge of language have gradually-developed characteristics (i.e., their modes of functioning, the nature of their perturbability, the types of transitions between their states), and these, in turn, depend in part on the anatomical differentiation history and in part on the history of perturbations that the developing system has incurred.

European neurophysiologists have been more interested in the structure of cerebral activity patterns and the internal interactions among such patterns than their colleagues on this side of the Atlantic. They have pointed out that a "cognitive act" has its own momentary history of formation; that it is the end result of patterned interactions—a topic that has been discussed under various headings, such as *Aktualgenese, Funktionsstruktur,* or *Wirkungsgefuege.* But no one, except Piaget, has even discussed the epigenetic history of these patterns.

In general, the problem of relating behavior or language to brain mechanisms is to find a model that relates aspects of *dynamic patterns* to the known anatomical and clinical or experimental facts in such a way that the phenomena of so-called plasticity (as shown, for example, by data on the age and rate of lesioning, or by the capacity to learn, forget or will to do things) become comprehensible without recourse to an implied demon that switches flows of impulses and makes decisions on where and how neuronal action is to take place. We do not yet have such a model. In casting around for possible explanations, we ought to keep two aspects of brain connectivity in mind.

1. It is possible that in certain limited tissues in the brain, cells are inter-connected randomly. If we consider this possibility, together with the fact that the number of synapses between neurons is many times larger than the number of neurons (by an order of magnitude of 10^3 to 10^4), then it becomes plausible to assume that neurons are not functionally autonomous in such areas but that the areas have their own characteristic cooperative behavior. Such behavior will be a function of each element's repertoire of behavior, the nature of the coupling between elements, the number of elements so connected, and the geometry of the assembly as a whole.

2. It is possible that the gross connections between nuclei and regions, which are highly regular and predictable (and therefore quite the opposite of random connectivity), are essentially channels through which the various structures per-turb one another. Assume that every histologically distinct structure in the brain has its own peculiar activity patterns; add to this the facts that just about every structure of the nervous system has a multiplicity of fiber systems that interconnect it (nonrandomly) to several other structures and that no nervous tissue is ever "idle;" then one is tempted to think that structures are not independent agencies that send messages to one another, but, rather, that the brain and its activities are in constant functional flux. Even when a steady state is reached, in the sense that the different activities in different parts of the brain are relatively constant, the equilibrium of the system as a whole is still precarious. Any alteration of activity in any part of the brain would cause chain reactions of new interactions and cross-perturbations that might take a long time to reach a new steady state. In other words, at any one moment, all the specialized activities in all the different parts of the nervous system can be viewed as a single configuration, and the activity patterns of the brain can be seen as a series of moment-to-moment transitions from configuration to configuration.

At present, neuroscientists are struggling with the formulation of new models for dealing with activity patterns such as those likely to occur in brains. Of special interest is the activity generated by systems that are composed of very large numbers of autonomously active but coupled elements (Elul, 1968; Freeman, 1972; Schmitt, 1969). The formalisms used in the description of fluid dynamics and their patterns are also under consideration for their possible application to brain func-tion (Eigen & De Maeyer, 1971; Katchalsky & Oster, 1969). Concepts such as that of the dissipative structures of nonequilibrium thermodynamics are beginning to interest the neurophysiologists (Blumenthal, Changeux, & Lefever, 1970) and may open new horizons for studying the brain and its dynamic patterns. The importance of these new endeavors lies in their potential for relating the structuralization of function to the structuralization of form (Eigen & De Maeyer, 1971; Glansdorff & Prigogine, 1971; Turing, 1952) and for explaining some of the plasticity phenomena briefly discussed in connection with language development. It is far too early to apply any of these concepts specifically to language mechanisms. But I think it is important to stress, even at this early stage, the existence of a conceptual framework and theoretical constructs that are based on well-defined physical, chemical, and mathematical notions and that are capable of elevating our picture of brain function from its present plane of switching diagrams to a new concept of four-dimensional dynamic patterns.

References

Bay, E. The classification of disorders of speech. *Cortex*, 1967, *3*, 26—31.

Bay, E. Aphasielehre und Neuropsychologie der Sprache. *Nervenarzt*, 1969, *40*, 53—71.

Blumenthal, R., Changeux, J.-P., & Lefever, R. Membrane excitability and dissipative instabilities. *Journal of Membrane Biology*, 1970, *2*, 351—374.

Bowden, D. M., Goldman, P. S., Rosvold, H. E., & Greenstreet, R. L. Free behavior of rhesus monkeys following lesions of the dorsolateral and orbital prefrontal cortex in infancy. *Experimental Brain Research (Berlin)*, 1971, *12*, 265—274.

Brodmann, K. *Vergleichende Lokalisationslehre der Grosshirnrinde*. Leipzig: Barth, 1909.

Brown, R. *A first language: The early stages*. Cambridge, Mass.: Harvard Univ. Press, 1974.

Buchsbaum, M., & Fedio, P. Visual information and evoked responses from the left and right hemispheres. *Electroencephalography and Clinical Neurophysiology*, 1969, *26*, 266—278.

Chomsky, N. *Aspects of the theory of syntax*. Cambridge, Mass.: MIT Press, 1965.

Conrad, K. New problems of aphasia. *Brain*, 1954, *77*, 491—509.

de Ajuriaguerra, J., & Tissot, R. Some aspects of psychoneurologic disintegration in senile dementia. In C. Müller & L. Ciompi (Eds.), *Senile dementia*, Berne: Huber, 1968.

de Reuck, A. V. S., & O'Connor, M. (Eds.) *Disorders of language*. CIBA Foundation Symposium. Boston: Little Brown, 1964.

Eigen, M., & De Maeyer, L. Carriers and specificity in membranes. *Neurosciences Research Program, Bulletin*, 1971, *9*, No. 3.

Elul, R. Brain waves. In K. Enslein (Ed.), *Data acquisition and processing in biology and medicine*. Vol. 5. Oxford: Pergamon, 1968.

Ertl, J., & Schafer, E. W. P. Cortical activity preceding speech. *Life Sciences*, 1967, *6*, 473—479.

Ertl, J., & Schafer, E. W. P. Erratum [ref. to Ertl and Schafer 1967]. *Life Sciences*, 1969, *8*, 559.

Freeman, W. J. Waves, pulses and the theory of neural masses. In R. Rosen & F. M. Snell (Eds.), *Progress in theoretical biology*. Vol. 1. New York: Academic Press, 1972.

Gazzaniga, M. *The bisected brain*. New York: Appleton, 1970.

Geschwind, N. Disconnexion syndromes in animals and man. *Brain*, 1965, *88*, 237—294, 585—644.

Glansdorff, P., & Prigogine, I. *Thermodynamic theory of structure, stability and fluctuations*. New York: Wiley (Interscience), 1971.

Goldman, P. S. Functional development of the prefrontal cortex in early life and the problem of neuronal plasticity. *Experimental Neurology*, 1971, *32*, 366—387.

Goldman, P. S., Rosvold, H. E., & Mishkin, M. Evidence for behavioral impairment following prefrontal lobectomy in the infant monkey. *Journal of Comparative and Physiological Psychology*, 1970, *70*, 454—463.

Goldstein, K. *Language and language disorders*. New York: Grune & Stratton, 1948.

Head, H. *Aphasia and kindred disorders of speech*. London: Cambridge Univ. Press, 1926.

Inhelder, B., & Piaget, J. *Genetic epistemology; The growth of logical thinking from childhood to adolescence*. New York: Basic Books, 1964.

Katchalsky, A., & Oster, G. Chemico-diffusional coupling in biomembrane. In D. C. Tosteson (Ed.), *The molecular basis of membrane function*, Englewood Cliffs, N.J.: Prentice-Hall, 1969.

Kimura, D. Left-right differences in the perception of melodies. *Quarterly Journal of Experimental Psychology*, 1964, *14*, 355–358.

Kimura, D. Functional asymmetry of the brain in dichotic listening. *Cortex*, 1967, *3*, 163–178.

Kling, A., & Tucker, T. J. Sparing of function following localized brain lesions in neonatal monkeys. In R. Isaacson (Eds.), *The neuropsychology of development*. New York: Wiley, 1968.

Lenneberg, E. H. *Biological foundations of language*. New York: Wiley Ch. 8, 1967.

Lenneberg, E. H. The effect of age on the outcome of central nervous system disease in children. In R. Isaacson (Ed.), *The neuropsychology of development*. New York: Wiley, 1968.

Luria, A. R. Brain disorders and language analysis. *Language and Speech*, 1958, *1*, 14.

Luria, A. R. *Higher cortical functions in man*. New York: Basic Books, 1966.

Luria, A. R. *Traumatic aphasia: Its syndromes, psychology, and treatment*. The Hague: Mouton, 1970.

McAdam, D. W., & Whitaker, H. A. Language production: Electroencephalographic localization in the normal human brain. *Science*, 1971, *172*, 499–502. (a)

McAdam, D. W., & Whitaker, H. A. [Reply to Morrell and Huntington, 1971.] *Science*, 1971, *174*, 1360–1361. (b)

Morrell, L. K., & Huntington, D. A. Electrocortical localization of language production. *Science*, 1971, *174*, 1359–1360.

Morrell, L. K., & Salamy, J. Hemispheric asymmetry of electrocortical responses to speech stimuli. *Science*, 1971, *174*, 164–166.

Piaget, J. *Biology and knowledge: An essay on the relations between organic regulations and cognitive processes*. Chicago: Univ. of Chicago Press, 1971.

Pick, A., & Thiele, R. Aphasie. In A. Bethe *et al.* (Eds.), *Handbuch der Normalen und Pathologischen Physiologie*. Vol. 15. Berlin: Springer-Verlag, 1931.

Rosen, J. D., Stein, D., & Butter, N. Recovery of function after serial ablation of prefrontal cortex in the rhesus monkey. *Science*, 1971, *173*, 353–356.

Schaltenbrand, G. The effects of stereotactic stimulation in the depth of the brain. *Brain*, 1965, *88*, 835–840.

Schaltenbrand, G., Spuler, H., Wahren, W., & Rümmler, B. Electroanatomy of the thalamic ventro-oral nucleus based on stereotactic stimulation in man. *Zeitschrift für Neurologie*, 1971, *199*, 269–276.

Schmitt, O. H. Biological information processing using the concept of interpenetrating domains. In K. N. Leibovic (Ed.), *Information processing in the nervous system*. New York: Springer Publ., 1969.

Sinclair, H. *Langage et opérations. Sous-systèmes linguistiques et opérations concrètes*. Paris: Dunod, 1967.

Sinclair, H., Boehme, M., Tissot, R., & de Ajuriaguerra, J. Quelques aspects de la désintégration des notions de temps à travers des épreuves morpho-syntaxiques de langage et à travers des épreuves opératoires chez des vieillards atteints de démence dégénérative. *Bulletin de Psychologie*, 1966, *247*, 8–12.

Smith, A. Speech and other functions after left (dominant) hemispherectomy. *Journal of Neurology, Neurosurgery, and Psychiatry*, 1966, *29*, 467–471.

Sperry, R. W. Plasticity of neural maturation. In M. Locke (Ed.), *The emergence of order in developing systems*. Developmental Biology, 1968, Suppl. No. 2.

Stein, D. G., Rosen, J. J., Graziadei, J., Mishkin, D., & Brink, J. J. Central nervous system: recovery of function. *Science*, 1969, *166*, 528–530.

Turing, A. M. The chemical basis of morphogenesis. *Philosophical Transactions of the Royal Society of London, Series B* 1952, *237*, 37–72.

Ueki, K. Hemispherectomy in the human with special reference to the preservation of function. *Progress in Brain Research*, 1966, *21B*, 285–338.

von Bonin, G. *Some papers on the cerebral cortex.* Springfield, Ill.: Thomas, 1960.

von Holst, E., & von Saint Paul, U. On the functional organization of drives. In S. E. Glickman & P. M. Milner (Eds.), *The neurological basis of motivation.* Princeton, N.J.: Van Nostrand-Reinhold, 1963. (Reprinted: 1969.)

von Monakow, C. *Die Lokalisation im Grosshirn.* Wiesbaden: Bermann, 1914.

von Weizsäcker, V. *Der Gestaltkreis.* Stuttgart: Thieme, 1950.

Wanderley, E. C., & Lefèvre, A. B. Afasia adquirida na infancia. *Arquivos de Neuro Psiquiatria,* 1969, *27,* 89—96.

Wood, C., Goff, W., & Day, R. Hemispheric differences in auditory evoked potentials during phonemic and pitch discrimination. *Science,* 1971, *173,* 1248—1251.

2. Ontogeny of Stable Speech Areas in the Human Brain

E. Bay

The use of language depends on the functioning of two unilaterally localized "speech areas" in the "dominant" hemisphere of the brain. These speech areas, and especially their unilateral location, are not based on genetically predetermined structures, but they develop functionally in one of the genetically equipotent hemispheres during childhood and in apparent simultaneity with the acquisition of speech.

So far, the scanty empirical data (particularly cases of acquired childhood aphasia) are not sufficient for definite and reliable statements about development and stabilization of the speech areas. As far as there are empirical data, they suggest the working hypothesis that the anterior (motor) speech area develops in conjunction with the appearance and stabilization of hand preference between 2 and 10 years of age. The temporal ("sensory") speech area seems to develop later than the anterior and more in correlation with acoustic and, possibly, conceptual aspects of language; its development and stabilization is also terminated at the age of 10.

Prior to the age of 2, both hemispheres are equipotent, and before the final unilateral stabilization of the speech areas there is a decreasing amount of plasticity with the possibility of shifting dominance from one hemisphere to the other.

However, a far greater amount of more reliable empirical evidence is required for final confirmation of these hypotheses.

Introduction

The normal use of language depends upon an undisturbed functioning of certain areas in the brain, the so-called speech areas. Damage to these speech areas in adults results in a characteristic disorder of speech, aphasia or dysphasia. Although this is evident, and although aphasia is a most common clinical syndrome, the interpretation of this fact is far from being clear, and disagreement about nearly every aspect of the aphasic disorder is considerable.

To begin with, there is controversy about whether there are several different types of aphasia (motor, sensory, etc.), or whether there is only a unitary aphasia modified by additional, nonverbal components (cf. Bay, 1962, 1964b, 1967). No less controversial is the exact pathopsychology of the disorder and the patho-physiological significance of the cerebral speech areas or "speech centers" for normal and pathological speech and language. In this respect, there exist only contradictory, speculative hypotheses. Even the exact site and size of the cerebral speech areas is not clear beyond doubt (Bay, 1964a, 1964c, 1969).

For our considerations here we can, fortunately, disregard most of the unsolved problems of aphasiology and confine ourselves to a few undisputed facts. There *are* cerebral speech areas, especially in the temporal lobe and in the frontal lobe, or around the Rolandic fissure. Destruction of such areas produces in normal adults characteristic disorders of speech. Posterior (temporal) lesions lead to an overall impairment of communication by language (aphasia), whereas anterior lesions (in the frontal lobe or Rolandic fissure) exclusively or predominantly affect expressive aspects of language; for our present purpose it is irrelevant whether one calls this condition "motor aphasia" or—as we prefer (Bay, 1962)—"dysarthria." I shall use the terms "speech area," "aphasia," and "dysarthria" (or "motor aphasia") only in this noncommittal sense.

The problem of ontogenesis of these speech areas is outlined by two well-known facts:

1. In the normal adult, damage to the speech area in one hemisphere, which we consequently call "dominant," produces aphasia or dysarthria, whereas damage to corresponding areas of the other, "nondominant" or "minor," hemisphere has no analogous effect on language performance. In severe and irreversible destruction of speech areas, the aphasic syndrome is also persistent. At least in the vast majority of adult cases, there is no reliable evidence of a transfer of speech functions to the other (minor) hemisphere.

In right-handed persons, the dominance of speech is, with few exceptions, in the left hemisphere. In the majority of left-handers speech dominance is also in the left hemisphere, but in roughly one third of left-handers it may be in the right. We shall come back to the problem of cerebral dominance in greater detail.

2. During development, prior to the acquisition of language, damage to the presumptive speech areas in either hemisphere neither produces aphasic speech nor impairs the normal acquisition of language (Basser, 1962). The insensitiveness of speech acquisition, and later on of speech performance, to unilateral damage to brain structures in early childhood is impressively demonstrated by the fact that hemispherectomy of a perinatally damaged hemisphere generally does not impair language. This is true for the left hemisphere as well as for the right (Basser, 1962).

Only bilateral brain damage severely impairs the acquisition of language and intellectual development. Such cases are frequently described as "developmental aphasia." This term, in our opinion, is a misnomer responsible for a good deal of confusion. The term "aphasia" was coined for the dissolution of already acquired speech functions leading to a distinct morbid pattern, the aphasic syndrome; it should be restricted to such cases of acquired aphasia (Critchley, 1967; Gloning & Hift, 1970; Subirana, 1961).

The concept of developmental aphasia is based on the hypothesis that impaired development of speech is caused by an early damage to pre-existing speech areas. However, contrary to the well-defined pattern of acquired aphasia, the term developmental aphasia refers to very different morbid states that are caused by very different pathogenetic conditions. It is applied to retarded or defective acquisition of speech due to mental retardation, or to hearing impairment, emotional problems, and so on. Of these different conditions, only cases of impaired language development due to bilateral brain damage might fit into the concept of developmental aphasia. In such cases, however, the disturbed acquisition of speech is combined with equally defective intellectual development, preventing a clear distinction between primarily linguistic and primarily intellectual troubles—at least at our present state of knowledge.

Therefore, for the problem of speech areas and their development, only cases of acquired aphasia are relevant—in children as well as in adults. Only they prove an involvement of specialized speech areas. It is evident, from these facts, that there exist fixed speech areas in one hemisphere of the adult brain, which cannot be replaced by other structures, especially not by corresponding areas in the minor hemisphere. These speech areas, however, are not unilaterally fixed as genetically determined structures, since both hemispheres are genetically equipotential regarding speech functions. Therefore, these speech areas must develop some time between birth and adolescence, with a great extent of plasticity during early life and rigid localization (lateralization) only in adults.

Development of Speech Areas and Aphasia in Children

When we try to describe more precisely the development of these stable speech areas during childhood, we meet some methodological problems. Since we are concerned with the pathology of human language, we cannot approach the problem by animal experiments, but must rely exclusively on human pathology, especially, on the occurrence, development, and outcome of childhood aphasia. The literature on childhood aphasia, however, is disappointing, because of the confusion caused by the term developmental aphasia. Most contributions in this field are concerned with abnormalities in the acquisition of speech for various reasons; papers on acquired aphasia are rare. So, in a bibliography prepared by the Information Center for Hearing, Speech, and Disorders of Human Communication (1968) on "Childhood aphasia", only 4 out of 137 references deal with acquired aphasia.

The small number of relevant papers is due to the rarity of pertinent cases. Therefore, there is no representative series of a single author large enough to solve the problem. Rather, we must rely on small numbers of cases published by different authors, investigated under varying conditions, and with generally poor clinical data that are insufficient for unequivocal inferences. Everyone who is aware of the controversies among aphasiologists about the interpretation of aphasic symptoms in adults, despite extensive language testing, will not be surprised that the poor data of speech performance in small children rarely allow an unequivocal interpretation. Especially ambiguous in children are the differentiation of expressive and receptive disorders and the distinction between the influence of general mental impairment on speech performance and the repercussion of disordered speech on mental development. We must, therefore, stress the statements of earlier investigators (Basser, 1962; Gloning & Hift, 1970; Tomkiewicz, 1964), that our present knowledge about the development of speech areas is largely based on guesswork, and that we need many more and better documented investigations for a definite solution of the problem.

The distinction between speech troubles following general mental impairment and specific speech disorders is particularly difficult in the attempt to define the earliest appearance of aphasia as a first indicator for the development of specialized speech areas. At this stage of speech development, we cannot expect such characteristic aphasic symptoms as paraphasia or grammatical distortions, which can only appear at a certain level of linguistic production.

Basser (1962), in his large and important collection of cases with subsequent hemispherectomy, has several children with an onset of "aphasia" at ages between 15 months and $2\frac{1}{2}$ years. The diagnosis, however, was made only retrospectively, after many years, when the patients came for hemispherectomy. All the children had a history of prolonged coma or repeated convulsions. Although they were speaking "single words" or "fairly well" prior to their acute disease, they stopped speaking for periods of from 3 weeks to 2 years, and there was some lasting intellectual impairment. These cases cannot be considered as reliable evidence for a specialized impairment of speech. Moreover, no case provides sufficient proof for the unilaterality of damage. A similar reserve is required about the diagnosis of acquired aphasia at the age of 2 years, 9 months, in two cases of Gloning and Hift (1970). In both cases the general intelligence was severely impaired or not testable, and there was bilateral damage in at least one case.

More convincing is a case described by de Rom (1935). A boy of 19 months with a depressed fracture of the left frontal bone due to a kick by a horse had right hemiplegia and "motor aphasia." Surgical intervention demonstrated laceration of the brain under the fracture. Three days after the operation he regained movement of the paralyzed limbs, and he began to speak after 11 days. Two months later his speech was normal again. This seems to be the only reliably documented case of acquired aphasia before the age of 3 years. As it was due to a laceration of the brain, and lasted less than 2 months, it might have been caused by widespread edema rather than by localized damage to a speech area (Riese & Collison, 1964).

It is important to note that the speech disorder in this earliest case was classified as "motor aphasia," with unimpaired comprehension of language. We shall have to come back to this point later one.

Opposed to such rather dubious evidence of aphasia prior to the third year are cases in which, at the same age, unilateral brain damage did not affect speech and speech development. Basser's material contains seven pertinent cases, five with damage to the right and two with damage to the left hemisphere. The cases are quite reliable regarding the absence of speech disorders; unsolved, however, is the problem of handedness. Afterwards, of course, handedness was determined by a lasting hemiplegia, which was present in all cases, and subsequent removal of the damaged hemisphere did not affect language.

These facts are too scanty to allow reliable conclusions, but they give little evidence for a lateralization of speech areas prior to the third year of life. In children older than three years, there is an increasing number of reports of isolated speech troubles after localized and unilateral brain damage.

More reliably determined can be the other borderline, namely, the age at which localized brain damage may produce irreversible aphasia, indicating that speech areas have become stable and unchangeable, as in adults.

Wenzel (1966) collected 110 cases of childhood aphasia, both from personal observation and from the literature. Irreversible speech disorders were observed at the age of 10 (Riese & Collison, 1964) and at 11 (Guttmann, 1942, two cases). Cases with an earlier onset of permanent speech disorders (e.g., some cases of Gloning & Hift, 1970) are not stringent, because of concomitant mental impairment or bilateral brain damage.

It seems to be a safe supposition, therefore, that the process of development and stabilization of speech areas is terminated after the age of 10 years. Between the ages of 3 and 10, the occurrence of acquired aphasia after unilateral brain damage indicates that specialized and lateralized speech areas are developing; the brain is still able, however, to compensate for isolated speech disorders completely. Ample experience with hemispherectomy proves beyond doubt that this compensation, if necessary, can be effected by transfer of speech functions to the other, originally minor, hemisphere.

The age of about 10 years marks the earliest limit of persistent aphasia; it also marks the development of definitely fixed speech areas. The stabilization of speech functions at this age is also illustrated by another well-known fact: children who lose their hearing before that age also lose their acquired language and become deaf-mute. When acquired later in life, deafness produces only some alterations in the prosodic qualities of speech; it does not produce loss of language. This coincidence is highly suggestive of an interdependence between the permanent acquisition of language (word memory) and the final fixation of speech areas.

Between 3 and 10 years of age, the child acquires the full command of human language. This period corresponds remarkably with the development of another aspect of hemispheric dominance, the development of hand preference. According to Gesell and Ames (1947), there is no consistent hand preference during the first two years. A clear, yet transient, hand preference occurs for the first time during the first half of the third year, followed by a lack of preference between $2\frac{1}{2}$ and $3\frac{1}{2}$ years of age. From the fourth year on, increasingly long periods of right-hand preference are interrupted by short spells of bimanual activity until right-hand preference is finally and consistently established after the age of 8. A correlation between delayed development of hemispheric dominance and retarded acquisition of speech is suggested by Dreifuss (1963), in cases of mild bilateral brain damage.

In this respect, it is interesting that there are significant differences in the types of speech disorders. All authors agree that acquired aphasia in infants results mainly in speech arrest or, in milder forms, in "unwillingness to speak," while comprehension of speech is undisturbed or, at least, fairly well preserved. Characteristics of "sensory" aphasia in adults, such as paraphasia, logorrhea, and jargon aphasia, do not occur in children (Basser, 1962; Guttmann, 1942; Tomkiewicz, 1964). As far as the authors differentiate between "motor" and "sensory" aphasia, the survey of Wenzel (1966) records 19 cases of "motor aphasia," ranging in age from 1 year, 7 months, to 12 years, including the case described by de Rom. Even without the latter case, there are still eight more occurring before the age of 6. Among Wenzel's cases without precise classification by the author, there are several where the scanty data suggest predominantly expressive disturbances. Gloning and Hift (1970) also find a strong prevalence of expressive disorders in their cases, which range in age from 2 years, 7 months, to 7 years. On the other hand, Wenzel reports only five cases diagnosed as "sensory aphasia;" these range from 6 to 14 years of age. In some of these it cannot be excluded that the receptive disorders may be due to loss of hearing.

The differentiation between "motor" and "sensory" aphasia, in our opinion, is ambiguous and of dubious value (Bay, 1967, 1969); moreover, the records are insufficient in most cases. Nevertheless, it is evident that aphasia in the vast majority of children between the ages of 6 and 10 (and perhaps exclusively between the ages of 3 and 6) concerns *expressive* speech, which frequently results in severe arrest. Together with the invariably concomitant hemiplegia, this is indicative of dysarthria (Bay, 1949, 1962). In most cases it is difficult to say whether—and, if so, how far—this dysarthria is accompanied by true (receptive) aphasia.

If this is true, then the organization occurring between the third and sixth year and the stabilization between the sixth and tenth year take place mainly in the anterior speech area, whether it is located in the frontal (Broca's) area of the inferior sensorimotor region (Bay, 1949). This brings in even closer connection the acquisition of (expressive) speech and the development of hand preference as related motor aspects of hemispheric dominance. This applies to the first manifestations of speech and of hand preference at the age of three and to their final stabilization after the age of 8. For the vast majority of cases with "normal" hemispheric dominance, this is certainly true. It must be remembered, however, that there are exceptions to this rule, especially in sinistrals, where hand preference and speech dominance are discordant.

Since the rare cases of childhood aphasia mainly concern the anterior speech area, little can be said about the functional development and unilateral fixation of the temporal speech areas responsible for real ("sensory") aphasia. We can only postulate that localization and, especially, lateralization occur at a later age or over a longer period of time, ending only at the age of 10. The parallel development of a unilaterally fixed temporal speech area and of a stable word memory, independent of further auditory input (p. 25), suggests speculations about neurophysiological bases of language—which are, however, beyond the scope of this discussion.

The concept of a gradually developing organization and localization (especially lateralization) of neurophysiological processes subserving speech in circumscribed speech areas, parallel to the acquisition of language, suggests correlations between age and the occurrence and course of speech disorders. In this respect, again, the available data are insufficient for a clear interpretation.

There exist no reliable data about the *frequency* of speech disorders relative to age. In the survey of Wenzel (1966), the majority of cases occurred before the seventh year. This, however, is not significant, because it represents a synopsis from quite diverse publications that had different aims and, therefore, different criteria for selection.

More material is available regarding the *course* of speech disorders relative to age. However, the duration of symptoms depends on many variables, particularly on the type and severity of the pathological process (Guttmann, 1942). Therefore, the very heterogeneous stock of available empirical data does not provide a clear answer to this question. Basser (1962) finds "an earlier age of occurrence of the lesion associated with a longer duration of speech loss." His series, however, contains several children between 15 months and $2\frac{1}{2}$ years of age, who cannot be considered aphasic (cf. p. 24). When we confine our considerations to indubitable cases of aphasia—for instance Wenzel's compilation of cases—we find a great variance of duration at every age. There is, however, a tendency to quick and complete recovery (within 3 months) before the age of 7; at a later age there is a higher proportion of cases of prolonged duration (1 year and more). Statistically, this result is far from being significant, but it supports the opinion of most investigators (Byers & McLean, 1962; Dreifuss, 1963; Guttmann, 1942) that recovery from aphasia is very rapid in early childhood. Cases of permanent aphasia occur only after the age of 9 years.

Such a distribution is in accordance with the theoretical expectations; but far more and better-documented cases are needed for definite conclusions.

Individual cases differ greatly in the occurrence, course, and extent of speech disorders, with differences dependent largely upon differences in the underlying pathology. Another source of this variance was suggested by Basser (1962), who promoted the theory that in some children speech areas develop directly in the left, or rarely, the right hemisphere, whereas in other cases both hemispheres participate in the development of speech, and lateralization in one hemisphere occurs only later. This theory is supported by the results of intracarotid amobarbital injections in aphasic adults (Kinsbourne, 1971; Milner, Branch, &

Rasmussen, 1966), which indicate that even in some adults the minor hemisphere still contributes to speech functions (Bay, 1973). But this theory, also, needs final confirmation.

Conclusion

When we try to sum up our present state of knowledge about the development of speech areas, we must first point out that the available data are insufficient. We can present a hypothesis consistent with them, but it is a hypothesis that needs final confirmation.

It is beyond doubt that the ability to use human language depends on the development of two "speech areas" in the brain: an anterior, at or near the cortical sensorimotor representation of articulatory muscles in the lower part of the Rolandic region (or in Broca's region); and a posterior, in the temporal lobe in connection with the auditory cortex.

Although in the normal adult, at least in the vast majority of cases, these speech areas are unilaterally in the dominant hemisphere, both hemispheres are genetically equipotential in this respect. Therefore, unilateral hemispheric damage in early infancy does not prevent a normal evolution of language or stabilization of speech areas (in the undamaged hemisphere), whereas bilateral damage interferes with both acquisition of language and intellectual development.

The anterior speech area, which is concerned with the motor aspects of speech, develops in conjunction with the appearance and stabilization of hand preference, thus establishing the main motor aspects of hemispheric dominance. Seemingly, this process begins with the appearance of the first speech sounds during the second and third year of life and continues with the progressive acquisition of articulatory skills. In the first stages of development, a transfer of functions to the other hemisphere is easily and promptly possible; but progressive lateralization of functions occurs with increasing complexity of functional differentiation. Final lateralization, however, is reached only after full acquisition of language at the age of about ten.

The development of the temporal speech area presents more problems. It seems to develop later than the anterior speech area and in closer correlation with acoustic and, possibly, cognitive and conceptual aspects of language. It is terminated at the age of ten, together with the stabilization of word memory. The increasing rigidity of lateralization here, again, corresponds to increasing functional complexity.

Normally, hand preference and the anterior and posterior speech areas are localized in the same dominant hemisphere. However, although there is no evidence for possible dissociated lateralization of the two speech areas, there may be a dissociation between speech areas and handedness, especially in left-handers. The causes for such dissociation are obscure.

In order to close the gaps in our knowledge and to confirm these speculations, we need far more evidence than is at present available. Such additional evidence might help, for example, to solve the problem of the possible contribution of the minor hemisphere to speech, or the correlated question of the fundamental differences in functional organization between dextrals and sinistrals and so-called ambidextrals.

References

Basser, L. S. Hemiplegia of early onset and the faculty of speech with special reference to the effects of hemispherectomy. *Brain*, 1962, *85*, 427—460.

Bay, E. Über die sogenannte motorische Aphasie. *Nervenarzt*, 1949, *20*, 481—490.

Bay, E. Aphasia and non-verbal disorders of language. *Brain*, 1962, *85*, 411—426.

Bay, E. Present concepts of aphasia. *Geriatrics*, 1964, *19*, 319—331. (a)

Bay, E. Principles of classification and their influence on our concepts of aphasia. In A. V. S. De Reuck & M. O'Connor (Eds.), *Disorders of language*. London: Churchill, 1964. Pp. 122—139. (b)

Bay, E. Problems, possibilities, and limitations of localisation of psychic symptoms in the brain. *Cortex*, 1964, *1*, 91—102. (c)

Bay, E. Probleme und Aufgaben der Aphasieforschung. In H. G. Bammer (Ed.), *Zukunft der Neurologie*. Stuttgart: Thieme, 1967. Pp. 247—254.

Bay, E. Aphasielehre und Neuropsychologie der Sprache. *Nervenarzt*, 1969, *40*, 53—61.

Bay, E. Der gegenwärtige Stand der Aphasieforschung. *Nervenarzt*, 1973, *44*, 57—64.

Byers, R. K., & McLean, W. T. Etiology and course of certain hemiplegias with aphasia in childhood. *Pediatrics*, 1962, *29*, 376—383.

Critchley, M. Aphasiological nomenclatures and definitions. *Cortex*, 1967, *3*, 1—25.

de Rom, E. Fracture du crane chez un enfant de 19 mois. *Journal de Chirurgie et Annales de la Sociéte Belge de Chirurgie*, 1935, *34*, 577—581.

Dreifuss, F. E. Delayed development of hemispheric dominance. *Archives of Neurology (Chicago)*, 1963, *8*, 510—514.

Gesell, A., & Ames, L. B. The development of handedness. *Journal of Genetic Psychology*, 1947, *70*, 155—175.

Gloning, K., & Hift, E. Aphasie im Vorschulalter. *Wiener Zeitschrift für Nervenheilkunde*, 1970, *28*, 20—28.

Guttmann, E. Aphasia in children. *Brain*, 1942, *65*, 205—219.

Information Center for Hearing, Speech, and Disorders of Human Communication. *Bibliography on childhood*. Baltimore: Johns Hopkins Medical Institutions, 1968.

Kinsbourne, M. The minor cerebral hemisphere as a source of aphasic speech. *Archives of Neurology (Chicago)*, 1971, *25*, 302—306.

Milner, B., Branch, C., & Rasmussen, T. Evidence for bilateral speech representation in some non-righthanders. *Transactions of the American Neurological Association*, 1966, *91*, 306—308.

Riese, W., & Collison, J. Aphasia in childhood reconsidered. *Journal of Nervous and Mental Disease*, 1964, *138*, 203—205.

Subirana, A. Nosological situation of so-called congenital aphasia. *Proceedings, 7th International Congress of Neurology*, 1961, *1*, 737—740.

Tomkiewicz, S. Aphasie chex l'enfant. *Revue de Neuropsychiatrie infantile et d'Hygiène mental de l'Enfance*; 1964, *12*, 109—122.

Wenzel, H. Die Aphasie im Kindesalter. I. D. (Thesis), Univ. Marburg, 1966.

3. The Naming Process and Its Impairment

L. S. Tsvetkova

The research described concerns the nature and mechanisms of the impairment of the ability to name objects in amnesic aphasia, occurring in lesions of the parieto-occipital areas of the dominant hemisphere.

Experiments confirmed the hypothesis about the *gnostic nature* of impairment of the naming process. It was demonstrated that disturbance of the cognitive basis of a word manifests itself in patients with this particular form of amnesic aphasia as an impairment of the ability to identify the features of an individual object, and in a tendency to equate the features of such an object with those of a group of similar objects.

To explain the mechanism of this disturbance, a disturbance of the identifying process at the level of the "standards" against which the perceived object is checked was postulated.

In this case, there may also be a disturbance of the identification pattern, the simultaneous presentation of "standard" images for checking against the hypothesis that arises being impossible because the memory traces are "weak" or "washed out," and successive presentation taking its place. This manifests itself at the level of speech in a retrieval strategy consisting of going through a series of words within one semantic field.

The Problem

The naming of an object is one of the most complex of speech processes. This problem has, at one time or another, exercised many of the greatest philologists and linguists, psychologists and neurologists, such as Sechenov, Potebnja, Vygotsky, Goldstein, Head, and others. From the pathologist's point of view, the mechanisms and the nature of disorders in the naming process are of particular interest, especially in cases where the nominative function has been impaired through local brain lesion, and there has been considerable controversy for many decades about the possible explanation.

The different aspects of the naming process are studied by various branches of science. What interests us are the nature and mechanisms of the process by which the subject finds the necessary name word. We have attempted to approach this problem via the pathology of the naming process, using a neuropsychological method of research. By studying disturbances of the nominative function, we feel we shall be able to penetrate to a deeper aspect of the naming process normally hidden from the researcher: first; its multi-level structure and the connection and interaction between these levels and, second, the interaction of speech with other psychological processes.

The mechanism of the naming process is distinct from that of the generation of sentences. The two sorts of speech activity pose different linguistic problems and the mechanims by which they are carried out are likewise different. In sentence generation, the process of seeking and finding the necessary word is a secondary process, subordinate to the main process of programming the utterance and giving it grammatical structure and also to the kinetic organization of the act of speech. Contextual connections are very important in the strategy of word retrieval, and selection of the necessary word is based on successive syntheses.

When the subject utters a name, there is, as a rule, no verbal context, and just one word is pronounced. The process of retrieval of the necessary name in this case entails the selection of a word from a series of other words not grammatically or syntactically linked but in all probability grouped together on the basis of semantic connections. The selection process is the primary process here and proceeds on the basis of simultaneous syntheses, that is, the words do not appear strung out in succession as in the first case, but simultaneously. One word has to be chosen from the whole group floating up into consciousness.

What is the mechanism by which the necessary word surfaces? Does it have an "internal" verbal context and if so, what is the word-context relationship? Is it only at the level of speech that the name appears, or is its appearance linked with other processes, gnostic processes in particular? What is the strategy of word retrieval? This is by no means a complete list of the questions that arise every time the problem of the psychology and psychopathology of the naming process is considered.

One of the tasks of this paper is to attempt to analyze the links between the name word and other words, to analyze the interaction of speech activity with cognitive processes, and to analyze the retrieval strategy.

The subject of our research was amnesic aphasia, which is a condition found in cases of focal brain lesion. The chief symptom of this kind of aphasia is impairment of the ability to find name words. This disturbance occurs in lesions of the more posterior areas of the brain (parietal, temporal, occipital), which are connected, chiefly, with the choice of words in speech, as distinct from the anterior (postero-frontal) areas, which are responsible for the successive organization of the act of speech, the establishment of intention and the programming of the oral utterance (Luria, 1969).

A characteristic of the amnesic aphasia syndrome is that the central pheno-menon, the impairment of the naming process, occurs, as a rule, while all other forms of speech—oral (receptive and expressive) and written—remain relatively unaffected. It is precisely this isolation of one symptom of speech impairment from others that has aroused the interest of many research workers.

The clinical picture of amnesic aphasia was established as early as the nineteenth century, and many of the greatest psychologists and neurologists (Wernicke, Lichtheim, Head, Goldstein, etc.) were subsequently concerned with it. Its study has posed researchers a number of problems over the course of the years. What is the nature and what are the mechanisms of the impairment of the naming function, what are the symptoms of straightforward "amnesia verbalis" and is this a separate form of aphasia? These and other similar questions are still unanswered today.

In this chapter, we shall touch on only one of these vexing questions, that con-cerning the nature and mechanisms of the impairment of the ability to name objects.[1] This question has been studied by many researchers, and each has come to a different conclusion.

In explaining the nature of amnesic aphasia and its mechanisms, the greatest neurologists of the nineteenth century started out from the concepts of narrow localizationism and associationism. Thus Wernicke, Lichtheim, Kussmaul, and others thought of amnesic aphasia as resulting from a disturbance of the links between the motor and sensory word image centers and the "center of concepts," whereas Kleist and Henschen considered that the disturbance resulted from derangement of the "word memory center."

In their treatment of amnesic aphasia, subsequent researchers in the first quarter of the twentieth century started out from gestalt psychology and thought of it as a consequence of the disturbance of "categorial" thought. They were thus of the opinion that people suffering from amnesic aphasia could not use words as symbols.

Goldstein's (1948) theory, which was very widespread at one time, regarded the naming process, as distinct from phrased speech, as an abstract form of activity. He wrote that in those suffering from aphasia "words cease to be abstract symbols of ideas, the abstract attitude is lost." He further wrote (Goldstein, 1948), "We have come to the conclusion that the difficulties in finding words experienced by this kind of patient are only the expression of an impairment of the abstract relation-ship [p. 258]."

The views of Soviet research workers on this matter are diametrically opposed to those of Goldstein.

---

[1] Our research concerns the primary disturbances of naming in amnesic and acoustico-mnesic aphasia.

Vygotsky (1956) thought that it was the path from the abstract to the concrete that was impaired in these patients, rather than the other way round. The work of Luria (1969) has shown that defects in naming result from an impairment of selection in the system of verbal connections; that is, when a patient has to name something (a phenomenon, an object), several alternatives that he finds equally valid come simultaneously to mind. This inability to choose the necessary word is the chief mechanism involved in disturbance of the naming process.

Kogan (1962), who has also been much concerned with this problem, concludes that amnesic disorders stem from the disorganization of the connections within the speech system. In his opinion, this disorganization may arise from difficulties relating either to verbal—visual concepts or to the possible multiple interpretations of a word. He considers the basic mechanism of impairment of the naming function to be the patient's persistent orientation toward a single type of connection between word and object, and his inability to switch over from one retrieval method to another.

Markova (1961), in investigating the clinical and pathophysiological aspects of this impairment, discovered that there was a disturbance of intersensory connections underlying this defect, since, according to her, difficulties in naming arise whether the signal enters through the auditory channel or the visual and tactile channels.

Thus, unlike Goldstein, Soviet researchers see the impairment of the naming function in amnesic aphasia as linked with speech and not with the general laws of the impairment of abstract intellectual activity. We find that researchers have differing points of view when they come to describe the mechanisms of impairment, some seeing a connection with visual object gnosis and others rejecting this point of view.

Davidenkov (1915) thought the impairment of the naming process in "visual" amnesic aphasia was caused by the inadequacy of the visual excitation to provoke the appearance of the verbal image. Many researchers observed the impairment of visual object images in this kind of patient. A. R. Luria (1969) pointed to the disturbance of the connections between the visual image and verbal denotations as a possible mechanism of the impairment of naming function in acoustico-mnesic aphasia. Kogan (1962) denies any connection between the impairment of the ability to name objects and gnostic processes. Kok (1967) considers this impairment a secondary phenomenon in relation to object cognition. A partial impairment of cognition is, in her opinion, the basis of the disturbance of the abstract ability in relation to any particular object.

From this very brief analysis of the approaches of various researchers to the problem of the nature and mechanisms of the impairment of the naming function, we can see the complexity of this problem and the abundance of unanswered questions.

The specific subject of our research was the nature and mechanisms of the impairment of ability to find a name word in amnesic aphasia.

Hypothesis

Before formulating a working hypothesis, we studied what had been written on the topic under consideration. We attempted first of all to clarify the psychological structure of the naming process.

In a number of psychological investigations, the process of naming an object is linked with the process of recognition. Sechenov (1952) pointed out this link and was the first to put forward a hypothesis about the naming mechanism. He said that recognition of objects is the result of the complex processing of repeated external influences, the result of the comparison of an actual impression with impressions already received. Recognition frequently depends on those features that already stood out as markers. The naming process is akin to this isolation of an object's distinguishing features in the process of comparison with a view to its recognition (Sechenov, 1952, p. 480).

The same idea is also found in contemporary Soviet research into the recognition (identification) process (Lomov, 1966; Rubakhin, 1966; Shekhter, 1967; and others). The researchers ascertain several levels in the identification process. Lomov, for instance, considers the basic elements of this process to be the formation of a perceived image, the checking of this image against a memorized set of "standards," and the selection from these of the one that suits the image (Lomov, 1966). Rubakhin (1966) attaches great importance to the analysis of an object's features in the formation of its image in the perception process.

Researchers are inclined to link the naming process primarily and directly with the identification of the object's essential features, although they point out that, more generally, naming is the result of all the levels operating together. In this connection, Shekhter (1967) writes: "The result of the collation process is a signal that evokes a response from the mechanisms of connections formed in past experience, for example connections between the characteristics of objects of a particular class and their verbal denotation [p. 42]."

Thus a word has a sensory basis, and the naming process is linked with the process of identification and primarily with the identification of the object's characteristics. Many researchers have pointed to the connection between a word and its sensory basis. As a denotation, the word is a specific unit of sensory and semantic content [Rubinshtein, 1958]. The denotative word isolates the essence of the object or phenomenon, generalizes it, and thus brings the phenomenon or object into the system of objects or phenomena.

All writers on aphasia further note the characteristic of amnesic aphasia, which is that patients experience particular difficulties in finding words to denote *objects.* Words to express the features and qualities, and so on, of objects are found much more easily. Our own practice confirms this.

One further important circumstance is also mentioned in literature on aphasia, and this is the presence of small defects in the visual gnosis of objects, frequently occurring in the syndrome of amnesic aphasia (Kok, 1967). In our practice, we have often encountered symptoms of this kind accompanying this form of speech defect. Lastly, anatomical and morphological information provides evidence of the existence of connections between the posterotemporal and infraparietal areas of the cortex and the occipital areas. All this raises the question as to whether this defect in the speech system, the defect in finding a word denoting an object, may not be linked with impairments of the gnostic level of the word, and, more precisely, with defects in the object-identifying process.

If this is so, another question arises: what level in the identification process must be disrupted to bring about impairment in the ability to find the necessary word?

We assumed that the nature of the impairment of the ability to produce the necessary word in amnesic aphasia was more probably linked with impairment of the word's gnostic basis than with the impairment of the patient's abstract behavior. Concerning the disruption of the mechanisms for choosing the necessary word from alternatives that present themselves, it may be an impairment at the level of selecting the object's characteristic distinguishing features.

The Methods and Results of the Experiment

To check our hypothesis, we carried out an experiment with patients suffering from amnesic and acoustico-mnesic aphasia.[2]

There were two parts to the experiment. First, we investigated the patients' ability to identify the essential features (a) of a class of objects and (b) of separate objects in a class at the level of the visual perception of the object or of its visual representation.

Two methods were employed for this purpose: the drawing method and that of the classification of stylized pictures (depicting animals). We wished to discover whether (a) the identification of the features of separate objects was impaired in the patients and (b) if so, which features, those generalized and characteristic of a whole class of objects, or more particular features, characteristic of separate objects within the class.

1. Drawing a specific object when given its name.

2. Drawing in particular details to complete the picture of a specific named object (in our test, details had to be added in order to make a rooster, a hen, or a chick). The patient was given a schematic drawing of a head and body (the parts common to a chick, rooster, and hen). Drawing in the details in fact took the form of identifying and adding those features that characterize and distinguish a chick, a cock, and a hen.

3. In the next series, the patient was required to draw in certain details so as to make some object or other belonging to a whole class whose name (that of the class) he was given. The patient, for example, was told that he had to complete a drawing to make some kind of "vegetable."

---

[2]The experiment was carried out jointly with N. G. Kalita.

4. In the next and last series, tests were made to see if the patient had visual object images and could actualize them by completing the drawing of a particular schematic element of an object.

Fourteen patients with amnesic aphasia were investigated, together with a control group of 20 healthy subjects, and 25 children of preschool and primary school age. The results showed that the drawings of all the patients, as distinct from those of the healthy subjects, were disturbed, not from the point of view of drawing technique, but from the point of view of being able to isolate the individual distinguishing features of objects. A qualitative analysis of errors (first series of tests) primarily revealed defects in the patients' visual object images. Eight patients out of 14 did not reproduce the characteristics of specific objects. The distinguishing features of a particular object were frequently confused with features belonging to a whole class of objects. For example, the rabbit was drawn by many patients with short ears and a long tail, the hen with four legs, and so on (Figs. 3—1 and 2). The second group of errors consisted in the distortion of the drawing until it was unrecognizable (Fig. 3—3). Finally, three patients did not carry out the test, explaining that they "couldn't think of anything." One said he "could not see" what he had to draw.

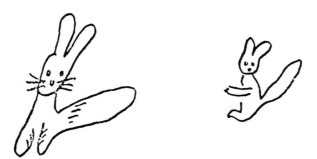

Figure 3—1. Drawing done according to verbal instruction (patient told the name word). (The instruction was to draw a rabbit and a squirrel). Patient S—va, age 38, higher education, acoustico-mnesic aphasia.

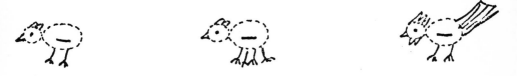

Figure 3—2. Completing a given element to make a "chick, hen and cock." (The details already given are shown by a dotted line.) Patient S—va.

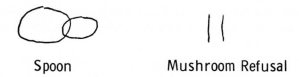

Spoon   Mushroom Refusal

Figure 3–3. Distorted drawings (patient told the name word). Patient *K*, age 40, amnesic aphasia.

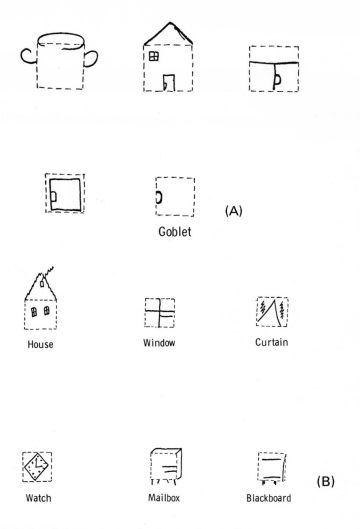

Goblet   (A)

House   Window   Curtain

Watch   Mailbox   Blackboard   (B)

Figure 3–4. Completing an abstract element to make any object.
(a) Patient *B—ev*, age 43, secondary education, acoustico-mnesic aphasia.
(b) Patient *K—va*, age 68, higher education, acoustico-mnesic aphasia.

In the second series of tests (drawing in details to make a hen, a rooster, and a chick), many mistakes were also detected. This task required the patients to produce the subtle distinguishing details of similar objects; that is, in this case, there had to be a subtle, differentiated analysis at the level of the visual images of objects evoked by the name. Analysis of the material showed that the chief error in the drawings consisted in defects in reproducing the subtle distinguishing features of the object. A kind of leveling out of distinguishing features was apparent.

Things went better in the third series of tests, where the patients were given drawings of parts of separate vegetables and were asked to draw in details to make a complete "vegetable." The whole group was called by the one word "vegetables." Most of the patients coped with this task successfully and correctly completed a cucumber, potato, radish, onion, and carrot.

In the fourth and last series, where the patients were asked to complete the drawing of a given abstract fragment so as to make it represent any item (object or phenomenon) they liked, the extremely poor quality of the visualization of objects could be seen. The patients frequently copied and tried to make the given fragment into something they had seen in the room; that is they made use of *visual perception* rather than of a *visual image* (Fig. 3—4a,b). The control group—patients with disturbance of the posterofrontal areas (with dynamic aphasia)—did all the drawing tests without mistakes (Figs. 3—5, 6, and 7).

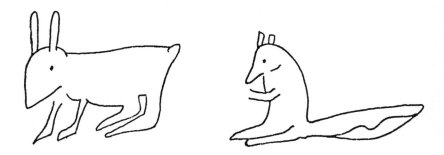

Figure 3—5. Drawing done according to verbal instruction (patient told the name word). (The instruction was to draw a rabbit and a squirrel.) Patient *P—ov*, dynamic aphasia.

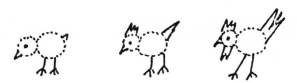

Figure 3—6. Completing a given element to make a "chick, hen and cock." Patient *P—ov*.

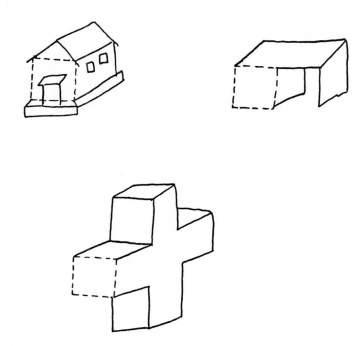

Figure 3–7. Completing an abstract element to make any object. Patient *P—ov*.

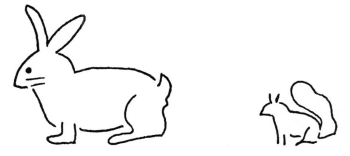

Figure 3–8. Drawing done according to verbal instruction (subject told the name word). (The instruction was to draw a rabbit and a squirrel). Subject *K—Na*, age 62, secondary education.

Thus in our experimental study of the level of visual object representation and their connection with words, we, in fact, as postulated, detected defects in isolating object-distinguishing features. We observe a certain leveling-out of the distinguishing features of an object belonging to any group and of distinguishing features of the whole group (class of objects).

This emerged particularly clearly in our test of completion of the drawings of

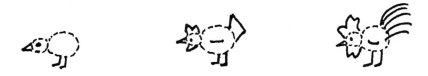

Figure 3—9. Completing given elements according to verbal instruction to make a specific object, i.e., to complete a "chick, hen and cock." Subject *K—Na*.

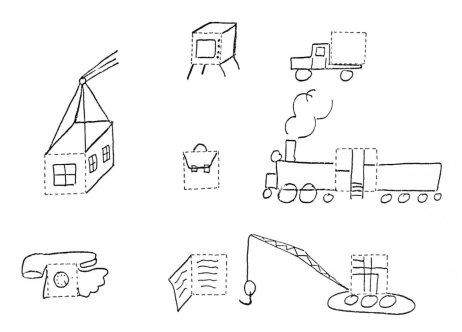

Figure 3—10. Completing a given abstract element, according to verbal instruction to make any object. Subject *E.Kh*, age 23, secondary education.

the hen, cock, and chicken. The patients ended up with average chickens, although the healthy subjects, even the primary school children, could produce in those tests clearly differentiated drawings (Figs. 8—12).[3] The patients have a set of distinctive features that were related more to the class of objects than to particular object of this class.

For these results of our experiment the question arose whether amnestic aphasic

[3] The experiments with children were carried out by the speech therapist T. M. Pirtshalaishvili.

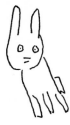

Figure 3—11. Drawing done according to verbal instruction (subject told the name word). (The instruction was to draw a rabbit and a squirrel). Child *K*, age 4.

Figure 3—12. Completing given elements according to verbal instructions, to make a specific object. Child *K*, age 4.

patients were able to isolate an object, distinguishing features at the level of visual perception. To determine this we have carried out an extra experimental series using the method of classifying the stylized (disguised) pictures, representing different animals (Fig. 3—13). These animals (mice, hares, cats, hedgehogs, pigs, dogs) were drawn in a variety of styles: ordinary, caricatured, or dotted ones, etc.

The usual shape and perspective of the animal representation, its colour and size were changed, but the basic features remained. The patients had to sort 50 pictures representing animals into groups. It was explained to the subjects that all the pictures had to be sorted but each group was to contain animals of only one kind. (The word "animal" was used only after the patient himself had looked at the drawing and said: "These are animals." The names of animals were not given.)

The results of this series of careful tests of the process of visual perception showed an impairment of fine visual differentiation in the whole group of patients. The defects showed themselves in a variety of ways. All the patients took longer to identify the objects; 56% of them made mistakes in attributing the animal to the right group (an animal from one group was put in another, e.g., the cat was put with the rabbits, and vice versa); 50% of the patients were unable to name some of the drawings, and last, 56% of the patients created a new group of animals.

Analysis of the patients' mistakes showed that there was an underlying difficulty in isolating the characteristic features of a particular animal. The distinguishing features of a particular object were confused in this series of tests, too, with the features of the more general group. For example, some patients put the stylized

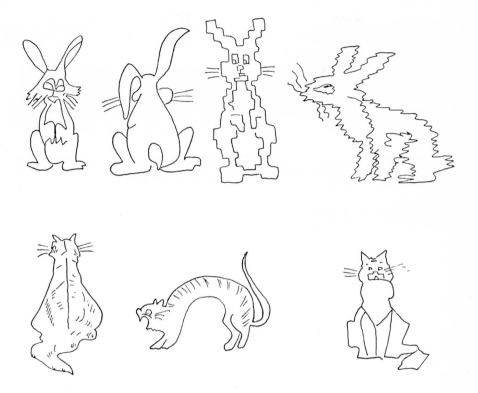

Figure 3—13. Stylized representations of animals.

rabbits in the cat group. In answer to the question "What is this?" they answered somewhat uncertainly, "A cat." In answer to the question why they thought it was a cat, the reply was always, "There are the ears, tail, and whiskers," although they agreed that these features were characteristic not only of cats but of all the other animals as well.

The control group of healthy subjects, both adults and children, and also those patients with lesions of the posterofrontal areas of the brain, made no mistakes in classifying the animals.

The first part of the experiment thus revealed that the patients with amnesic and acousticomnesic aphasia were suffering from an impairment of their ability to isolate the identifying features of a specific, individual object both at the level of visual perception and at the level of visual images. The process of isolating distinguishing features not belonging to a particular object but to the whole group of objects of the same kind (class of objects) was unaffected. Lastly, the word denoting the object was of no help in producing its image, as was demonstrated in the series of tests where an object had to be drawn from its name.

Our results show that underlying the kind of amnesic aphasia we are discussing there is apparently a disturbance in the sensory basis of the word, which leads to difficulty in the naming process.

The next question is therefore how this defect in the gnostic process expresses itself at the level of speech and what its manifestations are. We postulated that the patients would have more difficulty in finding words denoting specific objects than words denoting the properties and relationships of an object, which do not have the clarity and specific quality of the visual images proper to the objects of the real world.

To verify this hypothesis, we carried out a special test, which in fact confirmed our theory. Eight patients with amnesic and acousticomnesic aphasia took part in the test. They were shown 100 pictures representing (1) everyday articles, (2) items from children's vocabulary, (3) natural phenomena, (4) actions, (5) properties of an object (its color, taste, shape).

The pictures were shown to each patient ten times and the time taken by him to find each word was recorded. The results were subjected to quantitative analysis. The average time was worked out for (1) each word in the case of each patient, (2) each word in the case of all the patients. The time taken by all patients to find the words broke down as follows (in order of increasing difficulty):

1. Words denoting a property—average time 2.5 sec (1.4–7);
2. Words denoting action—average time 9.3 sec (2.6–20);
3. Words denoting objects—average time 15 sec (4–34).

Thus it was six times more difficult to find the names of objects than to find words expressing the more abstract phenomena of properties, and more than $1\frac{1}{2}$ times harder than for words expressing actions.

Thus whereas in the first part of the experiment we discovered impairment of the ability to identify the essential features of specific objects, the second part showed that the names of specific objects are found with considerably more difficulty than words expressing the properties and relations of objects, that is, those features of the real world of things that do not have as their basis complex visual forms. These facts, on the one hand, reconfirmed the theory about the link between impairment of the nominative function of speech and disturbance of the cognitive basis of the word and, on the other hand, showed that words designating the more general and abstract relationships of the material world are found more easily than words referring to objects.

The data from the first part of the experiment also make it possible to postulate that one of the possible mechanisms of this defect is an impairment at the level of the "standard images" against which the perceived image is compared. This is shown by the way in which the features of the individual object of a class are equated with the features of the class to which the object belongs, a frequent occurrence among patients, which replaces identification of distinguishing features.

The question is whether this peculiarity of visual perception is reflected at the level of speech, and, if so, how? To determine this, we submitted all the verbal reactions of our patients to qualitative and quantitative analysis. In searching for the necessary word, those with amnesic aphasia most frequently had recourse to the method of "going over" words, of repeatedly substituting one word for another. This "retrieval strategy" is characteristic of amnesic aphasia. These verbal reactions, as well as the methods of retrieval of the necessary word, were also submitted to psychological analysis.

In the quantitative analysis of the experimental data, a general trend was noted in the distribution of values, indicating the use by various patients of the following methods of searching for words. The commonest method (34% of all patients) was to start from a word of a related semantic group. The second most common method (16%) was to start from the object's function. In 12% of cases, patients used a combination of words in searching for the word they wanted.

We counted words denoting things (objects, phenomena) close in meaning as belonging to the same semantic group (e.g. *lightning*—not thunderstorm, not thunder, etc.; *fog*—not smoke, not dew, not cloud, etc.; *shelves*—not cupboard, not bookcase, not books; *cat*—not dog; *apple*—not pear, etc.).

Qualitative analysis of the verbal reactions (paraphasia) revealed a tendency among most patients to substitute a more general name for the specific name required.[4] E.g.:

1. *Shelves*—not a bookcase, not a cupboard, etc.;
2. *Thermometer*—not a watch, not an alarm clock, etc.;
3. *Teacup*—not a glass, not a teapot, etc.;
4. *Truck*—car, not really a car;
5. *Boy*—child;
6. *Rocket*—space;
7. *Reads*—studies;
8. They are *running*—not flying;
9. *Pistol*—shooting range.

Analysis showed that the patients search for the wanted word within the same semantic field and within a group of words denoting similar objects or phenomena.

Conclusions

Thus both the first and second parts of the experiment confirmed our hypothesis about the disturbance of the sensory basis of the word as the possible nature of the impairment of the nominative function of speech in patients suffering from amnesic aphasia.

---

[4] *Editors' note*: Evidently the order of generality of word meanings is sometimes difficult to preserve in translation from Russian to English.

Disturbance of a word's gnostic basis manifests itself in impairment of the ability to identify an individual object's features and in the tendency to equate the features of an individual object with those characteristic of a group of similar objects. It was for this reason that, in the series of tests in which they had to classify stylized objects (animals), the patients were unable to differentiate between objects similar in external appearance. In the drawing tests, the patients were unable to make accurate drawings and had recourse to a generalized image, and in the series of tests investigating the reflection of the world of objects at the level of language, all these defects likewise manifested themselves in difficulties in finding the exact word to denote a particular object and not some other closely related object.

For this very reason, the chief method of searching for a wanted word was to search within its semantic field by going through a whole range of words denoting things (objects, phenomena) in one semantic group.

The tendency noted among the patients to work from the more general word to the more particular, as shown by analysis of the examples of paraphasia, also supports the above hypothesis. All this makes it possible to doubt whether patients with amnesic aphasia suffer impairment of the "abstract categorial attitude" and whether the impairment of the ability to find a name is an impairment of the symbolic function. Our results with the group of patients we studied show that it is frequently more difficult to go from the abstract to the concrete than vice versa.

If, in the light of our information, we now look at the structure of the impairment of the naming process, the following hypothesis may be put forward. We said earlier that the naming process was linked with the process of identification, which includes a level of collating incoming information with the traces of images ("standards") of known objects recorded in the memory. In this process, there must be a prior stimulation of these traces or standards, involving the consecutive or simultaneous activation of the various memory traces (or systems of traces), that is, the postulation and checking of hypotheses. In normal subjects, the whole of this process is internalized, short, automatic, and unconscious. Only the end product of the complex process, in the shape of the name of the identified object, appears at the conscious level.

In pathological cases (amnesic aphasia) this process becomes externalized and prolonged, nonautomatic and conscious, precisely at the level of activating the traces and comparing them with the given object. The whole retrieval strategy— the method of going through a whole series of words—is evidence that the patient's memory traces are being activated and that hypotheses are being put forward and checked; one hypothesis is put forward in the form of a word and is rejected, a new hypothesis is put forward and the following word in the series appears, and so on.

As a physiological mechanism, it is possible to postulate here the presence of disagreement signals that arise when the incoming signals do not correspond with the neural model (E. N. Sokolov, 1959).

There can be a correct response to a stimulus only when the distinguishing features of an object encoded in the memory ("markers," to use the word of

Sechenov, 1952) coincide with the signaled distinguishing features of the stimulus object. Until they do coincide, identification cannot occur and hence the required word that indicates identification will not be produced.

All this gives grounds for supposing that our patients' naming process was impaired at the level of selection of a standard corresponding to the perceived image, the patient substituting for the normal process an extended strategy of repeated attempts to find the right standards. There may also be a disturbance of the pattern of interaction between perception and the producing of standards, that is, the interaction of the image perceived and the images playing the part of standards.

If we begin from the hypothesis found in modern literature on the subject, namely, that the visual identification of an object and the finding of the corresponding name may take place not only by means of the checking of successive hypotheses but also by means of the simultaneous switching-in of several standard images in answer to such a hypothesis (Nickerson, 1969; Potapova, 1970; Shekhter, 1968; and others), then we may suppose that it was precisely this pattern of identification that was disturbed in our patients. In this case, it may be considered that the disturbed standards ("washed out," "weak" traces) do not provide the necessary conditions for the simultaneous process of checking a hypothesis against the series of standards simultaneously presenting themselves. In the impairment of the naming process that we studied, therefore, a successive process takes the place of the simultaneous process of checking the hypotheses. At the level of speech, this disturbance manifests itself in the way the patient goes through successive names.

What we have said is not invalidated by those cases where the patient does not try to find the word in the same semantic field but proceeds from the functional significance of the object and resorts to going through a whole series of words and word combinations denoting the action of the object itself or what one does with the object. The patient, instead of saying "pen," says "Well, it's for writing, you take it and write," instead of "bread," says "You eat it, you bake it and eat it and they sell it in shops;" instead of "watch," says "Tick-tock, it goes, and it tells the time;" such functional descriptions refer equally well to a whole series of similar objects and one cannot tell which of them the patient has in mind (cf. pen and pencil, loaf and bread roll, watch and alarm clock). In one case, the patients use one type of substitution and in the other case a second type, but in both cases the search embraces several similar objects.

Naming is a complex mental process. It is certainly linked with cognitive processes (as developmental studies also show) and, like all the higher levels of mental activity, maintains its connection with the more elementary levels. Nevertheless, being intimately linked with the sensory basis, speech activity in the adult—naming, in particular—does not outwardly reveal this connection.

Figuratively speaking, it seems to us that the naming process is a vertical and not a horizontal one. Its "vertical" structure can be seen only in individual development and more clearly still in pathological cases.

Our experimental data and our hypothesis about the nature and mechanism of the impairment of the naming process call, of course, for further research and theoretical reflection.

References

Davidenkov, S. N. *Materials toward the study of aphasia*. Khar'kov Univ. Press, 1915. [In Russian.]

Goldstein, K. *Language and language disorders*. New York: Grune & Stratton, 1948.

Head, H. *Aphasia and kindred disorders of speech*. London: Cambridge Univ. Press, 1926.

Kogan, V. M. The dynamics of aphasia and the restoration of speech. Moscow: CYETYN Press, *Moscow*, 1962, [In Russian.]

Kok, E. P. *Visual agnosias*. Moscow: Meditsina, 1967. [In Russian.]

Lomov, B. F. On the structure of the processes of cognition. *Proc. 18th International Congress of Psychology, Moscow*, 1966, Symp. No. 16. pp. 135—142. [In Russian.]

Luria, A. R. *Higher cortical functions in man*. 2nd ed. Moscow: Moscow Univ. Press, 1969. [In Russian.]

Markova, E. D. The clinical and pathophysiological features of amnestic aphasia. Moscow: Meditsina, 1961. [In Russian.]

Nickerson, R. S. Binary-classification response times memory search and the question of serial versus parallel processing. *Report, 19th International Congress of Psychology, London*, 1969, p. 140.

Potapova, A. J. On the conditions impeding the parallel flow of cognitive process. *Voprosy Psikhologii*, 1970, No. 5. [In Russian.]

Potebnja, A. A. *Thought and language*. V. I. Kiev: Editions Ukrainian, 1926. [In Russian.]

Rubakhin, V. F. On the question of hypothesis selection in the identification of images. *Proc. 18th International Congress of Psychology, Moscow*, 1966, [In Russian.]

Rubinshtein, S. L. On thought and the means of its investigation. Moscow: Academic of Pedagogical Sciences Press, 1958.

Sechenov, I. V. The notion of an object and reality. In *Selected works*. Vol. 1. Moscow: State Academic of Sciences Press, 1952. [In Russian.]

Shekhter, M. S. *Psychological problems of recognition*. Moscow: Prosveshchenie, 1967. [In Russian.]

Shekhter, M. S. An hypothesis on parallel processes of comparison and their relation to the problem of intact recognition. *Proc. of the 3rd All Union Conference on Social Psychology, USSR, Moscow 1968*.

Sokolov, E. N. A nervous model of the stimulus. *Doklady APN RSFSR*, 1959, No. 4, p. 26. [In Russian.]

Vygotsky, L. S. *Selected psychological research*. Moscow: Academic of Pedagogical Sciences Press, 1956. [In Russian.]

Vygotsky, L. S. *Development of higher mental functions*. Moscow: Academic of Pedagogical Sciences Press, 1960. [In Russian.]

4. Basic Problems of Language in the Light of Psychology and Neurolinguistics

A. R. Luria

This chapter discusses some basic psychological approaches to the structure of verbal communication, as well as basic data obtained by observation of the alterations of this structure that are associated with local lesions of the human brain. These data are the start of a new branch of modern science—neurolinguistics— which provides an objective method for the study of the inner structure of language and speech and the underlying cerebral mechanisms.

The Problem

Linguistics, which over the last few decades has become one of the most accurate of the human sciences, uses primarily, if not exclusively, the structurological, or, what is almost the same thing, the hypotheticodeductive method in arriving at its conclusions.

When considering problems of vocabulary and semantics, linguistics does not, as a rule, go beyond the statement of the immediate meaning that it attributes to a word and the classification of these meanings into logical categories, separating the abstract and the concrete, the general and the particular meanings, and arranging them in a definite hierarchy. In considering the problems of the combination of words and syntax, linguistics limits itself to the classification of those combinations of words that give a definite meaning to a statement—to a description of those means employed by language to join separate words together into whole phrases. Structural, generative, and transformational linguistics are not an exception to the general rule; they are more an attempt to express the various forms of linguistic activity in definite formal models than to investigate either how the language process really works, or what potential systems of connections lie hidden behind each word, or what specific processes lead to the formation of a phrase or sentence.

This is why the particular branch known as *psycholinguistics* has grown up alongside general linguistics. Unlike ordinary linguistics, psycholinguistics sets out to study the specific processes of man's linguistic activity, to investigate the actual processes that lead to the formation of a word's meaning or the formation of a sentence, to distinguish its specific units and to describe those psychological (and psychophysiological) mechanisms that are part of this process.

Naturally enough, the structurological methods that suffice for general linguistics prove to be quite inadequate here, and the methods calling for the construction of separate models are replaced by completely different procedures.

These procedures include analysis of the process of development by which language is formed in ontogenesis and experimental psychological study of the conditions that underlie the formation of the meaning of individual words and phrases. They also include investigation of how each of these processes is impaired in pathological brain conditions and, in particular, in local brain lesions, which eliminate one or another of the factors underlying linguistic activity and so reveal those latent conditions for the formation of words and phrases that are invisible when the workings of speech are observed under normal conditions.

Each of these procedures, of course, leads to a more profound analysis of the actual processes underlying linguistic activity and to an investigation of those psychological conditions without an understanding of which the specific speech process remains concealed.

We shall attempt an analysis of this kind, limiting ourselves to a psycholinguistic analysis of the word and the statement, and bringing in each of the investigation methods to which we have just referred, giving particular attention to the branch that has come to be known as "neuropsychology" and which, in this case, could be called "neurolinguistics" (cf. Luria, 1970, 1973, 1974).

The Structure of the Word

It is a well-known concept in accordance with contemporary linguistics, that words, which are the main constituents of a language, designate, by convention, things, actions or qualities, events or relationships, or, finally, abstract ideas. It is also common knowledge that they make use of specific sound systems (phonetic and phonemic codes) and that they can be arranged in definite hierarchical systems beginning with the most specific and concrete and ending with the most general and abstract designations.

The fullest expression of a vocabulary is, of course, the dictionary, which expresses all possible variants of the meaning of words. But the most detailed analysis of the origin of words is found in historical (or diachronic) linguistics, which, with relative approximation, gives an analysis of how the meanings of words have changed in successive stages of a language's development.

It is quite natural that with such an approach, the actual use of a language's verbal wealth is reduced to a simple selection of the needed words from all the possible designations appearing in the dictionary, and is similar to the selection of a wanted card from a ready-made card index of lexical meanings.

To describe the actual process of choosing words in living speech like this is, however, a long way from the truth. It might have seemed plausible in the last century, when ideas of over-simplified associationism were current in psychology, but it hardly squares with the ideas that have taken shape in modern psychology as to the complex process by which words are actually used.

Modern psychology has deliberately rejected the idea of viewing every word as the simple designation of an object (things, actions, qualities, relationships, or concepts). In accordance with modern ideas, the word should be thought of rather as a multidimensional matrix of connections, and the use of each word as a process of selecting the wanted meaning from a large number of possibilities.

We shall clarify this idea, which greatly complicates our understanding of the way words are used, with the aid of a few examples.

Every word represents a definite sound complex, a small change in which may alter its meaning. Thus the word **koška** (*cat*) has the same general sound components as the word **kroška** (*crumb*), **kružka**, (*mug*), **kryška** (*lid*); and the word **skrepka** (*clamp*) as the word **skripka** (violin). Adequate understanding of any word, therefore, presupposes that the wanted word can be distinguished from all the words that sound like it; in other words, it implies a choice from among the number of likely compounds having a similar sound. If such a choice were not made, it would not be possible to understand the meaning of a word.

In addition, every word represents the designation not of one definite object, but of a whole series of possible objects. Thus the word *ručka* may designate a writing instrument (pen) and the small hand of a child, the handle of a door, the arm of a chair, and so on, and the word *časy* can at the same time mean an instrument for measuring time and time itself (**časy begut**, *time flies*). In some languages, of which English is an example, the multiple meanings of words are particularly evident—the word *to go* can at one and the same time mean "to walk, to run, to ride, to begin, to move forward," and so on. All this leads to the idea so frequently mentioned in linguistics that almost every word is, in practice, a homonym, and that using a word in its wanted sense implies a choice of the wanted meaning of the word from among a great number of possible alternatives.

Finally, every word represents a very complex formation that, alongside its designating function (or pertinence to an object), also includes a system of *generalizations* that is known in psychology as the word's meaning. Thus *ugol'* may mean either something that makes dirty, or something obtained by charring wood, or something for stoking fires, or the element carbon (C) of the periodic table, and so forth. As the eminent Soviet psychologist L. S. Vygotsky demonstrated (1934, 1956), the pertinence of a word to an object in ontogenesis may remain the same (**hleb** always designates *bread*, and **slon** always designates an *elephant*). However, the meaning of a word, that is, the system of generalizations lying behind it, does in fact change or develop; if the word **lavka** (*shop*) has an emotional significance for a child (a place where tasty things are bought), it subsequently takes on a specific, graphic meaning (a shop at the street corner), and, lastly, it changes into the complex idea of "commodity exchange system."

Naturally, even in this case, the use of a word in its required meaning also supposes a choice, which this time will be a choice from among the many likely semantic systems in which the word is included, the "decision making" underlying this choice taking place either according to the problem with which a person is faced, or according to the context, or to other factors.

All of this demonstrates that the use of words is a process incomparably more complex than the straightforward use of this or that unit of vocabulary, that it always entails a process of selection underlying which is the making of a decision, and that in different cases (depending on the level of development, personal experience, the task in hand, or the context) this selection process can take place in completely different ways.

Methods of Investigation

The question naturally arises as to what methods the psychology of speech (or psycholinguistics) has at its disposal for investigating the specific process we have just been describing, that of "making a decision" and choosing the wanted meaning of a word from among the many possible alternatives.

Are we able, by these means, to describe both the unequal composition of the various components of verbal connections and the changes brought about in them by such factors as age, intellectual development, individual peculiarities, the task in hand, or the general context of mental activities?

The first, fairly wide-known method, described in many psychological observations, is the recording of that enlarged sense in which words are used in early childhood, and in which a word given to a child is understood.

Psychologists are well acquainted with the observations of Darwin, whose grandson used the word *qua* for a duck, water, and a coin with a picture of an eagle on it, and those of Stumpf, whose son used one word for the cat that scratched him, warm furs, and a number of other widely varying phenomena.

Precisely the same facts were mentioned by Vygotsky who, in a well-known experiment with artificial words, showed that, in the early stages, every word has a compound meaning, possessing some feature or mark that is constantly found in the object, entering into its structure for a variety of reasons (Vygotsky, 1934).

Further research has confirmed that although at the early stages of ontogenesis an undifferentiated word such as **Tpru** (*Gee up! Whoa!*) could equally well signify an object, "horse," and an action ("Off you go" or "Stop"), if a noun suffix were added making it into *tpru-n'ka*, its range of meaning narrowed, and although still referring to an object (horse), it no longer signified an action or quality. We have made a more detailed analysis of this fact elsewhere (Luria & Yudovich, 1968).

Similar results have also been obtained in observations of the reverse process, when a child was given a word and it was then seen what specific meaning the word had at various stages of ontogenesis. As was demonstrated in a number of observations (Rozengrad-Pupko, 1948), if a 2-year-old child is given the word *bear* and asked to choose an object corresponding to it from among a group of objects not containing a bear, he will readily pick out a dog (the mark of an animal), a fur glove (the feature of hair and color), and so on. This diffuse meaning of a word disappears only at a subsequent stage, and is limited at first to a completely specific object, acquiring a more general significance later on. Other investigators have described findings similar to this concerning the change in the specific meaning of a word as age increases (Lublinskaya, 1959).

All of this led Vygotsky to the idea, already mentioned, that the meaning of words develops, and the whereas in the early stages the meaning of the word rests on an affective generalization, at later stages the visual image starts to be included with it, and later still, the abstract idea, too. The idea that the development that a word undergoes in ontogenesis expresses a profound change in interfunctional relationships, shifting the dominant role from emotional experience to visual memory and then to abstract logical codes, is related to a number of very profound ideas that Vygotsky introduced into psychology.

The second method, of investigating the actual system of links concealed behind a word, was applied considerably later than the first; it has all the advantages of a rigorous psychological experiment.

As we have already said, every word is a multidimensional matrix of connections (sound and semantic) from which the subject each time selects the appropriate meaning. The question remains, however, as to what objective means may be employed for establishing the specific connections underlying a word for a given subject and distinguishing between the dominant and the subordinate ("background") connections. In other words, how is it possible to establish in an objective way the "semantic field" of which every word forms a part? A method known as "semantic conditioning" was suggested some time ago for solving this problem (Razran, 1949a,b; Reiss, 1940; Schvarts, 1948, 1949, 1954). This involved establishing a conditioned reflex to a particular (test) word, after which tests were made to see what other words with semantic or phonetic similarity would elicit a similar conditioned reflex, and how strong the reaction evoked by such words would be.

We too have carried out a number of experiments along these lines, which demonstrated all the advantages of an objective approach to analyzing the system of specific semantic connections lying behind various words. These experiments, which have led to much further research (cf. Luria & Vinogradova, 1959, 1971; Vinogradova, 1956; Vinogradova & Ėjsler, 1959), were conducted in the following way. A subject in whom the vascular orienting reactions were first extinguished (narrowing of the vessels in the hand with widening of the vessels in the head, the latter being measured from the external temporal artery) was given a test word (e.g., *cat*), on hearing which he had to clench his right-hand (while the vascular reactions were being recorded with the aid of a finger mirror plethysmograph and the left-hand). After both reactions—the voluntary motor reaction and the involuntary orienting (vascular) reaction—to the test word had been well established, the problem was to find which words, although not eliciting a voluntary motor reaction, would still elicit an involuntary orienting reaction; or, in other words, to find what specific system of connections lay behind the test word.

The tests made it possible to reach quite clear conclusions. With normal subjects (children of 9—13 years of age) who were given the test word **koška**, *cat*, the homonyms **kroška** (*crumb*), **kryška** (*lid*), **kružka** (*mug*), **okoško** (*window*) did not elicit any orienting reaction, whereas words close in meaning to the test word (e.g., *kitten, mouse, dog, animal*), although not eliciting a voluntary motor reaction, nevertheless elicited for some time an involuntary orienting reaction, the strength of this reaction varying with the closeness of the connection between the given

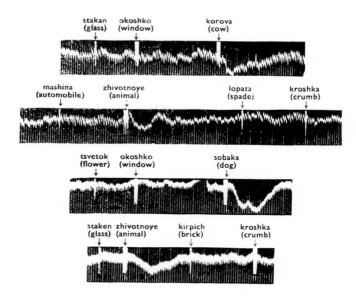

Figure 4—1. The nature of the reactions of normal school-children of 11—12 years of age to word stimuli. Words linked in meaning with the signal word **koška** (*cat*), **korova** (*cow*), **sobaka** (*dog*), **zivotnoye** (*animal*) evoke reactions; words similar in sound, **kroška** (*crumb*), **okoško** (*window*), have no effect. In the figure the plethysmogram of the finger in recorded. The moment of application of word stimulus is registered by vertical lines. The thin vertical lines are the recording of time in seconds.[1]

[1]Figures 4—1, 2, and 3 are taken from Luria and Vinogradova (1959).

word and the test word (Fig. 4–1). In mentally retarded children (defectives and imbeciles) of the same age, the same experiment gave different results. With these children, the involuntary orienting (vascular) reaction continued to be elicited both by words that were close to the test word in sound and by words close to it in meaning. The children with pronounced mental retardation had distinct orienting reactions to words close to the test word in sound (**kroška, kryška, kružka**), whereas words close in meaning (*mouse, animal*) did not elicit such reactions (Fig. 4–2).

This experiment convincingly demonstrates that the normal and the mentally retarded child have quite different systems of connections underlying words, and that the actual structure of semantic fields is different in each case. It is also interesting to note that the composition of these semantic fields may also reveal a definite dynamic. Thus if in the morning (when feeling fresh) a child with a medium degree of mental retardation (deficiency) has predominantly involuntary orienting reactions to words close in meaning, he has no such reactions to these words in the evening (when tired), but begins, on the contrary, to react to words close in sound (Fig. 4–3). This demonstrates not only that we have an

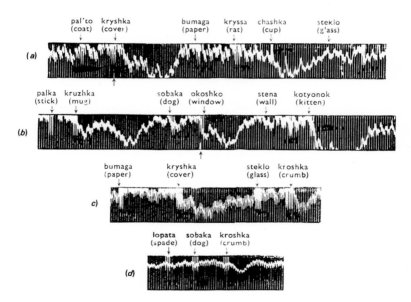

Figure 4–2. (*a*) The reaction to words of an imbecile (16 years). Not only vascular reactions but also arbitrary motor reactions are disturbed. Explanation given in the text. (The motor reaction is registered by a vertical line ↑ in the lower part of the tracing.) (*b*) and (*c*) are examples of vascular reactions in child oligophrenics (debiles of 12–14 years). While there is an absence of reaction to words having semantic connections with the signal word, reactions to words similar in sound to the signal are observed.

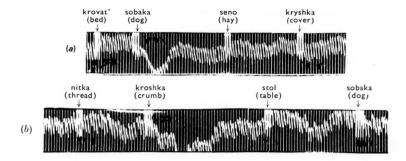

Figure 4–3. Effect of fatigue on the semantic system of an oligophrenic (a 17-year-old debile). Adequate semantic system gives way to primitive sound connections. (*a*) Before lessons; (*b*) after lessons.

objective method for discovering the system of connections that in fact underlies individual words in normal and abnormal subjects, but also that we are in a position to investigate the change in these connections as a function of the subject's condition.

The method we have just described made it possible not only to detect the existence of different kinds of connections underlying words but also to measure these connections, or, in other words, to carry out an objective analysis of the structure of the semantic field and the degree of kinship between its various parts. To do this, another variant of the method just described was employed.

A subject whose orienting reactions to words were extinguished in advance was given a particular test word (**skripka**, *violin*, in one series and **zdanie**, *building*, in another), accompanied by a painful irritation. In the end, each time the word was suggested, the conditioned reflex to the pain began (contraction of the vessels in the hand and the head). After this, the main test began, consisting of giving the subject neutral words (*window, sky*) and words close in meaning to the test words, such as *cello, balaika,* or *harp* in the first case, and *house, construction,* or *cottage* in the second.

The test revealed that reactions to the various words fell into three groups. Words close in sense to the test word continued for some time to evoke the specific pain reaction (contraction of the vessels of the hand and head). Those more distant in meaning began to evoke only a nonspecific orienting reaction (contraction of the vessels of the hand, dilation of those in the head). Lastly, the neutral words evoked no reaction at all.

By processing the findings (multiplying the intensity of the reaction by its length, or simply examining the type of vascular reaction), it was possible to determine the degree of these reactions and so to express how close the given word was to the test word.

The investigation carried out on normal adult subjects gave curves showing the degree of intensity of the specific or nonspecific reaction to words varying in their degree of closeness to the test word. In Fig. 4—4, we give a typical example of one such measurement of the degree of closeness of individual words included in the semantic field of the word *building*. It can be seen from this that the words *construction, premises,* and *house* evoked the maximum specific reaction (joint contraction of the vessels of the hand and head, similar to the reaction to the test word); the words *museum, theatre,* and *hut* evoked only a nonspecific orienting reaction; and, finally, neutral words (one of which in this case is the word *znanie,* which is close in sound to the test word) evoked no reaction at all.

It is easy to see what prospects this method opens up for the objective analysis of the structure of semantic fields and their modification under the influence of various factors (individual experience, problems to be solved, etc.). This will be of great value to psychology and psycholinguistics in the task of studying the specific connections between verbal elements in human consciousness.

We have, up to now, described the chief methods that have made it possible to analyze a word as a multidimensional matrix of connections. We have, however, not yet dealt with the procedures that could lead to an analysis of the role played by the various neurological mechanisms in maintaining normally operating semantic fields.

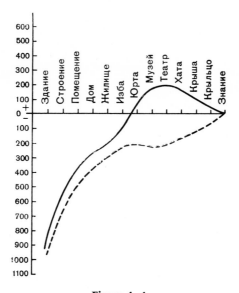

Figure 4—4.

For the third method of investigation, we must have recourse to the methods offered us by neuropsychology. It is a fact that normal use of semantic fields is possible only when the processes of stimulation are subject to a high degree of selectivity, which is a characteristic function of the brain's cortex. It is only in these conditions that it is possible to select the wanted meaning (or wanted connection) from all the possible systems of connections and to attribute to the selected meaning that durability that is characteristic of every *dominant* process.

It is a well-known feature of the physiology of the higher nervous processes that the basic condition that makes such a high selectivity possible is the normal relationship of the stimulating and inhibiting processes on the one hand, and their normal mobility on the other. Pavlovian physiology of higher nervous activity teaches that both these conditions are ensured by what Pavlov called "the law of strength," according to which strong or biologically significant stimulations evoke a strong reaction, and weak or biologically insignificant stimulations elicit a weak reaction.

The significance of this law for preserving a high selectivity in the course of mental processes can also be seen from the fact that when the tone of the cortex is lowered (in cases of marked fatigue or in the drowsy state before sleep), this law of strength changes, and the cortex begins to pass over into a *leveling phase*, when strong and weak, significant and insignificant stimulations begin to elicit one and the same reaction, or a paradoxical phase, when strong or significant stimuli begin to elicit only a weak reaction, and weak or insignificant stimuli elicit a strong one. It is not hard to see that in such circumstances, all selective activity by the cerebral cortex ceases to be possible, and there necessarily arises a unique condition—that in which the stimulation power of the various traces, that is, varying in strength, in any system is leveled out.

This can most clearly be seen in the change of structure of semantic fields that takes place in such circumstances. Everyone who has observed himself in a drowsy state (precisely the state that is characterized by phasic or inhibiting forms of cortical activity) well knows those strange and poorly coordinated connections evoked by various words, and the involuntary appearance either of secondary associations or of words close in meaning that never appear in the normal state.

One of the best descriptions of these unexpected appearances of secondary connections or words close in meaning comes from Tolstoy, in a scene from *War and Peace*, where one of the characters is on the borderline between sleep and waking:

> *On this knoll was a white patch which Rostov could not understand; was it a clearing in the wood, lighted up by the moon, or the remains of snow, or white horses? It seemed to him indeed that something was moving over that white spot. "It must be snow—that spot—**une tache**," Rostov mused dreamily. "But that's not a **tache**... Na... tasha, my sister, her black eyes. Na... tasha.*

Natasha . . . tasha . . . sabretache . . . yes! Natasha, attacks, tacks us, —whom?
The hussars. Ah, the hussars with their moustaches . . . . Along the Tversky
boulevard rode that hussar with the moustaches. I was thinking of him too, just
opposite Guryev's house . . ... Old Gurvey . . . . But that's all nonsense. The
great thing is not to forget somethingimportant I was thinking of, yes. Natasha,
attacks us, yes, yes, yes. Tha s right. [War and peace, *translation by C.*
Garnett, Part 3, Chapter 13, p. 249, Heinemann, London, 1961.]

One can easily see that the lowered (inhibited) state of the cortex with its chief feature, the leveling out of the probability of the appearance of various (in the normal state—variously probable) connections, can be a valuable means of studying those potential connections lying behind a word, consideration of which is vital for a careful analysis of speech in normal conditions.

Probably one of the most favored circumstances for such an investigation is the change of the vocabulary in the language of patients with local brain lesions.

Local brain lesions lead only relatively rarely to complete destruction of functionally integrated areas of the cerebral cortex. Most frequently they cause such areas to function in pathological ways, and one of the most important changes they cause is precisely the impairment of the normal law of strength and of the normal plasticity of the nervous processes, about which we spoke earlier.

It is a remarkable fact that these pathological changes do not spread subsequently to the whole cortex, but usually remain regional in nature. Thus in lesions of the parietal-temporal-occipital portions of the cortex, they reduce the most complex "tertiary" functions of the cortex to a pathological state, while leaving the visual or auditory areas and their functions relatively untouched. Lesions of the postcentral areas (tactual—visual integration) may, for instance, affect only somatosensory or kinaesthetic syntheses, while sparing primary visual sensory processes. This factor is of decisive importance when it comes to changes in the normal course of speech processes and, in particular, to the normal process of selecting wanted words.

In short, every word represents a multidimensional matrix of connections from which the wanted (adequate) connections are chosen while secondary connections are inhibited; in pathological conditions of the cortex, the very process of inhibiting secondary (inadequate) connections is impaired, and thus the appearance of any of the connections of this multidimensional matrix becomes equally likely. Competition between the equally likely connections leads to the phenomenon of "forgetting" and wanted word (amnesic aphasia) and to the appearance of inadequate connections or words (paraphasia) that resemble the wanted word either semantically or phonologically.

A single illustration will suffice. Patient B, with an arteriovenous aneurism within the temporal-parietal lobes of the left hemisphere, was giving an account of his illness. He very quickly began to experience difficulty in finding the wanted words, instead of which rival "side" connections easily appeared, and his account took the following form:

> *As I fill...full...fell ill. It was like this: things weren't so good...and I went right dawn...down...down. They took me off to the armoury—not it wasn't...it was to school—oh no! not school...into the Red Army...no, what am I saying...the Red Army!...it was, you know, where people go when they aren't well? To the infirmity?...that's it...the infirmary!*

It is easy to see that in this case, the word *infirmary*, which is being sought for, is first confused with a word having the same ending (*infirmary—armoury*) and then with a word designating another social establishment (*infirmary—school*), and then with the word *Red Army* linked with the words *Red Cross* being sought for along the chain, and the selective isolation of the wanted word becomes considerably more difficult.

If the lesion is in another zone of the cortex and causes a pathological condition of the auditory-motor integration of the left hemisphere, the understanding of words is impaired at another link in the chain. The secondary connections that appear involuntarily may have a different character, and instead of confusion of the wanted word with another close in meaning, there is inability to select the wanted sound, and a wrong phoneme appears, or the required articulant starts to be confused with a secondary one similar either in sound or articulation (literal paraphasia).

We shall give just two examples, the first of which is taken from observations of a patient with a focal lesion of the temporal (auditory-speech) areas of the left hemisphere (sensory aphasia), and the second from observations of a patient with a lesion of the lower portions of the postcentral (kinaesthetic) cortex and with apraxia of the speech organs (afferent motor-aphasia).

The example of the first kind of literal paraphasia, arising in cases of lesions of the left temporal lobe and acoustic-cognitive aphasia, shows the patient repeating the word **okno** (*window*) as **oglo...ono...ogno...sakno** (confusion of **okno** [*window*] with *steklo* [*glass*]), or the word **belka** (*squirrel*) as **beska...ljaska...liska**, which, after a lengthy effort, was replaced by the phrase: *Well, what's it like...a reddish fox.*

The example of the second kind of literal paraphasia shows a woman patient with a tumor of the left postcentral convolution and marked apraxia of the speech organs repeating **velosiped** (*bicycle*) as **voda...las...vola...svaja...voda...velo...svid...velo-ped...velosiped...velo-spit...velosvid,** and the word **škaf** (*cupboard*) as **naš...net...koz...net nož...ė-kstrof** (confusion with **ėtažerka** [*bookshelf*]). The same patient repeated the word **garderob** (*cloakroom*) as **ėlber...ėkvator,** the word **sobačka** (*doggy*) as **sv...sa...salnoška...sandežka...net sta...stanuška** and similarly other words.

Similar mistakes arise in the attempt to name objects; the only way out of the difficulties that occur is to try to produce the given word in a complete and continuous context. A considerable number of examples of this kind were analyzed in the work of E. S. Bĕjn (1947, 1957; Bĕjn & Ovcharova, 1970), and we shall not deal with them further here.

In the variants of the regional pathology of the cortex just described (embracing the posterior auditory, kinesthetic, and more complex synthesizing regions of the cortex of the left hemisphere), the pathological function impairs the normal process of selecting the wanted word from the multitude of possibilities, and it was precisely this that led to the discovery of the complex multidimensional matrix of connections that underlies every word.

As we have already said, the second condition for finding a wanted word is linked not with its direct selection from the matrix of possible connections, but with the speech context, which, in normal speech, is the most important selection factor. If the last word is left out of the sentence, *Winter came and the streets were deep with . . .*, there is no difficulty in supplying it according to the context, since all the necessary information is already given in what goes before. The word *snow* appears with a likelihood bordering on 100%. On the other hand, in the unfinished sentence *I went out to buy . . .*, the context does not give enough information to increase the likelihood of the appearance of one definite word, and there is a roughly equal chance of the words *a paper, some bread, some boots, a hat*, and so on, appearing. The help given by the context in the appearance of a wanted word has been the subject of a great deal of research in recent years. Most of these investigations, however, resulted from attempts to analyze the degree of redundancy of information and to assess its significance.

In this connection, we may point out that here, too, neuropsychological analysis offers as yet unexplored but promising possibilities.

In the three cases described above, the process of word selection according to general context not only remained intact, but was one of the most important ways of compensating for initial impairments (see also Jakobson, 1956, 1964, 1966). The difficulties the patients experienced therefore stemmed from the leveling-out of the likelihood with which the various connections of the word's multidimensional matrix made their appearance.

There is, however, another group of localized brain lesions in which no serious difficulty at all is experienced in selecting a wanted word from among many likely alternatives, and in which all the difficulties are shifted onto the process of selecting a wanted word according to the general speech context. This is caused by lesions in the anterior portions of the speech area of the left hemisphere, and is part of the general picture of "dynamic aphasia" described by us elsewhere (Luria, 1966, 1969, 1970; Luria & Tsvetkova, 1968a).

In these cases, the process of naming separate objects or, in other words, the process of selecting a wanted word according to a given specimen remains completely unaffected, and patients do not experience any perceptible difficulty whatever in choosing the wanted name from among several possibilities. On the other hand, considerable difficulties are observed when a patient has to find a wanted word in the context of a complete statement. It is precisely here that he is seen to have "gaps" as a result of which no words at all come to his mind; his active speech is impaired, and he is forced to have recourse to well-worn speech stereotypes, which begin to replace the impaired process of producing wanted words in a speech context.

We still know very little about the mechanisms underlying this kind of impairment. In other publications, we have put forward the idea that underlying these defects is to be found the impairment of inner speech, with its predicative role, and the associated impairment of the "linear pattern of the sentence" (Luria, 1969, 1970; Luria & Tsvetkova, 1968b; Riabova, 1970). However, a close study of the etiology underlying this kind of impairment in finding a wanted word is something for the future.

All the same, there is no possible doubt that psychological experiments and neuropsychological analyses are destined to bring to light many very important facts bearing on the actual mechanisms underlying the lexical aspects of speech.

The Structure of the Phrase

From an analysis of individual words and their meanings (vocabulary and semantics), linguistics goes on to analyze the fundamental laws governing combinations of words forming a proposition (grammar and syntax). These are, in fact, the branches of linguistics that have had most marked success, and together with structural linguistics and its separate divisions, generative and transformational grammar have come so near to being an exact science that they may be placed on an equal footing with logic and mathematics.

Nevertheless, despite these undoubted successes and the construction of fairly exact models, the question as to how, in fact, the process of forming a phrase or sentence proceeds, what are its components, what is the relation of its component parts to the general structural laws governing a statement, and of its linguistic components to its extralinguistic components, has remained largely unanswered.

In addition, practically no work has been done until recently on specific psychological processes such as those that lead to the *formation* of a statement and those that underlie the *understanding* of a statement, with its superficial meaning and its concealed, interior sense. Along with a study of the structural linguistics, it was essential to study the psychological construction, which would come closer both to the process of forming the statement (codifying thought into speech) and to the processes involved in its understanding (decoding the speech structure and converting the statement or series of statements into their underlying meaning).

There is no doubt that contemporary psychology has greatly advanced the study of these problems also. The research of G. A. Miller into the structure of the communication process in adults (Miller, 1967, 1970) and the work on the process of sentence formation in children and on the change-over from the one-word sentence accompanied by a wealth of extralinguistic "sympactical" means (Bühler, 1934; Luria & Yudovich, 1968) have provided important material that throws light on the specific structure of both the processes mentioned—the formation of a statement and its decoding.

Linguistics has satisfactorily described the main aspects of the construction of a sentence. It has long distinguished a whole series of various structural devices, beginning with a simple exclamation or a one-word statement in which the thought is conveyed by an accompanying extralinguistic (intonational and sympractical) context, and ending with the most complex system of subordination of words to one another, by means of inflections, connectors, and word order, whereby, in the words of Bühler (1934), language is made into a system adequate for the independent expression of any thought. Linguistics makes a clear distinction between those kinds of statements that express visual events and those that express complex logical relationships. This differentiation of the "communication of events" and the "communication of relationships" was first propounded by Svedelius (1897) and has been fully confirmed by contemporary language studies. Lastly, linguistics knows quite well in what cases grammatical structure is able to remain incomplete, and when a complete and detailed use of all language codes is called for. The extended work on oral and written language, on the language of drama and the language of epos, carried on by Bühler (1934) and Vygotsky (1934), makes it possible to describe this dimension quite accurately. Also, the introduction into linguistics of the methods of information theory brings that science closer to a position where it can evaluate the surplus components of language and analyze those conditions that determine them.

There is great disparity between the methods for discovering the complex process by which thoughts are embodied in language, on the one hand, and, on the other, the methods for discovering the meaning concealed behind words. It is precisely this disparity that justifies our efforts to describe here only one (relatively novel) approach to research on this subject: the neuropsychological method, with its analysis of both structure and meaning.

The process of verbal expression—the turning of a thought into a statement or system of statements—undoubtedly comprises a number of steps and requires a series of conditions.

First, a statement must result from a *motive*. (Skinner, 1957, distinguishes between two response types, the -*mand* (demand) and the -*tact* (contact), to which we may add the -*cept* (concept), each of which may be presumed to have its own motive.)

Second, a thought must precede the statement (although, as in an exclamation, the thought may not be verbally represented or, as in question-and-answer dialogue, may be reduced to a minimum).

The third step, as yet little studied, is the transformation of the thought into organized speech. Following Vygotsky (1934), this phase is usually termed "inner speech;" It is abbreviated in structure, predicative in function, and conceals within itself the potential linear pattern of the sentence to come. (This phase has recently attracted considerable attention as part of the study of generative grammar.)

The final step, of course, is the embodiment of the prepared content in the form of organized, external speech; this uses a variety of grammatical language codes and is distinguished by varying degrees of completeness, including intonational and prosodic features that serve to connect separate semantic units into a more general semantic whole.

The decoding (or understanding) of an organized statement, of course, works the other way; starting with a series of phrases received by the hearer (or reader), it goes on to combine these units into groups, to sort out the most important of them, and to decipher the ways in which one is subordinate to another. At the end of this process, in which grammatical and prosodic features play their part, the hearer is ready for the next stage, that of abbreviating the organized statement into "inner speech;" from here, he either synthesizes the general, abstracted thought of the whole, or reconstructs the underlying intentions and, ultimately, the motives of the speaker.

Methods of psychological inquiry capable of tracing the component parts of this very complex process step by step, and showing the place each occupies in the task of decoding a communication, are as yet unknown to us. A sufficiently full analysis of the specific processes of encoding and decoding communications is doubtless a matter for the future. For the present, therefore, and bearing in mind all the inadequacies of our knowledge, we must seize every opportunity to map out the components of each stage and to clarify the role played by each component.

One way to do this is afforded by neuropsychology, which means analyzing the ways in which the process of forming or interpreting a communication changes in the event of lesions to various areas of the brain. It is common knowledge that a local lesion of the dominant (left) hemisphere not only brings about a familiar pathological condition in the cortex, but suppresses one of the factors needed for the normal working of one or another functional system, in our case impeding the normal functioning of speech activity (cf. Luria, 1966, 1969, 1970, 1973).

It is natural, therefore, that the process of forming or decoding a statement, including as it does a whole chain of links and factors, is adversely affected in a variety of ways according to which link of the process has been impaired. It is precisely this that makes it possible to use the neuropsychological method to analyze these component parts and to see exactly what happens to a statement when one or another of its component parts is removed.

Let us arrange this brief survey of our material in the order in which statements are formed (as described earlier). As we have already remarked, the formation begins with a *motive*, which prompts a man to speak, and with an *intention or thought*, which must be embodied in organized speech.

Both of these driving forces depend on a significant extent on the integrity of the frontal portions of the brain, which are intimately related to the formation of motives and intentions and to the establishment of projects or thoughts underlying the speech formula. As we have shown in detail elsewhere (Luria, 1962, 1966, 1969, 1970, 1973; Luria & Homskaja, 1966), patients with massive lesions of the prefrontal sections of the brain are easily diverted by any secondary stimulus, and display pathologically heightened and hard-to-inhibit orienting reflexes, but prove unable to establish independent motives or intentions (in the formation of which, apparently, the patient's own external and internal speech plays a decisive role); neither do they submit to the programming influence of received oral instructions. Such patients normally cannot formulate any active statements (it makes no difference whether they come under the -*mand* system or under the -*tact* system), since they are quite unable to formulate an intention or a thought; at the very best, they answer questions either by echoing the words or by using monosyllables.

The fact that these patients still retain intact the grammatical structure of the language (they can repeat a given sentence or even, immediately, a short story) shows that the impairment of their active speech is of an extralinguistic nature; this kind of impairment cannot be studied within the context of the present article.[2]

Impairment of speech takes on quite a different character in cases of lesions of the anterior sections of the speech zones of the left hemisphere (the lower portions of the posterior frontal section and their connections with the anterior temporal sections). These impairments, which produce a picture of "dynamic" (or to use the classical term, "transcortical motor") aphasia, have been sufficiently well described, although their underlying mechanisms are still almost completely unstudied, and ideas about them have still not progressed beyond the stage of hypotheses.

An important feature of these cases is not only that the incitement to speak is impaired, but that the structure of speech is impaired, as well, which gives a priori grounds for relating these impairments to the corresponding linguistic ones and makes it possible to use observations about them to clarify some of the important conditions necessary for the formation of a phrase or sentence.

As is well known, lesions of the anterior sections of the speech zone cause no impairment of the nominative function of speech, and the naming of separate objects remains perfectly feasible. The first distinct symptoms appear in these cases when one goes on from naming separate objects to connected, contextual speech.

In the most serious cases of such impairment, the patient may speak only in separate words, and is incapable of finding the predicate forms (verbs) to link them. Thus he talks in a "telegraphic style;" all his speech is limited to the designation of individual objects and never turns into complete, full-fledged state-

---

[2] We shall not dwell here on all the evidence pointing to the fact that the impaired ability to decipher language in patients of this group is unique in character. This theme is dealt with in a special paper entitled "Towards a neuropsychological analysis of the decoding of communications," which is being prepared for press.

ments. The prosodic components are also impaired, and the intonational and melodic organization of speech completely disappears. Patients of this group have a typical way of speaking, as illustrated by the following attempt of a veteran to tell how he was wounded:

> *So . . . the battalion . . . the front . . . well . . . how was it? . . . and then . . . it was . . . a hospital . . . and so, oh dear, oh dear, oh dear . . . and then . . . better, better . . . talking . . . nothing at all . . . .*

It is easy to see that the chief characteristic of speech that is affected in such cases is the predicative structure. This suggests that underlying the predicative structure of speech are quite different brain mechanisms from those that regulate its nominative function.

The second form of dynamic aphasia (distinguished from the first by Luria & Tsvetkova, 1968b; Riabova, 1970a) does not cause the whole of speech to be reduced to just the nominative function alone, and the connected character of the statement remains intact to a far greater degree, but all the patient's spontaneous speech is replaced either by repetition of the statements made to him or by a stereotype well rooted in previous experience. The independent formation of a statement is seriously impaired in these cases, and the patient can neither reproduce a fairly lengthy story nor, still less, make an "oral composition," forming the necessary sentences independently, but is forced to "grope for" the separate nominative components of the sentence

> *Well then . . . about the war . . . well then . . . again . . . how I was wounded . . . and then . . . about the hospital . . . .*

or to substitute ready-made stereotypes for an independently constructed statement. I shall never forget the occasion when one of these patients, in answer to a suggestion that he should say something about "the north," said *In the north there are bears,* and, after a long pause, added, *which I must bring to your attention.* A similar observation was made in the case of another patient who, having completely failed at the same talks, said, after a long pause:

> *In the wild north there grows alone*
> *A pine tree on a barren crest*

substituting for an independent sentence a well-established stereotype of a poem he had previously learned.

We still do not know the mechanisms underlying either form of dynamic aphasia. There is much that suggests that underlying the phenomena we have described is impairment of inner speech, which, as noted above, is abbreviated in structure, predicative in function, and affords the most important means for converting thought into the linear pattern of the sentence (cf. Luria & Tsvetkova,

1968b). The fact that the basis of organized speech must be sought for precisely in inner speech is increasingly beginning to attract the attention of the proponents of generative grammar; we have every reason to think that a careful analysis of such impairments will one day provide valuable material for a better understanding of the important process of the generation of grammatical speech. We can do no more here than refer in passing to the evidence that points to impairment, not of formation (encoding) of a communication, but of understanding (decoding). There has been practically no investigation of the problem of impairment of the understanding of speech in various kinds of expressive (motor) aphasia; in the thousands of publications describing this kind of aphasia, we find scarcely more than two or three that give an analysis of how receptive language is impaired in such cases.

It was long thought that the impairment of expressive speech characteristic of the cases described brought about no impairment of receptive speech, and that the understanding of information received was not affected in such cases. However, as careful observations have shown (the collection and publication of which are not yet complete), this supposition cannot be considered entirely correct; impairments in the formation of contextual speech are accompanied by similar (although more attenuated) impairments in the decoding of contextual structures.

In such cases, the patient is frequently unable to transmit a complex communication consisting of a whole series of statements, because the sense of one statement does not "flow" automatically into that of the succeeding statement; this process, which L. S. Vygotsky (1934) named the "confluence (in-flowing) of sense,"[3] is gravely impaired. It is precisely for this reason that the prosodic structure of the sentence, in which the change of intonation can, in a decisive fashion, influence the meaning of what is being said, is also inadequately received; the patient, who is himself unable to impart to a sentence the necessary intonational and melodic structure, is accordingly unable to distinguish clearly between the expressions "*I* am going to the movies," "I am *going* to the movies," and "I am going to the *movies*"; or "The *husband* shot his wife," "The husband *shot* his wife," and "The husband shot his *wife*." The ability to understand sentences differing both in intonation and stress pattern and in punctuation is a matter requiring further careful investigation in patients of this group; it is highly probable that important discoveries will be made in this direction.

We have one more piece of evidence, which has by now been well established. As we shall demonstrate later, patients with lesions of the posterior (parietal-occipital) sections of the speech areas are unable to comprehend immediately the sense of several logical and grammatical structures that come under the heading of "communication of relationships," although they understand contextual grammatical structures perfectly. For example, they are unable to distinguish between

---

[3]"The flowing of the sense of one statement into the interior sense of the succeeding statement [Vygotsky, 1974]."

the father's brother and *the brother's father*, or to say which of the two sentences is correct; *The earth lights the sun* or *The sun lights the earth*.

In patients with lesions of the anterior portions of the brain, the situation is completely reversed. The patients, while experiencing no difficulty at all in decoding communications of relationships of the kind just described, are faced with marked difficulties when given the task of evaluating the correctness of contextual grammatical structures or, in other words, those forms that link together the elements of a statement into a single, concrete whole. Patients of this kind find it extremely difficult, for example, to say which of the two sentences is correct, *The steamer is going along the river* or *The steamers is going along the river*, or to say which statement is in accordance with the rules of connected discourse, *I am writing along the papers* or *I am writing on the paper*. The well-known phenomenon of the "feel of the language," which is the consequence of successfully automatized organized speech, suffers severely in this kind of patient, and this impairment can be clearly observed both in expressive and receptive language.

As we have already said, careful analysis of this kind of speech disorder is only in its infancy, but it is quite certain to contribute much that is new to the solution of the mystery surrounding a number of the conditions necessary for the formation of grammatical speech.

A completely different form of disruption of the component parts of a statement appears in cases of lesion of the systems of the left temporal region, the upper part of which is, of course, the central apparatus for auditory-speech analysis and synthesis (cf. Luria, 1966, 1969, 1970, 1973). It is common knowledge that lesions of these areas do not impair motivation or intention, and also spare the apparatus of inner speech, including the ability to form the "linear pattern of the sentence." The prosodic components of speech also remain intact, even when lesions in this area are massive. Considerable impairment occurs in these cases either in the capacity for distinguishing the differentiating elements of auditory speech—the phonemes (sensory or acoustic-cognitive aphasia)—or in the ability to retain a sufficiently wide band of audio-speech records and to keep them free from pathologically heightened inhibition (audio-mnesic aphasia) (cf. Luria, 1970, 1971b).

This primary impairment has a marked effect upon the retention in memory of the essential content of the sentence and, hence, on the construction of the whole statement.

A patient with the type of lesion described may not understand the meaning of a word that sounds strange to him, confusing it with words close in sound—**golos** (*voice*), **kolos** (*ear of corn*), **holost** (*bachelor*), **kolhoz** (*collective farm*)—and thus the lexical elements of the whole sentence may totally fail to reach him. In trying to find an individual word, he may have real difficulties in choosing it from the multidimensional matrix and substitute a word close in meaning, giving rise to verbal paraphasia (e.g., saying *crow* or *magpie* instead of *jackdaw*), or experience difficulty in finding the accurate sound construction of a given word, giving rise to phonemic paraphasia (instead of **golub** [*pigeon*], saying **gorod** [*town*], **gorov**,

grolov, godlov, etc.). In such a patient, however, the general intonation and stress pattern of the sentence usually remains intact, as may the general sense of the sentence, which he actively reconstructs from several preceding (particularly predicative) components. The capability to reconstruct in this way is in proportion to the general activity factor, the factor relating to the prosodic structure of the remaining speech.

We may illustrate this point by showing how patients with a tumor in the temporal language area of the left hemisphere attempt to repeat a sentence or story read to them.

Patient K, when asked to repeat the sentence, *Spring came and the leaves came out on the trees,* responded, *Well . . . it was already warm, and it turned very nice.* The sentence *A policeman is standing on the wet roadway* was repeated as *Well . . . It's in the street . . . rain and there goes a soldier.*

Patient Vi, when asked to repeat the familiar story of "The Jackdaw and the Pigeons," began:

> *Well, this . . . crow . . . no . . . a* grey one *. . . no* says *. . . came up to the birds . . . no to these . . . ants* (murav'jam) *. . . no to the sparrows* (vorob'jam) *. . . they ate very well . . . and it also recognized her . . . she says . . . no shrieks . . . and they chased her away . . . well you shouldn't do that . . . so that it's something else. . . .*

It is easy to see that although the lexical content of speech has completely collapsed, there is retention of the ability to comprehend the general meaning; retained also in these reproductions are the essentials of stress and intonation patterns. The general structure of individual sentences of stories remains intact, even though the patients cannot reproduce the individual words (except for some verbs). This relative independence of general semantic structure of a statement from its lexical components indicates that these two aspects are dependent upon different brain structures. This may be of very great interest to psycholinguists, and will doubtless lead to a more serious analysis of those "deep structures of language" (Chomsky, 1957, 1965), whose description is of special interest for structural and transformational linguistics.

It remains for us to speak about the last form of localized brain lesions, in which the fragmentation of the structure of the statement occurs in completely different ways and whose study affords an opportunity for the description of new parameters of language structure.

As we have noted earlier, and shown elsewhere, lesions localized in the tertiary zones of the lower temporal and temporal-occipital areas of the left hemisphere lead directly to the breakdown of the ability to transform a temporal sequence of elements into synchronic and, in particular, spatial patterns. These impediments affect particularly the structures of "asymmetric space," in other words, space that includes the features of "right" and "left," the two sides being marked by nonequivalence (cf. Luria, 1946a, 1966, 1969, 1970, 1973).

Patients with such lesions continue to grasp simple forms and representations without difficulty. However, if they are asked to find out about the arrangement of the hands on a clock or the co-ordinates of a map, they are completely unable to do so, and confuse left and right, east and west, precisely as a result of this defect. They are unable to do work involving interpretation of designs, and have difficulty in naming the fingers of their hand, and so forth. They also have defects in counting; although they can grasp single figures, they easily lose track of a complex number, and cannot correctly carry out arithmetical calculations that presuppose the preservation of the interior quasi-spatial distribution of numerical elements.

Such patients naturally display very evident speech defects. These defects, however, are markedly different from all those that have been mentioned above. The patients in this group evince no defects in steps one and two (motive and thought or intention) of the process of verbal expression, and the basic thought remains intact. The transition from intention to contextual speech (the phase of inner speech) remains unimpaired in these patients, and we do not detect the slightest hint of impairment in the predicative function of inner speech or in the linear pattern of the sentence.

In a number of cases, these patients show clear defects in choosing a wanted word from its multidimensional matrix, experiencing the difficulties we described at the beginning of this chapter. These defects, however, are evidently linked with those cases in which the lesion has extended to the temporal regions of the left hemisphere; they do not appear to be the principal defects.

The main defect in the organization of speech processes among these patients is something completely different. Although they retain contextual speech to the full, they are unable to use those logical and grammatical codes that are the verbal expression of the "communication of relationships" and for the mastery of which the "asymmetrically ordered space" factor is necessary.

For this reason, in these patients, all grammatical forms of speech fall into either of two categories. Forms that do not call for the asymmetric ordering of space and whose meaning does not stem from a sequentially ordered chain of words or images remain fully intact. On the other hand, these patients are either completely or to a very large extent unable to use those grammatical structures for which the principle of the asymmetric ordering of space is needed.

Patients of this group can easily understand such sentences as *The house is on fire* or *The dog bit the boy*, but they are unable to understand constructions like *the father's brother* or *the brother's father*, *Summer is before Spring* or *Spring is before summer*, and in attempting to interpret the latter constructions they rely more readily on their habitual contextual sound than on their logical and grammatical organization, which remains inaccessible to them. Thus, comparing the constructions *the father's brother* and *the brother's father*, they observe that the words *father* and *brother* appear in both, and that their meaning is evidently linked, but the essential difference between these constructions is beyond them.

Patients in this category can easily understand a long sentence like *Father and mother went out to the theatre, and grandma and the children stayed at home*, but are quite unable to understand the equally long sentence *Olga went from the factory to the school that Katya attends, to tell what she had seen in the woods.* Interrelating the elements of the latter sentence, arranging them in a single cluster of quasi-spatial co-ordinates, and transforming the text given them in the process of doing so, is quite beyond these patients; they cannot understand where the first and the second girls in the sentence were or who exactly was saying something and who was the listener.

It is natural that the meaning of constructions similar to Burtt's famous test, *Olga is fairer than Sonja but darker than Katya,* is quite beyond patients of this category, and even lengthy attempts to work out what it means come to nothing, because of the impairment of their ability to turn information received sequentially into synchronic quasi-spatial arrangements; these disturbances are the primary result of these lesions.

It is easy to see that identification of the factor just described, which underlies several grammatical constructions and to an even great extent underlies the ability to divide all grammatical constructions into two completely different groups according to its presence or absence, is of very great significance for linguistics; the method just mentioned, which makes it possible to differentiate between these constructions in an objective way, is, for linguistics, an important auxiliary procedure. There is no doubt that the methods propounded in recent years by transformational linguistics will make it possible to go even deeper into the differences just described, and that the part played by neuropsycholinguistic analysis in making it possible to identify these forms objectively will number among the major contributions to the general field of language research.

Conclusions

We have dealt with only a few spheres in which neuropsychology has been successfully applied to the solution of linguistic problems. We saw that together with genetic and experimental psychology, this method, which with good reason may be called "neurolinguistics," opens up new and important possibilities for the analysis of those speech processes that it has been thought impossible to analyze until now; we may now advance from the formal description of linguistic structures, using mainly the hypothetico-deductive method, to an analysis of specific speech processes as they pass from thought to linguistic statement and from linguistic statement back to thought.

The task of describing the main components of this complex process and of isolating those factors that underlie specific forms of linguistic activity should be regarded as one of the most important tasks awaiting both linguistics and the psychology of speech. The methods we have described, in particular the neuropsychological analysis of linguistic processes, afford one possible approach to this task, and they may, at the same time, provide an answer to the very thorny problem of precisely what the study of the functional organization of the brain is able to tell us with regard to verbal behavior. Thus neurological investigations will be of great assistance in the solution of linguistic problems.

References

Bĕjn, E. S. Psychological analysis of sensory aphasia. Unpublished doctoral dissertation. Univ. 1947. [In Russian.]

Bĕjn, E. S. Basic laws of the word structure and the grammatical structure of speech in the aphasias. *Voprosy Psikhologii*, 1957, No. 4. [In Russian.]

Bĕjn, E. S., & Ovcharova, P. A. *The clinic and the treatment of aphasia. 1970.*

Bühler, K. *Sprachtheorie.* Jena: Fischer, 1934.

Chomsky, N. *Syntactic structures.* The Hague: Mouton, 1957.

Chomsky, N. *Aspects of the theory of syntax.* Cambridge, Mass.: MIT Press, 1965.

Jakobson, R. Two aspects of language and two types of aphasic disturbances. In R. Jakobson & M. Halle (Eds.), *Fundamentals of language.* The Hague: Mouton, 1956.

Jakobson, R. Towards a linguistic typology of aphasic impairments. In A. V. S. De Reuck & M. O'Connor (Eds.), *Disorders of language.* Ciba Foundation Symposium. London: Churchill, 1964.

Jakobson, R. Linguistic types of aphasia. In L. Carterett (Ed.), *Brain functions.* Vol. IV. *Speech, language and communication.* Berkeley & Los Angeles: Univ. of California Press, 1966.

Lublinskaya, A. A. *Essays on the psychological development of the child.* Moscow: Izd. Akad. Pedagog. Nauk, 1959. [In Russian.]

Luria, A. R. *The study of aphasia in the light of brain pathology.* Vol. 1. *Temporal Aphasia.* (Vol. 2. *Semantic Aphasia.* : MS, 1940. [In Russian, not published].

Luria, A. R. On disturbances of grammatical operations in brain disease. *Izvestiya Akademii Pedagogicheskikh Nauk RSFSR,* 1946, No. 3. [In Russian.] (a)

Luria, A. R.*Traumatic aphasia.* Moscow: Izd. Akad. Meditsin. Nauk SSSR, 1947. [In Russian.] (Engl. transl.: The Hague, Mouton, 1970.)

Luria, A. R. *Higher cortical functions in man.* Moscow: Izd. Moskov. Univ., 1962. (2nd ed., 1969.) [In Russian.] (Engl. trans.: New York, Basic Books, 1966.)

Luria, A. R. *The human brain and psychological processes.* Vol. 1. Moskow: Izd. Akad. Pedagog. Nauk, 1963. [In Russian.] (Engl. transl.: New York, Harper, 1965.)

Luria, A. R. *The human brain and psychological processes.* Vol. 2. Moscow: Izd. Prosveshchenie, 1970. [In Russian.]

Luria, A. R. *The lost and recovered world.* Moskow: Izd. Moskov. Univ., 1971. [In Russian.] (a)

Luria, A. R. Memory disturbances in local brain lesions. *Neuropsychologia,* 1971, 9, 367–375. (b)

Luria, A. R. Objective research in the dynamics of semantic connections. In *Semantic structure of words.* Moscow: Izd. Nauka, 1971. [In Russian.] (c)

Luria, A. R. *The man with a shattered world: The history of a brain wound.* New York: Basic Books, 1972.

Luria, A. R. *The Working Brain.* New York: Basic Books, 1973.

Luria, A. R. Basic problems of neurolinguistics. In Th. Seboen (Ed.) *Current trends in linguistics.* Vol. 12. Pp. 2561–1599. The Hague, Mouton & Civ.

Luria, A. R. *Basic problems of neurolinguistics.* The Hague: Mouton & Civ (in press).

Luria, A. R. *Neuropsychology of memory.* Washington: Scripta Publishers (in press).

Luria, A. R., & Homskaja, E. D. (Eds.) *Frontal lobes and the regulation of mental processes.* Moscow: Izd. Moskov. Univ., 1966. [In Russian.]

Luria, A. R., & Tsvetkova, L. S. The mecanisms of dynamic aphasia. *Foundations of Language,* 196' 4,   (a)

Luria, A. R., & Tsvetkova, L. S. *Neuropsychological analysis of problem solving.* Moscow: Izd. Prosvehchenie, 1968. [In Russian.] (b)

Luria, A. R., & Vinogradova, O. S. An objective investigation of the dynamics of semantic systems. *British Journal of Psychology*, 1959, *50*(2), 89–105.

Luria, A. R., & Vinogradova, D. S.   Objective study of the dynamic of semantic systems. In *semantic structure of the word*. Moscow: Nauka Publish. House. 1971. Pp. 27–82 [Russian].

Luria, A. R., & Yudovich, F. Y. *Speech and the development of mental processes in the child*. London: Staples, 1968. (Reprinted: Penguin Education, 1971.)

Miller, G. A. Psycholinguistic approaches to the study of communication. In D. L. Arm (Ed.), *Journeys in science*. Albuquerque: Univ. of New Mexico Press, 1967.

Miller, G. A. Four philosophical problems in psycholinguistics. *Philosophy of Science*, 1970, 37, No. 2.

Razran, G. Semantic, syntactic and phoneticographic generalizations of verbal conditioning. *Journal of Experimental Psychology*, 1949, *39*, (a)

Razran, G. Stimulus generalization of conditional responses. *Psychological Bulletin*, 1949, *46*, (b)

Riess, B. F. Semantic conditioning involving the galvanic skin reflex. *Journal of Experimental Psychology*, 1940, *26*.

Riabova, T. V. Psycholinguistic and neuropsychological analysis of dynamic aphasia. Candidate dissertation, Moscow Univ., 1970. [In Russian.]

Rozengrad-Pupko, G. L. *Speech and the development of perception in early childhood*. Moscow: Izd. Akad. Meditsin. Nauk, 1948. [In Russian.]

Schvartz, L. A. The role of the word and its acoustic image as a conditioned stimulus.] *Byulleten Eksperimental'noi Biologii i Meditsiny*, 1948, *25*, 1949, *27*. [In Russian.]

Schvartz, L. A. The word as a conditioned signal. *Byulleten Eksperimental'noi Biologii i Meditsiny*, 1954, *38*, Nos. 15–18. [In Russian].

Skinner, B. F. *Verbal behavior*. New York: Appleton, 1957.

Svedelius, C. *L'analyse de langage*. Uppsala, 1897.

Vinogradova, O. S. On some features of the orienting reactions to second signal system stimuli in normal and mentally retarded school children. *Voprosy Psikhologii*, 1956, No. 6. [In Russian.]

Vinogradova, O. S., & Ejsler, K. A. The appearance of verbal connections in the registration of vascular vascular reactions. *Voprosy Psikhologii*, 1959, No. 2.

Vygotsky, L. S. *Thought and language*. Moskow: Stosekgiz, 1934. [In Russian.] (Engl. transl.: Cambridge, Mass., MIT Press, 1962.)

Vygotsky, L. S. *Selected psychological research*. Moscow: Izd. Akad. Pedagog. Nauk, 1956. [In Russian].

5. Methods for the Description of Aphasic Transformations of Language[1]

André Roch Lecours

An outline is presented of the postulate that language production is the result of the articulation of less complex linguistic units into more complex ones, which combine in turn to constitute progressively more complex units. The usefulness of that postulate in aphasiology is underlined, and methods for the description of paraphasic and paragraphic transformations of language are proposed and illustrated. Formal and semantic similarities between linguistic units are said to play an important role in the genesis of paraphasias and paragraphias; ways of measuring the degree of formal similarity between different types of linguistic units are suggested. The fact that comparable sequential structures are to be found in transformations involving units of different levels of complexity—phonemic paraphasias, neologisms, verbal paraphasias—is discussed. The notions of dyssyntaxia and incoherence, as applied to jargonaphasic language, are reviewed in relation with that of verbal paraphasia.

Description and Analysis of Aphasic Transformations

The existence of ("pure") cases of aphasia, in which a particular aspect of linguistic behavior—for instance, the realization of speech sounds through the combined activities of the different muscles of the buccophonatory apparatus; the choice of some of these sounds (phonemes) and their serial integration into more complex linguistic segments; the capacity for producing grammatical sen-

---

[1] The author's research activity is supported by the Medical Research Council of Canada.

tences, and so forth—is selectively imparied, or nearly so, in relation to the presence of a focal brain lesion, permits a clearer definition of some of the facts for which an exhaustive theory of language should account. The specific contribution of neurologists to the formulation of such a theory is to provide data on the aphasias and to suggest physiological interpretations of these data. Their purpose in venturing into the taxonomy of aphasic transformations of language, hopefully in collaboration with linguists and psycholinguists, is thus two-fold: to establish correlations between a class of pathological linguistic behaviors and the topography of the different brain lesions resulting in these behaviors and to gain a better insight into the physiology and physiopathology of language production and comprehension.

The different parameters that can be taken into consideration in describing aphasic language are often delineated by pathology itself, that is, by a comparison of abnormal to normal linguistic behavior. Aphasic language may differ from conventional language in prosody, fluency of speech flow, relative availability of the different types of linguistic units, comprehension of spoken or written language, and so forth (Alajouanine & Lhermitte, 1960; Howes, 1964; Howes & Geschwind, 1962; Lhermitte, 1965). The particular aspect of the aphasias that is the subject of this chapter is the linguistic structure of aphasic language when it results from an acquired brain lesion in the adult, or, in other words, when it results from the dysfunction of damaged parts and of the adaptation of remaining uninvolved parts in an organism that, prior to focal disease, could govern normal linguistic function. Although one might find arguments in favor of describing aphasic language per se, at least in certain types of disturbances (agrammatism, for instance), we will thus consider aphasic language as a transformation of normal language and propose ways of describing the former by reference to the latter.

Description of aphasic language by reference to normal language can, on the one hand, be done by comparing a linguistic segment transformed by an aphasic subject to its (precisely identified) normal counterpart. This is frequently impossible when one is studying conversational language, since it is exceptional that one can be reasonably sure of the one correct form that the subject was presumably attempting to produce; when aimed at gathering data on large samples, such comparisons are therefore limited to the description of linguistic material produced in repetition and reading tests and, to a certain degree, in naming tests and in narration. Comparison can be established, on the other hand, between a given sample of language produced by an aphasic patient and samples produced by normal subjects of a corresponding sociocultural level. This method is particularly useful in studying narration and conversational language. Whether through comparisons between transformed linguistic segments and their specifically identified normal counterparts, or through comparisons between samples of aphasic conversation of a given type and samples of conversational language produced by normal speakers, descriptions repeated at intervals provide objective criteria to assess the longitudinal evolution of aphasic deficits. The results of re-education might be evaluated in that manner.

Substitution of one linguistic segment for another is common in the oral and written language of aphasic subjects. For instance:

(1)	/v-ε-r-t-i-ʒ/	→	/f-ε-r-t-i-ʒ/	(R)[2]
(2)	F-O-U-R-N-I-R	→	E-O-U-R-N-I-R	(D)
(3)	L'armée/frɑ̃s-εz/ ...	→	L'armée/frɑ̃s-jεl/ ...	(C)
(4)	... de faire l'**aumône**.	→	... de faire l'**arôme**.	(R)
(5)	Elle portait **le panier** [à sa grand'mère].			
	→	Elle portait **le sac** ... **la bourse** ... **le sachet** ...		(N)
(6)	... **un agent de police** ... → ... **l'argent du peuple** ...			(R)

The following are basic characteristics of such transformations by substitution: arthric and graphic anomalies may be and often are completely absent, that is, although erroneously chosen, the replacing segment may be and often is correctly formed; both the replaced and the replacing segments are conventional units of the speaker's community's language, and they are of comparable levels of linguistic complexity; varying with patients, or with time and types of production (see footnote 2), the level of linguistic complexity of the involved units can be different. In (1), replacement of one phoneme by another results in a *phonemic paraphasia*,[3] in (2), replacement of one letter by another results in a *literal paragraphia* (see Footnote 3); in (3) replacement of one affix by another results in a *monemic* (*morphemic*) *paraphasia* (see Footnote 3), in this case a type of *neologism* (Lecours, in press; Lecours & Lhermitte, 1972); in (4) and (5), replacement of one word by another results in a *verbal paraphasia* (see Footnote 3); and in (6), replacement of one phrase by another results in a variety of compounded verbal paraphasia for which no particular name has yet been proposed.

The very existence of aphasic transformations bearing unambiguously on units of different levels of linguistic complexity confers, in our opinion, a certain physiological credibility to the linguistic postulate that the production of language is

---

[2]Numbers (in parentheses to the left of each example) will be used throughout this chapter to refer to corresponding examples. In most cases, both the conventional segment and its aphasic counterpart are given; the arrow between the two then means "is transformed into." When the sequence resulting from a transformation of spoken language does not figure in the (French) dictionary, the transcription is made using the symbols of the International Phonetic Alphabet (IPA), as listed in Juilland's *Dictionnaire Inverse de la Langue Française* (Mouton, The Hague, 1965); oblique bars always delineate such sequences. Dysorthographic transformations are transcribed in capital letters, and hyphens are used to separate the constitutive units of a segment given as an example. The units directly involved in a transformation are in bold face type. Isolated letters in parentheses (right of each example) identify the type of linguistic production: (R) for *reading*; (P) for *repetition*; (N) for *narration* (Little Red Riding Hood); (C) for *conversational language*; (D) for *writing to dictation*; and (W) for *written essay*. The aphasic transformations given in the examples were produced by adult subjects seen at la Salpêtrière, in Paris, and at l'Hôtel-Dieu de Montréal.

[3]Phonemic paraphasia, literal paragraphia, monemic and verbal paraphasia or paragraphia: aphasic transformations which, considered in the linguistic context in which they occur, can be described in terms of deletion, addition, displacement, or substitution of, respectively, phonemes, letters, monemes (morphemes), or words (Lecours, Dordain, & Lhermitte, 1970).

integrated on several levels and is economical (Buyssens, 1967; de Saussure, 1966; Martinet, 1967); simple units, the number of which is restricted (by the physical limits of the apparatus responsible for their production), are combined to constitute stocks of progressively more complex units, the potential number of which becomes greater with each *level of articulation*. The number of levels of articulation and of *types of linguistic units* to which one refers in describing linguistic sequences varies, within certain limits, with one's point of view and interests. Study of the linguistic productions of aphasic patients, in conversational language and in narration as well as in naming, repetition, reading, and so forth, has led us to accept a scheme in which the *trait* or *feature* (a definite state of given parts of the buccophonatory apparatus), considered as a descriptive and not as a distinctive element (Martinet, 1967), is the simplest (useful) linguistic unit (Lecours *et al.*, 1970).

From the trait to the sentence, three levels of articulation are easily identifiable through analysis of aphasic language. Each of these can be disorganized in a predominant or even in a selective manner by different types of aphasic disturbances. They are (1) a *phonetic* level, defined as the choice of a certain number of *traits*[4] and their integration into a unit of a higher order of complexity, the *phoneme* (see Footnote 4) (Malmberg, 1966); (2) a *phonemic* level, defined as the choice of a certain number of phonemes and their integration into units of a higher order of complexity, the *monemes* (see Footnote 4) (Martinet, 1967); and (3) a *morphological–syntactical* level, defined as the choice of a certain number of monemes and their integration into progressively more complex segments, the *syntagms* (see Footnote 4) (Martinet, 1967). Whatever the considered level, the choice of each unit of lesser complexity, as a component of a given unit of greater complexity, supposes the exclusion of a certain number of other units of lesser complexity. And the integration into a unit of greater complexity is performed according to a learned set of community-accepted conventional rules (phonetic, phonological, morphological, and syntactical systems); the integration is nearly cotemporal at the phonetic level and is sequential at the phonemic and morphological–syntactical levels. Aphasic disorganization of the phonetic level leads to the phonetic disintegration syndrome (*syndrome de désintégration phonétique*—Alajouanine, Ombredane, & Durand, 1939), which can exist in pure or nearly pure form (Alajouanine & Lhermitte, 1960; Pierre Marie, 1926); aphasic disorganization of the phonemic level leads to a production of phonemic transformations—phonemic paraphasias and certain types of verbal paraphasias as in example (4); and aphasic disorganization of the morphological–syntactical level may lead to the production of verbal transformations—monemic

---

[4] The following definitions are incomplete but sufficient in the context of this chapter: *Trait* (or *feature*): a peripheral event resulting from the action or lack of action of different muscles of the buccophonatory apparatus; *phoneme*: an audible event, resulting from near concomitant realization of several traits, that can be produced and recognized by all normal members of a given linguistic community; *moneme* (or *morpheme*): a "minimal sign" (Martinet, 1967), that is, the smallest linguistic segment that conveys a particular meaning; *syntagm*: a group of monemes serially ordered following the syntactic convention of a given linguistic community—syntagms can be of different orders of complexity (Lecours *et al.*, 1970).

and verbal paraphasias as in examples (3), (5) and (6), dyssyntactic transformations, and "incoherence" which will be described later. Although jargonaphasic language usually includes both phonemic and verbal transformations, there are cases in which one or the other form is predominant or exclusive (Alajouanine, Lhermitte, Ledoux, Renaud, & Vignolo, 1964; Lecours & Lhermitte, 1969). The different sublevels of the morphological—syntactical level have not been treated separately because no cases of predominant or exclusive involvement of one of these sublevels have been reported; in analyzing jargonaphasic or agrammatic language, it is nevertheless important to keep in mind that monemes enter into the constitution of simple syntagms and that both these types of units, the monemes and the simple syntagms, combine to constitute progressively more complex syntagms (Companys, 1968).

It is also of some importance to know that a short sequence of linguistic units can occasionally behave like a single unit, that is, presumably, correspond to a single choice of the speaker (Martinet, 1967). This fact is probably related to a very high or to a more or less exclusive incidence of association. Such segments, which can occur at each of the levels of articulation, are referred to as *joint units*. In the following paragraphia, for instance,

(7)   **PH**-*A*-*R*-*M*-*A*-**C**-*I*-*E* → **PH**-*A*-*R*-*M*-*A*-**PH**-*I*-*E*   (D)

it is likely that the correct description is substitution of $(PH)^5$ for (C) rather than substitution of (P) for (C) with the addition of (H), or substitution of (H) for (C) with the addition of (P).

Repeatedly observed in aphasic transformations by simple substitution is the high degree of similarity between the replaced and the replacing units, whatever their level of linguistic complexity. In (1), for instance, the involved units share all but one of their constitutive traits; in (4) and in (6), they share several of their constitutive phonemes. In (5), the similarity is no longer between forms but between meanings: the name of a container, *basket*, is successively replaced by the names of other containers, *bag*, *purse*, and *satchel*. Since it might, on the one hand, provide clues concerning the mechanisms of selection of units in language production (Lashley, 1951; Lhermitte, Lecours, & Bertaux, 1969) and, on the other hand, permit quantitative appreciation of the degree of recuperation achieved by a given patient, knowing more about this descriptive parameter of aphasic language, that is, devising methods for measuring the degree of similarity between replacing and replaced units in transformations by substitution, becomes a problem of interest.

The degree of similarity, or *paradigmatic distance* (PD), between replaced and replacing units in interphonemic substitution, is easily expressed in terms of the

---

[5] When a group of two or more letters correspond to a single phoneme, that is, constitute a grapheme, these letters often behave as joint units in dysorthographic transformations. Certain associations between a lexical moneme and an affix, particularly in nouns and in adjectives, also tend to behave like joint units (Martinet, 1967); this is also true of certain locutions, usually composed of one simple syntagm (coined expressions).

number of traits that are not shared by the two phonemes. In this measurement, the smaller the distance, the greater the degree of similarity (Lecours & Lhermitte, 1970; Poncet *et al.*, 1972). Early in the evolution of aphasic patients whose language production is characterized by a predominant or exclusive production of phonemic paraphasias identifiable as such, approximately half of the interphonemic sub-stitutions usually involve phonemes that differ by only one of their constitutive traits: the proportion of substitutions at PD = 1 was found to be 50.5% in studying 1624 phonemic transformations produced by seven such patients in repetition and reading tests (Fig. 5—1).[6]

In studying verbal paraphasias or paralexias, it is also relatively easy to define a *formal similarity index* (FSI) taking into account the number of phonemes or letters common to both the replaced and the replacing words, and the number of common units appearing in comparable positions in the two words. In this measurement, the greater the index (maximal FSI value = 10), the greater the degree of similarity

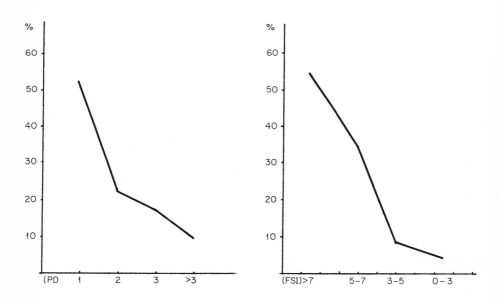

Figure 5—1. *Left:* Similarity between replaced and replacing units in phonemic substitutions. Bears on 1624 phonemic transformations produced by seven patients; repetition and reading tests (isolated words). PD = 1 in 50.5% of the substitutions, PD = 2 in 22.2%, PD = 3 in 18%, and PD > 3 in 9.3%. *Right:* Formal similarity between replaced and replacing words in verbal substitutions (purely gram-matical words excluded). Bears on 610 verbal transformations produced by one patient; reading test (isolated words). FSI > 7 in 54% of the substitutions, FSI between 5 and 7 in 33.5%, FSI between 3 and 5 in 9%, and FSI between 0 and 3 in 3.5%.

---

[6]None of these patients had arthric difficulties, i.e., taken individually, the phonemes they uttered were correctly realized and therefore adequately transcribed through use of the IPA symbols.

(Lecours & Lhermitte, 1970). The proportion of substitutions at FSI > 7 was found to be 54% in studying 610 verbal transformations produced by an aphasic patient in reading isolated lexical words (words containing at least one lexical moneme) (Fig. 5–1). Although theoretically feasible through semantic analysis (Greimas, 1966; Katz & Fodor, 1964; Mounin, 1972), calculation of a *semantic similarity index* would, in our opinion, yield few physiologically interesting data because of the important variations, from one individual to another, of the semantic value of all but the most concrete words. It is nevertheless interesting to determine, when analyzing a corpus of verbal substitutions, the proportion of those transformations in which an unambiguous semantic relationship exists between replaced and replacing words.

When there is little or no similarity between replaced and replacing units in aphasic substitutions involving linguistic units of any level of complexity, the replacing unit is often identical (8–15) or similar (16, 17) to a post-positioned (8–11) or to a pre-positioned (12–17) unit of the immediate context.

(8)	/v-j-ɔ-**l**-a-**s**-e/	→	/v-j-ɔ-**s**-a-**s**-e/	(R)
(9)	R-E-**C**-O-U-**V**-E-R-T	→	R-E-**V**-O-U-**V**-E-R-T	(W)
(10)	... **inform**ations antérieurement **acquis**es.			
	→ ... **acquis**itions antérieurement **acquis**es.[7]			(C)
(11)	On voit même l'**armée** allemande **attaquer** l'Est de la France.			
	→ On voit même l'**attaque** allemande **attaquer** l'Est de la France.[7]			(W)
(12)	/i-n-a-**k**-t-i-**f**/	→	/i-n-a-**k**-t-i-**k**/	(R)
(13)	**F**-O-U-R-**N**-I-R	→	**F**-O-U-R-**F**-I-R	(D)
(14)	... qui sont très différents de ce qu'on a appris à des **gosses**. On leur a appris des tas de **choses**.			
	→ ... qui sont très différents de ce qu'on a appris à des **gosses**. On leur a appris des tas de **gosses**.[7]			(C)
(15)	**La Belgique**, alliée de la France et de l'Angleterre, fait ce qu'elle peut. Elle le fait bien mais cela n'arrive pas à arrêter **les Allemands**.			
	→ **La Belgique**, alliée de la France et de l'Angleterre, fait ce qu'elle peut. Elle le fait bien mais cela n'arrive pas à arrêter **la Belgique**.[7]			(W)
(16)	/ʃ-œ-m-i-**n**-e/	→	/ʃ-œ-m-i-**ʒ**-e/	(P)
(17)	Elle garde notre **fille** à la **maison**.			
	→ Elle garde notre **fille** à la **petite**.[7]			(C)

Besides transformations in which there exists a high degree of similarity between replaced and replacing units (1–6) and transformations in which the replacing unit is identical or similar to another unit of the immediate context, one frequently notes substitutions in which both of these factors enter into play. Examples are the following two phonemic paraphasias, in which the replacing unit is both identical to

---

[7] In (10), (11), (15) and (17), the subject corrected himself, thus providing the conventional form corresponding to the produced transformation; in (14), the conventional form is obvious.

another unit of the context and shares all but one of its constitutive traits with the replaced phoneme:

(18)	/p-*i*-*s*-**t**-ɔ-*l*-ɛ/	→	/**t**-*i*-*s*-**t**-ɔ-*l*-ɛ/	(R)
(19)	/d-ɛ-*r*-**n**-*j*-*e*/	→	/d-ɛ-*r*-**d**-*j*-*e*/	(R)

One may propose the following description of transformations (8) to (17): reduplication (8–15) or near-reduplication (16, 17) of a unit with replacement of a pre- or post-positioned unit of the immediate context by the additional unit (doublet) thus generated. This description, separating the addition phenomenon from the substitution phenomenon, is validated by the existence of transformations in which addition by reduplication occurs without the additional unit replacing another unit of the sequence. For instance:

(20)	/*d*-*e*-ã-**b**-*y*-*l*-ã/	→	/*d*-*e*-**b**-ã-**b**-*y*-*l*-ã/	(R)
(21)	B-O-U-**R**-G	→	B-O-**R**-U-**R**-G	(D)
(22)	/*t*-**i**-*g*-*r*/	→	/*t*-**i**-*g*-*r*-**i**/	(R)
(23)	**M**-A-T-I-N	→	**M**-A-**M**-T-I-N	(D)

Transformations (8) to (23), including (18) and (19), illustrate an important fact for one interested in describing phonemic and literal as well as verbal or more complex aphasic transformations of language: although the influence of the units of the immediate context is probably negligible in a certain proportion of transformations by substitution, description of aphasic transformations cannot be adequate without systematically taking the units of the immediate context into consideration. The role played by units of the immediate context may indeed be, at least at first sight, quite intricate. Let us consider, for instance, the following seven phonemic paraphasias produced by one of our patients:

(24)	/*d*-ɛ-*s*-ã-*d*-ã/	→	/*d*-ɛ-*s*-*d*-ã/	(R)
(25)	/*p*-*u*-*l*-**a**-*j*-*e*/	→	/**a**-*p*-*u*-*l*-*j*-*e*/	(R)
(20)	/*d*-**e**-ã-**b**-*y*-*l*-ã/	→	/*d*-*e*-**b**-ã-**b**-*y*-*l*-ã/	(R)
(26)	/*s*-**e**-*k*-**y**-*r*-*i*-*t*-*e*/	→	/*s*-**y**-*k*-*r*-*i*-*t*-*e*/	(R)
(27)	/*s*-ɔ-**l**-*i*-*d*-*a*-*r*-*i*-*t*-*e*/	→	/*s*-ɔ-**l**-*e*-*d*-*a*-*r*-*i*-*t*-*e*/	(R)
(28)	/*a*-**v**-*i*-*k*-*y*-*l*-**t**-œ-*r*/	→	/**v**-*a*-**t**-*i*-*k*-*y*-*l*-**t**-œ-*r*/	(R)
(29)	/*a*-**b**-ɔ-**m**-*i*-*n*-*a*-**b**-*l*/	→	/*a*-**m**-ɔ-**n**-*i*-*n*-*a*-**b**-*l*/	(R)

Quite different as to their linear structures, these transformations may nevertheless be described by the definition of only three basic operations: (a) the deletion of the first of a pair of identical units, illustrated in its pure form by (24); (b) the displacement of a unit, with pre-positioning, illustrated by (25); and (c) the addition by reduplication of a unit, with pre-positioning of the additional doublet, illustrated by (20). Transformations (26) to (28) represent combinations of two of these basic rules, each combination resulting in a different type of substitution: in (26), the first of a pair of identical units is deleted, as in (24), and it is replaced by displacement of another unit, with pre-positioning, as in (25); in (27), the first of a pair of identical units is again deleted, as in (24), but this time it is replaced by reduplication of another unit, with pre-positioning, as in (20); in (28), there is displacement of a unit, with pre-positioning, as in (25), and the original position of the displaced unit is filled by reduplication of another unit, with pre-positioning, as in (20). Transformation (29) represents a combination of the three basic operations: the first of a pair of identical units is deleted, as in (24); the deleted doublet is replaced by displacement of another unit, with pre-positioning, as in (25); and the original position of the displaced unit is filled by reduplication of still another unit, with pre-positioning, as in (20) (Fig. 5—2). One should note, in (29), besides the above described sequential factor, the fact that replaced and replacing phonemes are similar in the two interdependent substitutions realized by the transformation (PD = 1 in both cases).

Examples (24), (25) and (20) illustrate three of the nine basic operations from which a model of reference has been elaborated for the description of phonemic paraphasias (Lecours and Lhermitte, 1969). Examples (26) to (29) illustrate some of the possible combinations of these three basic operations. The structure of phonemic transformations, at least in the productions of certain patients in repetition and reading tests, and that of literal paragraphias in certain subjects with acquired or developmental dysorthographia (Lecours, 1966), is indeed systematic enough to permit computer description through prevision of all possible combina-

	DELETION OF THE FIRST OF A PAIR OF IDENTICAL UNITS	DISPLACEMENT OF A UNIT WITH PRE-POSITIONING	ADDITION BY REDUPLICATION OF A UNIT WITH PRE-POSITIONING
24	+		
25		+	
20			+
26	+	+	
27	+		+
28		+	+
29	+	+	+

Figure 5—2. Description of seven phonemic paraphasias. One of three basic operations occurs in isolation in (24), (25) and (20); combinations of two of these three basic operations occur in (26), (27) and (28); a combination of all three basic operations occurs in (29).

tions between two, three or four of these nine basic rules (Fig. 5—3). Computer description remains possible even when a single word or short syntagm is the site of several transformations, a frequent phenomenon illustrated by the following two examples:

(30)   /**m**-**a**-**l**-**a**-*b*-*i*-*l*/   →   /**a**-**m**-**a**-**l**-**a**-*b*-*i*-**m**/   (R)

(31)   A-**G**-*R*-**I**-*C*-**U**-*L*-**T**-**U**-*R*-*E*   →   A-**G**-*R*-**U**-*C*-**T**-**U**-*L*-**G**-**U**-*R*-*E*   (D)

In (30), there is an addition of the same type as that in (20) (reduplication of a unit with pre-positioning of the doublet), and there is a substitution of a type similar to that in (27) (reduplication of a unit with post-positioning of the doublet which replaces the second of a pair of identical units). In (31), there is a first substitution of the same type as those in (8) to (11) (reduplication of a unit with pre-positioning of the doublet which replaces another unit of the sequence), and there is a second substitution of a type similar to that in (28) (displacement of a unit by pre-positioning and its replacement by a doublet generated by reduplication and post-positioning of another unit of the sequence). Stating that a single word or short syntagm is the site

(1-):	DELETION OF A UNIT FIGURING *ONLY ONCE* IN THE STIMULUS.
(3-):	DELETION OF THE FIRST OR SECOND OF TWO IDENTICAL UNITS FIGURING IN THE STIMULUS. [(3_1-) and (3_2-)]
(-2):	ADDITION OF A UNIT THAT DOES NOT FIGURE AT ALL IN THE STIMULUS.
(-4):	ADDITION BY REDUPLICATION OF A UNIT FIGURING IN THE STIMULUS. [(-4_A) and (-4_R)]
(-5-):	CHANGE OF POSITION OF A UNIT OF THE STIMULUS. [$(-5_{A2}-)$, $(-5_{R1}-)$ and $(-5_?-)$]

DASH RIGHT OF NUMBER = "NEGATIVE VALENCE" [AN OPEN POSITION]

DASH LEFT OF NUMBER = "POSITIVE VALENCE" [A POSSIBILITY OF FILLING AN OPEN POSITION]

"EXCHANGE OF VALENCES" = SUBSTITUTION

FIRST ORDER: [NO EXCHANGE OF VALENCES]

/k-$\tilde{3}$-p-1-ϵ-k-s	→	"k-$\tilde{3}$-p-1-ϵ-s"/	(3_2-)
/a-k-u-r-$\tilde{a}$	→	"a-k-r-u-r-$\tilde{a}$"/	(-4_A)
/d-e-k-a-1-a	→	"e-k-a-1-a-d"/	$(-5_{R1}-)$
/t-a-r-t	→	"t-r-a-t"/	$(-5_?-)$

SECOND ORDER: [ONE EXCHANGE OF VALENCES]

/p-i-s-t-ɔ-1-ϵ	→	"t-i-s-t-ɔ-1-ϵ"/	$(1-4_A)$
/i-n-a-ʀ-t-i-f	→	"i-n-a-k-t-i-k"/	$(1-4_R)$
/a-m-i-k-a-1	→	"i-m-i-k-a-1"/	(3_1-4_A)
/d-i-m-i-n-y-$\tilde{a}$	→	"d-y-m-i-n-$\tilde{a}$"/	$(3_1-5_{A2}-)$
/p-s-i-k-ɔ-1-ɔ-3-i	→	"p-s-i-k-1-ɔ-s-ɔ-3-i"/	$(-5_{A2}-4_R)$
* /f-i-n-i-s-ϵ	→	"f-i-s-i-n-ϵ"/	$(m=n)$

THIRD ORDER: [TWO EXCHANGES OF VALENCES]

/k-a-t-e-d-r-ɐ-1	→	"a-k-e-t-r-a-1"/	$(1-5_{R1}-5_{R1}-)$
/a-b-ɔ-m-i-n-a-b-1	→	"a-m-ɔ-n-i-n-a-b-1"/	$(3_1-5_{A2}-4_A)$
/t-r-a-d-y-k-t-œ-r	→	"d-r-a-k-y-t-œ-r"/	$(3_1-5_{A2}-5_{A2}-)$
* /p-a-p-i-j-$\tilde{3}$	→	"p-$\tilde{3}$-p-a-j-i"/	$5-5 \atop 5$

FOURTH ORDER: [THREE EXCHANGES OF VALENCES]

/d-ɐ-k-a-1-œ-r-$\tilde{3}$	→	"k-ɐ-r-a-d-œ-1-r-$\tilde{3}$"/	$(-5_{R1}-5_{R1}-5_{A2}-4_A)$
(C-U-L-T-I-V-A-T-E-U-R	→	"C-U-R-V-I-L-A-T-E-U-R")	$(3_1-5_{A2}-5_{R1}-4_A)$

Figure 5—3. *Left:* Nine basic rules permitting the description of phonemic paraphasias or literal paragraphias in cases where comparison can be made between a transformed word and its precisely identified conventional counterpart. *Right:* Illustrative examples with description. No substitution in first order transformations; one substitution in second order transformations; two interdependent substitutions in third order transformations; three interdependent substitutions in fourth order transformations. From a descriptive point of view, the examples marked by an asterisk may be considered as intermediary forms between the second and the third, and the third and the fourth orders.

of several transformations does not mean that there exist no linear relationships between these transformations; it means that the reference model is not powerful enough to account for such relationships if any.

Besides automatically writing and classifying linear descriptions of phonemic transformations, this analysis provides data on several other parameters. It calculates the paradigmatic distance in all substitutions (Fig. 5−1); it gives the incidence of *selection* as opposed to *seriation* errors (the former being the simple replacement of a unit by a similar one and the latter a transformation in which there is destruction or creation of at least one pair of identical or similar—PD = 1—units) (Lecours, 1966; Lecours & Twitchell, 1966); in pair destructions and pair creations, it determines the number of units intervening between the doublets (proximity factor); it calculates the relative importance of the pre- and post-positioning phenomena; it studies the effect of the length of words and of their structural difficulty (presence of clusters of consonants, recurrence of identical or similar phonemes, etc.) on the production of phonemic transformations; it compares the different transformations produced in response to multiple presentations of a single stimulus; and it provides data concerning the susceptibility of individual phonemes in relation to their phonetic characteristics (voiced, nasal, continuant, etc.) (Lecours *et al.*, 1973; Lecours & Lhermitte, 1969, 1970; Poncet *et al.*, 1972).

Because of the necessity of a unit-to-unit comparison, the reference model outlined here for the description of aphasic transformations of language has been automated only for the description of phonemic paraphasias and of literal paragraphias. As shown by several of the examples already used to illustrate this argument (3−6, 10, 11, 14, 15, 17), it is nevertheless useful in attempts at more systematic descriptions of aphasic transformations involving linguistic units more complex than the phoneme or the letter and grapheme.

There is, on the one hand, a type of aphasic neologism, observed so far with a high incidence in the conversational language of only two jargonaphasic patients by this author, in which segments of words corresponding for the most part to monemes are the involved units. In both of these patients, most of the neologisms were used in place of a noun (80%) or of an attribute (15%). Transformations (32−35) are abstracted from the transcription of a conversation with one of these patients; the sample included 317 such neologisms, that is, 42 per 1000 words of conversation. Nearly all of the 317 neologisms are constituted of two easily identified monemes, a lexical one and an affix, hence the suggested label *monemic paraphasia* (Lecours, in press, Lecours & Lhermitte, 1972). In the four examples cited here, one of the constitutive monemes is borrowed from the immediate context:

(32)   *Ce que je donne ne donne pas les* /**prɔm**-yr/ *que j'ai* **prom**us.   (C)

(33)   *Je pourrais vous le dire sans me* **tromp**er, *mais je n'ose même pas dans ce* /**trɔ̃**baʒ/.   (C)

(34)   *On rem**ball**ait à l'arrière; c'était un* /**bal**-aʒ/ *assez dur.*   (C)

(35)   *L'artill**eur** a son* /blãʒ-**œr**/ *très différent, beaucoup plus dur que le Français.*   (C)

Although there is no way to identify the conventional word, if any, that is replaced by a neologism in these transformations, it remains that the structure of (32), but for the fact that the involved unit belongs to a higher level of linguistic complexity, is comparable to that of (8), and the structure of (33) to (35) is comparable to that of (12) (reduplication of a unit with anticipation of reiteration).

Given the possibility of a more or less precise reconstitution of the conventional form of jargoned sentences, through use of contextual indices or of spontaneous corrections by the aphasic speaker or writer, certain relatively complex verbal transformations may, on the other hand, be described by reference to the model outlined earlier. Let us consider, for instance, the following sentences abstracted from the transcription of a conversation concerning his professional life with the jargonaphasic ex-director of a brick manufacturing plant[8]:

> *On fabrique de la brique avec de la terre cuite. Ce n'est pas vrai d'ailleurs.*
> *On fabrique de la brique avec de la terre qui n'est pas cuite d'une façon*
> *et puis avec de la terre qui n'est pas cuite de l'autre. Il y a deux qualités*
> *de brique: une plus claire et une plus foncée.*
> *Ces deux élements sont arrivés à se joindre et, suivant la proportion et*
> *suivant la proportion que je peux indiquer, moi, eh bien! il est indiqué*
> *que nous arrivons à faire la proportion.*
> *Moi, je fais de la brique foncée, de préférence, mais on fait de la brique*
> *claire également.*

(36) *La brique claire, elle est déplorable parce qu'elle est claire; et puis elle*
     est foncée parce qu'elle est mieux.   (C)
     Moi, je préfère la foncée parce qu'elle est plus belle au point de vue
     présentation. Ça fait une brique qui a de l'allure, qui a de la classe et
     puis qui a de la présentation.

The surrounding context of (36) is rich enough for one to propose the following as an approximate reconstitution of the corresponding conventional form:

(36)   *Pale brick is deplorable because it is "negative attribute,"*
           and dark brick is better because it is "positive attribute."

It is, of course, impossible to ascertain that the above is the only possible correct reconstitution of (36), but it is reasonable to assume that any reconstitution should be made of two opposed propositions including, in this order:

(36.1)   *—pale—deplorable—"negative attribute"*
(36.2)   *—dark—better—"positive attribute"*

In the verbal transformation produced by the patient, these two propositions include:

---

[8] In a 15-min sample of conversation, this patient produced no phonemic paraphasias.

(36.1)	—pale—deplorable—pale	(C)
(36.2)	—nil—dark—better	(C)

The disorder in choice and serial integration of words, in (36.1), is thus comparable to the disorder in choice and serial integration of phonemes in

(12)	/i-n-a-**k**-t-i-**f**/ → /i-n-a-**k**-t-i-**k**/	(R)

and the disorder in choice and serial integration of words, in 36.2., is comparable to the disorder in choice and serial integration of phonemes in

(37)	/**k**-a-t-e-**d**-r-a-l/ → /a-**k**-e-t-r-a-l/	(R)

A few general comments on verbal transformations of language in aphasia may be derived from this description of a particular sequence of jargonaphasic language. The most obvious one concerns the definition itself of verbal paraphasia, which generally includes little more than the notion of simple word substitution. A more complete definition of verbal paraphasia may, in our opinion, be formulated by establishing a parallel between the respective structures of phonemic and verbal transformations. It should include the following notions: the substitution of one word for another is to be considered in the context of the sentence, in the same manner as the substitution of one phoneme for another is considered in the context of a word or short syntagm; the replaced and the replacing words may be formally or semantically similar to one another; the replacing word may be identical or similar, as in (17), to another word of the immediate context; the description of the linear structure of verbal paraphasias must take into account the possibility of *deletion, addition,* and *displacement,* as well as of *substitution* phenomena, as in (38) and (39); in the same manner that several interdependent phonemic substitutions may result from a single phonemic paraphasia (29, 37), several interdependent word substitutions may result from a single verbal paraphasia (see 36.2); the units involved in verbal paraphasias may be of a level of complexity greater than that of the single word (6)—as in (40), such segments may often be considered as joint units (see earlier).

(38)	*Avec quoi fabrique-t-***on*** de la brique?*	
	→ *Avec quoi* **on** *fabrique-t-***on*** de la brique?*	(C)
(39)	*Tout aussitôt se développe un* **assaut** *et cet* **assaut** *est* **brutal** *et violent.*	
	→ *Tout aussitôt se développe un* **assaut** *et ce* **brutal** *est violent.*[9]	(W)

(40)	*J'ai un hélicoptère comme* **tout le monde** *qui était avec* **tout le monde**	(C)

[9] In (39) and (45), the subject corrected himself, thus providing the conventional form corresponding to the produced transformation. Note, in (45), conservation of the reflexive pronoun.

A second point is that the semantic incoherence of jargonaphasic speech, which sometimes precludes nearly all possibility of linguistic communication with the subject, is not necessarily the behavioral manifestation of a conceptual deficit. In other words, no one would deny the existence of severe comprehension difficulties in a large proportion of jargonaphasic subjects, but the incoherence of their linguistic productions might nevertheless result from an expressive rather than a conceptual disorder. To the hearer, sequence (36), which formally states among other things that pale brick is dark, is no doubt quite incoherent; but its significance as to the speaker's linguistic deficit might indeed be of the same order as that of a mere phonemic paraphasia (Denny-Brown, 1963, 1965; Geschwind, 1971).

The problem of the description of dyssyntactic transformations in aphasic language, which necessarily merges with that of the description of semantic transformations, may also be (partly) clarified by studying the relations between verbal paraphasias and dyssyntactic transformations (paragrammatism), especially since one can confidently state that the latter, up to a point, constitute an accidental variety of the former. Verbal paraphasias bearing on grammatical monemes, for instance, *ipso facto* create dyssyntactic transformations.

(41)   *Elle portait une galette* **à** *sa grand'mère.*
         → *Elle portait une galette* **sur** *sa grand'mère.*   (N)
(42)   *Ma sœur, elle travaillait* **chez** *un docteur.*
         → *Ma sœur, elle travaillait* **dans** *un docteur.*   (C)

The same is usually true in the very rare cases when a word belonging to one lexical category replaces a word belonging to another lexical category. As in (43), this phenomenon is observed almost exclusively in seriation errors (see earlier).

(43)   *Il n'y a pas à* **dire**, *c'est* **drôle**.
         → *Il n'y a pas à* **drôle**, *c'est* **drôle**.   (C)

Whether bearing on lexical or on grammatical units, verbal transformations other than those resulting in a simple substitution often realize dyssyntactic transformations (38, 39). This is particularly true of transformations by simple addition, as in

(44)   *Moi, dans quelques mois, je* **partirai** *parce que je dois* **partir**.
         → *Moi, dans quelques mois, je* **partirai** *parce que je dois*
         partirai.   (C)

Most samples of jargonaphasic and jargonographic language contain a certain number of transformations, which, depending on one's point of view, may be considered dyssyntactic or, on the contrary, be taken as evidence of a preservation of the syntactic system. Such is the case in (45), where an adjective is reduplicated and pre-positioned, the anticipated doublet replacing the predicate and taking, correctly from a morphological point of view although such a verb as *difficiler* does not exist in French, its morphological mark.

(45) *Les Norvégiens font leur guerre, se* difficilent (as in (5), p. 77)
      autant qu'ils peuvent mais, malgré l'envoi de militaires anglais et même
      de militaires français, ce n'est pas un long et difficile *combat.*   (W)

As opposed to agrammatism, paragrammatism thus cannot be considered as a specific involvement of syntax. In most cases of jargonaphasia, syntax is indeed surprisingly respected if one considers the number of verbal transformations resulting in nonsensical sentences that are perfectly well structured from a syntactical point of view. The following comment of a patient on the last U.S. presidential election illustrates this point:

(46) *On s'est surtout occupé de la partie intérieure, et on s'est aperçu que,*
      partout ailleurs, ils ont mis des petits colporteurs, et qu'ils ont pu, avec
      des poudres et du veston, avec un manteau colporté de la meilleure
      poudre, former de suprêmes jugements.   (C)

This relative preservation, in spite of an important production of verbal transformations, of the rules of association between words in the formation of sentences, reminds one of the still more definite preservation, in patients whose aphasia is characterized by an important production of phonemic paraphasias, of the rules of association between phonemes in the formation of words (Lecours & Lhermitte, 1969). The fact that transformations resulting in addition or deletion of a unit, without replacement, are more frequent at the phonemic (20, 22, 24, 26, 28, 30, 37) than at the verbal level (38, 39, 44) might be related to the frequent possibility of making such transformations without going against the corresponding set of conventional rules of association (integration into a unit of greater complexity) at the former but not at the latter level.

However interesting because of the clues they may yield on language cybernetics, descriptions of verbal transformations of language in jargonaphasia following the procedure outlined here—which was originally devised for computer description of phonemic and literal transformations—remain, since they cannot be automated, fragmentary and time-consuming in the best of cases. Hence the attempts made at la Salpêtrière and at l'Hôtel-Dieu de Montréal to devise a method for computer comparisons between large samples of conversational language in jargonaphasic and normal subjects.

Each sample consists of 15 min of (tape recorded) oriented conversation.[10] The recordings are meticulously transcribed in their entirety, then each word or locution is rewritten as a 4-digit code-number indicating its lexical or grammatical category, its syntactic function in the context where it appears, its conventional or neologistic nature, and so forth. The code is built in such a manner that a particular set of indices permits segmentation of the text into syntagms of different levels of complexity (clauses, phrases and sentences) and delineation of repetitive segments which, as illustrated by (47), are common in the conversational language of all jargonaphasic subjects.

[10]The proposed themes were: the disease, the family, the work, the last vacation, the military experience if appropriate.

(47)   *Alors, ce ... celui-là est beaucoup ... est tout à fait différent entre le ...*
       les ... le ... les /ãsyl/, si vous voulez, entre les ... les ... les ... les artil-
       leurs, les artilleurs /italar/ qui sont ... qui ont de ... des /rãsjal/,
       des ... qui ont des ... des /rãsjɔl/ différentes avec des ... des /ar/ ...
       des artilleurs.   (C)

Thus coded, the texts are submitted to a first computer analysis, which gives
the incidence of each code number and regroups them following different linguistic
criteria. This first analysis also detects and counts certain varieties of aphasic errors
and transformations: lack of gender or number concordance, errors concerning
the tense and mood of verbs, verbal paraphasias, neologisms, and so forth. The
latter, for instance, are found in several cases to replace nouns and attributes in a
nearly specific manner (Lecours, in press), as a rule in sentences of which they are
essential components (32–35, 48).

(48)   *Bon, alors, mon âge actuel, c'est /vɛrsje/, si vous voulez, et je suis*
       comme /fɔrsaʒ/ comme tous les soldats en /bɔrsaʒ/ en France, avec un
       /fɔrsjal/ comme tout le monde, qui n'a rien de spécial, mais enfin qui
       n'est pas un /lɔraʒ/ particulier, quoi! Il est /fɛrsil/ mais c'est tout,
       quoi! Il n'a pas de /vɔrsjal/ pour moi, si vous voulez, quoi!   (C)

All repetitive segments are then computer identified and eliminated from the
text. What would be left of sequence (47), after this operation, would, for instance,
correspond to

(47)   *Alors, celui-là est tout à fait différent entre les artilleurs /italar/ qui ont des*
       /rãsj⊃l/ différentes avec des artilleurs.

The text is thereafter automatically rewritten in terms of phrases (or short
syntagms: nominal, prepositive, predicative, etc.) and submitted to an analysis
giving the incidence of each type of phrase and regrouping them following different linguistic criteria. This second analysis also detects and counts certain
varieties of aphasic anomalies: phrases missing an essential component, misplace-
ment of a word within a phrase, phrases structured around a neologism, and so
forth.
   A third program of analysis bears, this time, on the sentence level. The texts, as
rewritten prior to the second analysis, are studied by reference to a normative
grammar. Besides providing data on the length of sentences—to be related to
data on frequency of pauses and on fluency—this third analysis should permit
the detection of errors and transformations specifically at the sentence level:
abnormally high incidence of recurrent similar syntagms within the same sentence
(see 47: *entre les artilleurs* and *avec des artilleurs*—compare with 8–15); lack of an
attribute or of a direct object following a predicate requiring one; serial mis-
placement of a shorter syntagm within a sentence; unfinished principal proposition

after production of an included subordinate or relative; and so forth. Bizarre dyssyntactic transformations, sometimes obviously resulting from the *télescopage* of two sentences (49), should also be detected at this final stage of the description.

(49) *Le plus que je possible.*[11]   (C)

Different indices and ratios can be extrapolated from these analyses, some of which would be of interest in studying jargonaphasic (paragrammatic) as opposed to agrammatic conversational language: proportion of lexical versus grammatical words (before and after elimination of the repetitions), of *I*s or *me*s versus other personal pronouns, of infinitives versus other verbs, and so forth. Likewise, they permit the definition of a quantitative index of *manque du mot* (word finding difficulty) (Lhermitte, 1965) as it is manifested in conversational language (Table 5−1).

TABLE 5−1[a]

	Case 1	Case 2	Case 3	Control 1	Control 2
Number of words in 15 min of conversation:	1345	772	1613	2802	3104
Hesitations (*euh*):	20.8	14.2	15.5	2.0	2.7
	(280)	(110)	(250)	(57)	(84)
Repetitions of articles, prepositions, etc.:	12.2	4.8	4.3	1.8	0.7
	(164)	(37)	(69)	(50)	(23)
Incomplete sentences:	4.2	5.7	1.4	1.0	1.0
	(56)	(44)	(22)	(28)	(30)
Word-finding difficulty index:	37.2	24.7	21.1	4.8	4.4
	(500)	(191)	(341)	(135)	(137)

[a] *Definition of a quantitative index of word-finding difficulty (*manque du mot*) as it is manifested in conversational language. Naming of images and objects was paraphasic in Case 1 and normal in Cases 2 and 3. The comparatively smaller number of words produced in 15 min. of conversation by the three patients as compared with the two controls was related to frequent and long hesitations in the former; in Case 2, an arthric difficulty also played an obvious role. Verbal paraphasias were relatively frequent in Case 1 and nearly absent in Cases 2 and 3; the same was true of comprehension difficulties. Neither of the patients was logorrheic. Three phenomena were taken into consideration and cumulated in calculating the index: hesitations as marked by the utterance of one or several* euh; *repetitions of articles, prepositions, actualizers (e.g.,* c'est), *etc., nearly always prior to production of a noun or of an attribute; sentences from which an essential lexical component was missing. In the four lower lines: the second figure (in parentheses) is an absolute number and the first figure represents the incidence of the phenomenon per 100 words of conversation.*

[11] Obviously a concatenation of *le plus que je peux* and *le plus possible*. Transformations of similar structure are occasionally observed at a level of lesser linguistic complexity, e.g., *animal* + *mammifère* → /mamimal/, *Algérie* + *Amérique* → /alʒerik/, etc.

Summary and Conclusion

Methods for the description of aphasic transformations of language have been outlined and illustrated. They all are based on acceptance of the linguistic postulate that language production is integrated on several levels and is economical; the structure of several types of aphasic transformations of language were said to confer on this postulate a certain physiological credibility.

A methodology was suggested that is aimed at systematic comparisons between given segments of aphasic language and their precisely identified normal—or conventional—counterparts; whatever the level of linguistic complexity of the involved units, description is then performed by reference to a model providing for the structures of different transformations by elision, addition, displacement or replacement of units. Intricate transformations were described as combinations of simpler ones. Identity or similarity between linguistic units was said to be an important parameter in the description of aphasic transformations of language, and ways of measuring the degree of formal similarity between different types of linguistic units were suggested. The possibility of automating the descriptions in the cases of phonemic and literal transformations was mentioned (Lecours, Deloche, Lhermitte, 1973).

The fact that comparable structures can be observed in transformations involving units of different levels of linguistic complexity was underlined. It led to labeling certain types of aphasic neologisms as monemic paraphasias, and to reconsidering the definition of verbal paraphasia on a parallel with that of phonemic paraphasia. The notion of dyssyntaxia and that of incoherence, as applied to jargonaphasic language, were then reviewed in relation to the definition of verbal paraphasia.

A methodology for automated comparative descriptions of conversational language in aphasic versus normal subjects was briefly discussed. It is restricted to studying the organization of words into sentences, and it consists of an attempt to segment the samples into progressively more complex units and to study, for each sublevel, the incidence of normal and of erroneous or transformed units characteristic of that sublevel.

So far, these methods have been used to describe the linguistic productions of a few normal adults and of several patients, also adults, whose aphasic deficits were the result of focal brain damage. It is to be noted that most of the types of language transformations discussed in this chapter do occur in the productions of normal subjects, obviously related, as a rule, to fatigue, distraction, haste, and so forth, or in relation to the "parasiting" of language behavior by parallel mental activities (Freud, 1962). With some modifications, these methods might also prove of interest for the description of the language of children of different ages. If interested in comparing the language productions of children to those of aphasics, however, one should keep in mind the essential difference between the developing child and the adult aphasic: the former's linguistic production represents the behavioral output of a maturing system, that is, of a system actively involved in learning processes, whereas the latter's represents the behavioral output of what is left, after focal lesion, of a mature system, that is, of a system whose function was the manipulation of learned data rather than the learning of new data. Hence the difficulty in the interpretation of certain structural similarities between the linguistic productions of aphasics and those of children, similarities which in our experience are very seldom more than fragmentary. To state that such similarities indicate that aphasia constitutes a regression of the aphasic to an earlier stage of linguistic ontogeny would be the equivalent of stating that, because of destruction of certain anatomical regions or pathways, the aphasic is brought to use other anatomical regions or pathways that governed language production during childhood and were more or less given up at a later stage. Even if not utterly implausible, the cases of aphasia in which such an interpretation could be brought forward are certainly not very frequent.

Acknowledgments

The author is indebted to Professor François Lhermitte and to Madame Blanche Ducarne, whose knowledge of aphasia and of aphasics has often contributed to discussions concerning the research summarized in this chapter.

Bibliography

Alajouanine, T., & Lhermitte, F. Les troubles des activités expressives du langage dans l'aphasie; leurs relations avec les apraxies. *Revue Neurologique*, 1960, *102*, 66—91.

Alajouanine, T., Lhermitte, F., Ledoux, R., Renaud, D., & Vignolo, L. A. Les composantes phonémiques et sémantiques de la jargonaphasie. *Revue Neurologique*, 1964, *110*, 5—20.

Alajouanine, T., Ombredane, A., & Durand, M. *Le syndrome de désintégration phonétique dans l'aphasie.* Paris: Masson, 1939.

Buyssens, E. *La communication et l'articulation linguistique.* Paris: Presses Universitaires de France, 1967.

Companys, E. Les jonctions. *Le Français dans le Monde*, 1968, *57*, 20—24.

de Ajuriaguerra, J., & Hécaen, H. *Le cortex cérébral.* Paris: Masson, 1966.

Denny-Brown, D. The physiological basis of perception and speech. In L. Halpern (Ed.), *Problems of dynamic neurology.* Jerusalem, 1963. Pp. 30—62.

Denny-Brown, D. Physiological aspects of disturbances of speech. *Australian Journal of Experimental Biology and Medical Science*, 1965, *43*, 455—474.

de Saussure, F *Cours de linguistique générale.* Paris: Payot, 1966.

Freud, S. Slips of the tongue and slips of the pen. In J. Strachey (Ed.), *The standard edition of the complete psychological works of Sigmund Freud.* Vol. 6. London: Hogarth Press & Inst. Psychoanalysis, 1962.

Geschwind, N. Aphasia. *New England Journal of Medicine*, 1971, *284*, 654—656.

Goodglass, H., Quadfasel, F. A., & Timberlake, W. H. Phrase length and the type and severity of aphasia. *Cortex*, 1964, *1*, 133.

Greimas, A. J. *Sémantique structurale.* Paris: Larousse, 1966.

Hécaen, H., Dubois J., & Marcie, P. Critères neurolinguistiques d'une classification des aphasies. *Acta Neurologica et Psychiatrica Belgica*, 1967, *67*, 959—987.

Howes, D. Application of the word-frequency concept to aphasia. In A. V. S. De Reuck & M. O'Connor (Eds.), *Disorders of language*. Ciba Foundation Symposium. London: Churchill, 1964.

Howes, D., Geschwind, N. Quantitative studies of aphasic language. *Research Publications, Association for Research in Nervous and Mental Disease*, 1962, *42*, 229–244.

Jakobson, R. Towards a linguistic typology of aphasic impairment. In A. V. S. De Reuck & M. O'Connor (Eds.), *Disorders of language*. Ciba Foundation Symposium. London: Churchill, 1964. Pp. 21–64.

Jakobson, R., & Halle, M. *Fundamentals of language*. The Hague: Mouton, 1956.

Katz, J. J., & Fodor, J. A. The structure of a semantic theory. In J. A. Fodor & J. J. Katz (Eds.), *The structure of language: Readings in the philosophy of language*. Englewood Cliffs, N.J.: Prentice-Hall, 1964. Pp. 479–518.

Lashley, K. S. The problem of serial order in behavior. In L. A. Jeffress (Ed.), *Cerebral mechanisms in behavior*. New York: Wiley, 1951.

Lecours, A. R. Serial order in writing: a study of misspelled words in developmental dysgraphia. *Neuropsychologia*, 1966, *4*, 221–241.

Lecours, A. R. An essay on the notion of neologism in aphasic language. *Proceedings, 3rd International Symposium of Aphasiology, Oaxtepec, 1971*, in press.

Lecours, A. R., Deloche, G., & Lhermitte, F. Paraphasies phonémiques: Description et simulation sur ordinateur. In *Colloque IRIA—Informatique Médicale*. Rocquencourt: Institut de Recherche d'informatique et d'Automatique, 1973. Pp. 311–350.

Lecours, A. R., Dordain, G., & Lhermitte, F. Recherches sur le langage des aphasiques. 1. Terminologie neurolinguistique. *L'Encéphale*, 1970, *59*, 520–546.

Lecours, A. R., & Lhermitte, F. Phonemic paraphasias; linguistic structures and tentative hypotheses. *Cortex*, 1969, *5*, 193–228.

Lecours, A. R., & Lhermitte, F. Recherches sur le langage des aphasiques. 2. Mesure des relations de similarité entre unités linguistiques et modèle de référence pour la description des transformations aphasiques. *L'Encéphale*, 1970, *59*, 547–574.

Lecours, A. R., & Lhermitte, F. Recherches sur le langage des aphasiques: 4. Analyse d'un corpus de néologismes; notion de paraphasie monémique. *L'Encéphale*, 1972, *61*, 295–315.

Lecours, A. R., & Twitchell, T. E. Sequential errors in written language: their form, occurrence, and nature. Communication presented to the 18th annual meeting of the American Academy of Neurology, Philadelphia, April 1966.

Lhermitte, F. Sémiologie de l'aphasie. *Revue du Praticien*, 1965, *15*, 2345–2363.

Lhermitte, F., Derouesné, J., & Lecours, A. R. Contribution à l'étude des troubles sémantiques dans l'aphasie. *Revue Neurologique*, 1971, *125*, 81–101.

Lhermitte, F., Lecours, A. R., & Bertaux, D. Arousal and seriation of linguistic units in aphasic transformations. In L. D. Proctor (Ed.), *Biocybernetics of the central nervous system*. Boston: Little, Brown, 1969. Pp. 389–417.

Lhermitte, F., Lecours, A. R., & Ouvry, B. Essai d'analyse structurale des paralexies et des paragraphies. *Acta Neurologica et Psychiatrica Belgica*, 1967, *67*, 1021–1044.

Malmberg, B. *La phonétique*. Paris: Presses Universitaires de France, 1966.

Martinet, A. *A functional view of language*. London & New York: Oxford Univ. Press (Clarendon), 1961.

Martinet, A. *Eléments de linguistique générale*. Paris: Collin, 1967.

Mounin, G. *Clefs pour la sémantique*. Paris: Seghers, 1972.

Perceau, L. *La redoute des contrepèteries*. Paris: Briffaut, 1963.

Pierre Marie, P. *Travaux et mémoires*. Vol. I. Paris: Masson, 1926.

Poncet, M., Degos, C., Deloche, G., & Lecours, A. R. Phonetic and phonemic transformations in aphasia. *International Journal of Mental Health*, 1972, *1*, 46–54.

Ranschburg, P. *Die Lese- und Schreibstörungen des Kindesalters*. Halle: Carl Marhold Verlagsbuchhandlung, 1928.

Sabouraud, O., Gagnepain, J., & Sabouraud, A. Aphasie et linguistique. *Revue du Praticien*, 1965, *15*, 2335–2343.

Tissot, R. *Neuropsychopathologie de l'aphasie*. Paris: Masson, 1966.

6. The Relation of Nonverbal Cognitive Functions to Aphasia

O. L. Zangwill

A short account is given of the nature of aphasia, with particular reference to the extent to which it transcends mere disorder of speech. The degree to which aphasic patients remain capable of nonverbal communication, for example, in the form of gesture or pantomime, is assessed, and the relation of defect in musical accomplishment to disorder of language is reviewed. The capacity of aphasic patients to express themselves by drawing or modeling and the extent to which they are able to maintain adequate spatial orientation are considered. Finally, the relation of language to thinking and problem-solving is discussed, with special reference to the extent to which aphasic patients can cope with abstract issues. Some implications for rehabilitation are briefly outlined.

Introduction

The term *aphasia* is traditionally used to denote loss or defect of speech resulting from a focal lesion of one hemisphere of the brain, as a rule the left, but very occasionally the right. This definition, however, is often regarded as too narrow. In the first place, speech is seldom, if ever, affected in isolation. There are commonly associated defects in reading, writing, and calculation, although these skills are not necessarily affected to the same extent as spoken speech. In the second place, many people today regard the disorder in aphasia as essentially one in the realm of signs and signification. As Hughlings Jackson (1878) long ago remarked: "There is, at least in many cases, more than loss of *speech*; pantomime is impaired; there is often loss or defect in symbolizing relations of things in any way [p. 159]." In consequence, his pupil, Sir Henry Head (1926), was led to specify the basic defect in aphasia as one of symbolic formulation and expression. Although not everyone accepts the view that there is in aphasia a general disturbance of symbolic communication, few today would restrict the disorder exclusively to the reception and expression of oral speech.

The aim of this chapter is to ascertain, in so far as this may be possible at the present time, the extent to which aphasic patients manifest disorder in spheres of activity that cannot be regarded as primarily dependent on language. Among them are gesture and pantomime, music, drawing and modeling, spatial orientation, abstract classification, and performance on psychometric tests of the kind commonly described as "nonverbal." Apart from its theoretical interest, the extent to which nonverbal activities are affected in aphasia is of considerable practical importance. For if the disorder is truly restricted to language, the aphasic patient should be at no greater disadvantage than a healthy individual endeavoring to communicate in a language with which he is imperfectly acquainted. Despite his linguistic handicap, such an individual is in no way affected in his thinking or judgment or in the execution of skills making little or no demands on language. But if, on the other hand, the disorder transcends language and involves activities that can properly be described as nonlinguistic, the position of the patient is clearly very much graver. In such a case, doubt might well be entertained as to his intellectual integrity and judgement in the practical matters of daily life. While everyone agrees that aphasia is not dementia, the issue of whether or not there is an intellectual defect is a crucial one for all concerned with the rehabilitation and resettlement of patients with central disorders of language and communication.

Gesture and Pantomime

Are aphasic patients in general capable of nonverbal forms of communication? Can, for example, such a patient express by gesture or pantomime an idea or intention that he cannot, as we say, put into words? Clinical experience discloses that this is indeed often the case, especially in patients whose speech disorder is predominantly expressive and who have good insight into their linguistic deficiency. Critchley (1939) cites the case of a girl rendered almost entirely speechless by a cerebral embolism, who evolved so subtle a language of gesture that "she could inform her friends each day what doctors and visitors had seen her [p. 27]." Alajouanine and Lhermitte (1964) tell of the owner of a racehorse stable who, unable to explain the meaning of the word *gelding*, resorted to an expressive gesture of cutting something. But these dramatic instances of successful gesture language are perhaps somewhat exceptional. While gestures tend in general to be better preserved than verbal utterances, pantomime is often scanty and symbolic gestures poorly performed. In such cases, is the gestural deficiency part and parcel of the general disorder of language or is it, on the other hand, due to a breakdown of a separate communication system only indirectly related to language?

Although the evidence is equivocal, it does appear that a breakdown in gestural communication is not necessarily a direct outcome of a disorder of spoken language. In his pioneer studies of *apraxia* (loss or defect of purposive action in the absence of paralysis or sensory loss), Liepmann (1908) showed that failure to imitate or perform symbolic gestures on command is on occasion present in the absence of aphasia. More recently, Goodglass and Kaplan (1963) devised a useful series of tests to assess the adequacy of pantomime and gestural communication. Although performance was undoubtedly worse in a group of aphasics than in a comparable group of brain-injured patients without aphasia, no relation was found between the severity of aphasia and the degree of gestural deficiency. The authors therefore concluded that disorders of gesture language do not necessarily form part of a general disturbance of symbolic formulation and expression.

Goodglass and Kaplan's findings provide some support for the proposal that it might be possible to retrain severely aphasic patients by teaching them a system of gestural communication, such as sign language as taught to the deaf. The fact that a chimpanzee has been successfully taught a considerable vocabulary (Gardner & Gardner, 1969) adds further credence to the idea. Indeed, Gazzaniga (1971) has already reported some pilot experiments on re-training aphasics using a nonverbal procedure adapted from the work of Premack (1971) with a chimpanzee. Such methods might well find application in the re-training of motor aphasics, who do not as a rule exhibit gross defect in expressive movement.

Music

Aphasic patients with some degree of musical accomplishment are not uncommon, and when studied from this point of view, are often found to be less impaired in their musical performance than in expressive speech. Indeed, the ability to sing, hum, or whistle familiar tunes is often preserved in spite of severe expressive aphasia, although there is often difficulty in initiating vocalization, and attempts to utter the appropriate words may render performance even worse (Head, 1926). It is noteworthy, too, that in the one case of excision of the left hemisphere for glioma in a right-handed man that has been at all carefully studied (Smith, 1966), the patient retained some capacity to sing and even to vocalize the words in spite of otherwise almost total aphasia. Such observations have led to the suggestion that music is less fully lateralized than speech and may be sustained, to some considerable extent at least, by the nondominant hemisphere.

As with aphasia, amusia can be present as predominantly receptive, that is, as a failure to recognize tones or melodies or to read musical notation, or as predominantly expressive, that is, as difficulty in producing tones or melodies either by singing or performance on a musical instrument (Weisenburg & McBride, 1935). Indeed, the fact that expressive and receptive disorders of musical accomplishment are so well differentiated has been adduced to support the analogous distinction in the sphere of language (Feuchtwanger, 1930). Amusia, however, appears to result from lesions of the dominant hemisphere less predictably than does aphasia, and is also more common in association with lesions of the nondominant hemisphere. A surprising case of persistent amusia with only mild and transitory expressive aphasia following right hemisphere lesion in a right-handed man has been described (Botez & Wertheim, 1959).

In an unpublished thesis, Dorgeuille (1966) carefully examined musical abilities in 26 brain-damaged patients, in 22 of whom the damage was focal. Amusia without aphasia occurred in four cases (in two of which the lesion was right-sided) and aphasia without amusia in three. In general, there was a parallel between the type of language disorder (predominantly expressive or predominantly receptive) and the type of amusia, though no consistent relation was found between severity of impairment in the two spheres. Like gesture language, therefore, musical accomplishment appears to be in part, at least, independent of language and may survive the destruction of expressive speech.

A study of aphasia in a celebrated composer (Alajouanine, 1948) revealed that creative capacity was virtually annulled. Whether this is a necessary consequence of aphasia is uncertain, but from the point of view of rehabilitation it is important to bear in mind that the more creative the activity, whether literary or musical, the greater the handicap likely to result from a lesion of the dominant hemisphere. At the same time, the relative independence of disorders of language and of musical accomplishment gives hope of a measure of rehabilitation in some professional musicians stricken by aphasia.

Drawing and Modeling

The graphic arts are conventionally regarded as modes of expression independent of language and might therefore be expected to escape destruction in any of their practitioners who develop aphasia. Indeed, artistic expression is reported to have remained at a relatively high level in, at all events, one well-known artist stricken by aphasia (Alajouanine, 1948). None the less, aphasic patients often seem to experience difficulty in drawing, especially when asked to reproduce common objects from memory (Head, 1926) or drawings of human figures (Weisenburg & McBride, 1935). Maps and plans may also be very poorly drawn (Head, 1926), although it should be borne in mind that this may be found in cases of right hemisphere lesions without aphasia (Paterson & Zangwill, 1944). Although the nature of the drawing disability appears to vary somewhat according to the hemisphere affected, a careful study (Warrington, James & Kinsbourne, 1966) has revealed no essential difference in its severity as between left-sided and right-sided lesions. It might seem, therefore, that disorders in drawing are essentially unrelated to disorders of speech.

At the same time, there is a good deal of evidence that ideational deficits in aphasia may be reflected in performance on tests of drawing and modeling. In this connection, Bay (1962) has taken the poor performance of his patients on such tasks to indicate a conceptual deficit. The "idea" of the object is poorly reflected in the drawing, and salient features may be omitted. Bay has also reported that patients who are unable to name a missing feature in an incomplete drawing are also unable to complete it. This interesting observation might suggest that anomia is an amnesic defect rather than one of classification, as had been held by Goldstein (1948). Although individual differences are considerable, aphasic patients are seldom able to express their ideas by drawing in a completely normal fashion, suggesting that the disorder in some sense transcends the realm of language to embrace nonverbal forms of communication.

In a recent study, de Renzi, Faglioni, Scotti, and Spinnler (1972) have shown that the ability to represent the colors of familiar objects, such as a cherry, a banana, or a mail box, is commonly defective in aphasic patients despite the fact that there is no defect of color discrimination or failure in color recognition as such. Indeed, of the 18 patients in their series of 166 giving the poorest results, all but one were aphasic. The authors do not regard this defect as a direct result of the disorder of language, but rather as the outcome of an underlying failure of associative memory. This failure to associate color with form, they suggest, is comparable to the analogous inability seen in some cases of aphasia to associate objects with the sounds they produce or with their appropriate uses. This hypothesis of a relatively specific intellectual deficiency, which is to be ascribed neither to general intellectual loss nor yet to a specifically linguistic incapacity, is reminiscent of the view of Pierre Marie (1906), which has more recently been revived by Bay (1964).

Despite this evidence of defect in various aspects of nonverbal expression, it would be premature to conclude that attempts to train aphasic patients to make greater use of graphical expression are contraindicated. Indeed, progress along these lines is often more rapid than in speech re-education proper. Indeed Hatfield and Zangwill (1974) have shown that some severely aphasic patients are able to communicate their intentions and experiences in a limited way by serial drawings ("picture stories"), suggesting that far greater use might be made of visuomotor techniques, particularly in the case of patients with predominantly expressive defects who are unlikely to exhibit marked difficulties in drawing, copying, or constructional skill.

Spatial Orientation

Orientation in space is, as a rule, well preserved in aphasia, although on occasion it may be disturbed in patients with posterior unilateral (and in particular bilateral) brain damage. In such cases, the patient may have difficulty in following routes formerly well known to him or in recognizing familiar landmarks. Difficulties in using maps or in drawing or working with plans are likewise by no means uncommon (Head, 1926), although it should be borne in mind that such difficulties are just as common, and perhaps even more disabling, in cases of right hemisphere injury unaccompanied by any disorder of language (Paterson & Zangwill, 1944). Commonly, too, aphasic patients are handicapped in spatial orientation as a direct consequence of the language difficulty. Even when the speech disorder is relatively mild, the patient may find it virtually impossible to give directions to others, especially when these involve compass directions or distinctions of right and left (Benton, 1959), or to formulate his topographical knowledge in a communicable form. Some loss of topographical memory has occasionally been described.

In experiments on spatial orientation using specially designed visual or tactile maps, Teuber and his colleagues have found that, in general, aphasic patients perform more poorly than patients with comparable brain damage but without aphasia (Semmes, Weinstein, Ghent, & Teuber, 1963). They do not, however, regard language pathology as either a necessary or a sufficient condition for decrement on their orientation tests.

Abstraction

It has been argued by many who have taken a psychological approach to aphasia (e.g., Goldstein, 1948; Head, 1926; Pick, 1931; van Woerkom, 1925) that the basic disturbance lies not so much in language per se as in the underlying thought processes. In general, the higher the level of abstraction, the greater the resulting deficit. Further, it should be possible by the use of appropriate techniques to demonstrate this deficit in nonverbal performance. Hence the stress that has been placed on the value of tests of sorting, classification, and the like in the assessment of brain-injured patients (see, e.g., Goldstein & Scheerer, 1941).

The results are not, however, altogether easy to assess. Although significant defects on nonverbal abstraction tests have been reported by some workers (de Renzi, Faglioni, Savoiardo, & Vignolo, 1966), others have reported no greater incidences of defect in aphasic patients than in control groups of brain-damaged patients without aphasia (Bauer & Beck, 1954; Meyers, 1948; Zangwill, 1964). Yet there seems little doubt that performance on such tests is especially sensitive to lesions of the dominant hemisphere (de Renzi *et al.*, 1966; McFie & Piercy, 1952), which are, of course, frequently associated with aphasia. De Renzi and his associates make the interesting suggestion that the areas of the left hemisphere subserving language may also be those specialized for the carrying out of intellectual tasks of a symbolic nature.

At the same time, it should be borne in mind that classification tests are often performed satisfactorily by aphasic patients, particularly those with anterior brain lesions and primarily executive language disorder. Where, however, defect is apparent on such tests, the prognosis with regard to occupational resettlement must evidently be guarded.

Problem Solving

The term "nonverbal" is often used of psychometric tests the performance of which does not obviously depend on language. Such, for example, are the Raven

Progressive Matrices (Raven, 1938), a test of educing logical relationships presented in diagrammatic form, or the Picture Completion, Picture Arrangement, and Block Design subtests of the Wechsler-Bellevue Scale (Wechsler, 1958). To call such tests "nonverbal," however, is certainly not to say that language plays no part in their solution or that performance is in no way impaired by linguistic handicap. None the less, it has been known since the work of Weisenburg and McBride (1935) that in aphasia, performance on "nonverbal" intelligence tests is far less impaired than on "verbal" intelligence tests, and the use of the former in assessing the intellectual competence of aphasic patients is now standard practice.

At the same time, performance even on nonverbal tests is apt to be affected to some extent. Weisenburg and McBride clearly demonstrated that aphasic patients, as a group, showed a significant decrement on a variety of nonverbal tests in relation to the performance of a healthy control group. If, however, the control group consisted of patients with right hemisphere damage without aphasia, the inferiority of the aphasic group was no longer found. Although at the time this result was somewhat unexpected, we now know that right hemisphere lesions are apt to produce significant decrement on many types of nonverbal performance, especially those depending upon spatial judgement and constructional skill (Newcombe, 1969).

What are the reasons for defective performance on nonverbal tasks in aphasia? There is no easy answer to this question. Performance on such tasks may be affected by a variety of factors—sensory, motor, perceptual, and linguistic—and it is often hazardous to surmise whether poor performance on any particular task is to be attributed to general intellectual loss or to some more specific disability or combination of disabilities. None the less, it is reasonable to ask whether aphasic patients show difficulties in problem solving that are to be ascribed to intellectual rather than to sensory, motor, or linguistic handicap.

In trying to answer this question, the first point to bear in mind is that high-level perceptual or motor disability can produce gross decrement on nonverbal intelligence tests, whether or not there is associated aphasia. According to Alajouanine and Lhermitte (1964), it is only those patients in whom aphasia is associated with apraxia who give really poor results (IQ below 80) on the Wechsler-Bellevue Performance Scale. Zangwill (1964) has called attention to gross defects in performance on the Raven Progressive Matrices of patients with constructional apraxia, which may or may not be associated with aphasia. Whether constructional apraxia is properly to be regarded as an "intellectual" disorder is uncertain (see Warrington, 1969), but at all events it is one that may present quite independently of disorders of language.

Teuber and his associates have made several attempts to devise tests that are genuinely nonverbal, modeling their procedures to a large extent on the kinds of task that have been devised to study discrimination learning and problem solving in subhuman primates. One such is the "hidden figures" test, adapted from the work of Gottschaldt, in which the patient is required to identify a specific geometrical figure when it is embedded in the context of a more comprehensive design that largely masks it (Teuber & Weinstein, 1956). Although the test might appear to be one of visual rather than of verbal ability, impairment among brain-injured veterans was found to be significantly related to the presence of aphasia, this deficiency being still apparent when intelligence (as measured by the Army General Classification Test) was equated in the aphasic and nonaphasic groups. Another task in which aphasic subjects were found to do particularly poorly was a "conditional reaction" test, inspired by a method much used in animal experiments (Weinstein, Teuber, Ghent, & Semmes, 1955). Here the subject is presented with a square and a circle on one or the other of two backgrounds, one with vertical and the other with horizontal stripes. The circle must be chosen if the background is striped horizontally, the square if it is striped vertically. As monkeys can learn to solve this type of problem, it is reasonable to suppose that its solution is independent of language. Faced with it, however, aphasic patients appear to encounter exceptional difficulty.

To explain this result, it could be argued—following Vygotsky (1962)—that in man, thinking has become so predominantly a matter of language that any linguistic disorder is bound to reduce its efficiency. Hence confronted with the embedded-figure or conditional-reaction task, the healthy subject will make much use of verbal analysis to guide his strategy. Denied this, the aphasic will be clearly at a disadvantage. A similar explanation might be given of the failure of aphasic patients to solve the more difficult items of the Progressive Matrices test, in which verbal analysis undoubtedly plays an important part (Zangwill, 1964). There is, indeed, electrophysiological evidence of subvocal activity accompanying the solution of these harder problems (Sokolov, 1972). If this explanation is correct, failure on the part of aphasic patients to solve nonverbal problems could be regarded as a direct consequence of the language deficiency.

Yet many who have worked with aphasics find it hard to explain away the whole of the patient's difficulty in problem solving as a secondary consequence of his language handicap. As Weinstein (1964) has remarked: "An important aspect of aphasia is defective organization and selection of material, linguistic as well as non-linguistic, and disturbance is manifested only partly in the obvious difficulties with linguistic reception, expression and memory [p. 159]." If he is right, we must accept that there is a genuine limitation of thought and action going beyond mere linguistic incapacity. The aphasic is not merely "lame in thinking," as Hughlings Jackson so aptly put it; he has in some sense forgotten how to think.

Speech and Thought

Let us pursue this metaphor. Clearly, the devastation of intellectual life consequent upon aphasia is greatest wherever effective performance calls for the intelligent use of language, explicit or implicit. As Weisenburg and McBride (1935) pointed out, limitation of intellectual capacity is shown principally in performances that require the intelligent development of the language formulation as a whole. Elvin and Oldfield (1951), in a valuable analysis of the essays written by a dysphasic university student over a 2-year period, noted a close parallel between the restitution of intellectual and linguistic competence. Zangwill (1964) has called attention to the severe difficulties encountered by patients with very minimal speech disorders in explaining the meaning of well-known idioms, proverbs, or figures of speech. Here the disability is apparent only in the intellectual applications of language; its function in ordinary social communication remains intact. From a clinical point of view, language defect at this high level may appear too inconspicuous for serious attention; yet for those, such as writers and journalists, who "trade in words" for their livelihood, it may prove truly catastrophic.

Although, in general, degree of speech and of intellectual incapacity run parallel, intelligence may on occasion remain at a surprisingly high level despite gross defect or confusion of speech. Some patients who are speechless, or virtually so, perform well on nonverbal intelligence tests and show little or no defect of abstraction. In such cases, one may surmise, implicit or "inner" speech is adequately preserved. Again, patients with jargon aphasia may perform relatively well on tests such as the Progressive Matrices (Kinsbourne & Warrington, 1963), yet the reasons they give for their decisions are totally incomprehensible. Here the reasoning process is substantially intact; it is only its verbal formulation that is deficient. This may perhaps be due to the fact that the understanding of relations embodied in pictorial or diagrammatic form is vested in the nondominant rather than the dominant hemisphere and hence escapes destruction in aphasia.

Conclusion

Can any conclusions of practical import be drawn from this short survey of nonverbal functions in relation to aphasia? In the present state of our ignorance regarding the basic mechanisms of thought and speech, the assessment and rehabilitation of patients with speech disorders is inevitably very much an ad hoc affair. None the less, a brief summary may perhaps be of use to those who seek to base measures of re-education so far as may be possible on the findings of relatively systematic observation and experiment.

1. Pantomime and gesture are affected to some extent in aphasia, although there is little correlation between the severity of the speech disorder and the degree of gestural deficiency. The possibility of training severely aphasic patients to use sign language is worthy of exploration.

2. Defect in the sphere of music (amusia) is often, although not invariably, present in cases of aphasia, although here again there is no consistent relation between the severity of aphasia and the loss or defect in musical accomplishment. Singing, with or without the use of words, is often better preserved than articulate speech. Amusia is more common than aphasia in association with lesions of the nondominant hemisphere, suggesting that the lateralization of musical accomp-

lishments is less complete than that of spoken language. There might therefore be greater possibility of re-education in music than in speech after lesions of the dominant hemisphere.

3. Drawing and modeling often give difficulty to patients with aphasia, apparently due to an ideational rather than to a perceptual or motor disability. In particular, the representation of colors of familiar objects may be strikingly at fault. The extent to which aphasic patients can express themselves by drawing varies considerably from case to case, but might in some cases be developed appreciably further by compensatory training.

4. Spatial orientation is for the most part unaffected in aphasic patients, who seldom lose themselves in a familiar locality. On the other hand, difficulties often arise if the patient is requested to give or follow directions, especially when mention is made of right and left or of points of the compass. Constructing or reading maps and plans may likewise give difficulty, especially in cases with posterior hemisphere lesions. Special tests of spatial orientation under laboratory conditions are poorly performed by aphasic subjects, although language pathology as such does not appear to be either a necessary or a sufficient condition for such failure.

5. As a group, aphasic patients perform poorly on tests of classification or abstraction, though good results are sometimes obtained in individual cases, particularly those in which the speech disorder is predominantly expressive. Loss of "abstract attitude" appears to be correlated with lesions of the dominant cerebral hemisphere rather than with the presence of speech pathology per se.

6. Scores on nonverbal intelligence tests as a rule show decrement in aphasia, particularly if there is associated visuospatial or constructional disability. Problem-solving tasks of a kind much used in animal experiments also tend to be performed less well by aphasic patients than by otherwise comparable brain-injured patients without aphasia. It cannot, however, be concluded that these findings necessarily indicate reduced intellectual competence in practical affairs such as, for example, testamentary capacity.

7 The relative superiority of aphasic patients on nonverbal as opposed to verbal intelligence tests may be due to the fact that visuospatial and perhaps also soma-esthetic skills are in all probability executed under the predominant control of the nondominant cerebral hemisphere. It follows that the development of visuomotor and manipulative skills based primarily on nondominant hemisphere function would seem an obvious target for rehabilitation in aphasia.

References

Alajouanine, T. Aphasia and artistic realization. *Brain*, 1948, *71*, 224—241.

Alajouanine, T., & Lhermitte, F. Non-verbal communication in aphasia. In A. V. S. De Reuck & M. O'Connor (Eds.), *Disorders of language*. Ciba Foundation Symposium. London: Churchill, 1964. Pp. 168—182.

Bauer, K., & Beck, D. Intellect after cerebro-vascular accident. *Journal of Nervous and Mental Disease,* 1954, *120,* 379–395.

Bay, E. Aphasia and non-verbal disorders of language. *Brain,* 1962, *85,* 411–426.

Bay, E. Principles of classification and their influence on our concepts of aphasia. In A. V. S. De Reuck & M. O'Connor (Eds.), *Disorders of language.* Ciba Foundation Symposium. London: Churchill, 1964. Pp. 122–142.

Benton, A. L. *Right-left discrimination and finger localization.* New York: Hocker-Harper, 1959.

Botez, M. I., & Wertheim, N. Expressive aphasia and amusia following right frontal lesion in a right-handed man. *Brain,* 1959, *82,* 186–202.

Critchley, M. *The language of gesture.* London: Arnold, 1939.

de Renzi, E., Faglioni, P., Savoiardo, M., & Vignolo, L. A. The influence of aphasia and of hemispheric side of the cerebral lesion on abstract thinking. *Cortex,* 1966, *2,* 399–420.

de Renzi, E. Faglioni, P., Scotti, G., & Spinnler, H. Impairment in associating colour to form, concomitant with aphasia. *Brain,* 1972, *95,* 293–304.

Dorgeuille, C. J. Introduction a l'etude des amusies. Thèse pour le Doctorat en Medicine, No. 443, Dactylo-Sorbonne, Paris, 1966.

Elvin, M. B., & Oldfield, R. C. Disabilities and progress in a dysphasic University student. *Journal of Neurology, Neurosurgery, and Psychiatry,* 1951, *14,* 118–128.

Feuchtwanger, E. *Amusie:* Studien zur pathologischen Psychologie der akustischen Wahrnemung und Vorstellung und ihrer Strukturgebiete besonders in Musik und Sprache *Monographien Aus Dem Gesamtgebiete Der Neurologie Und Psychiatrie.* Berlin: Springer, 1930.

Gardner, R. A., & Gardner, B. T. Teaching sign language to a chimpanzee. *Science,* 1969, *165,* 664–672.

Gazzaniga, M. Language training in brain-damaged humans. *Federation Proceedings, Federation of American Societies for Experimental Biology,* 1971, *30,* 265.

Goldstein, K. *Language and language disorders.* New York: Grune & Stratton, 1948.

Goldstein, K., & Scheerer, M. Abstract and concrete behaviour: an experimental study with special tests. *Psychological Monographs,* 1941, *53,* 151.

Goodglass, H., & Kaplan, E. Disturbance of gesture and pantomime in aphasia. *Brain,* 1963, *86,* 703–720.

Hatfield, F. M., & Zangwill, O. L. Ideation in aphasia: the picture-story method. *Neuropsychologia,* 1974, *12,* 389–393.

Head, M. *Aphasia and kindred disorders of speech.* London: Cambridge Univ. Press, 1926. 2 vols.

Jackson, J. Hughlings. On affections of speech from disease of the brain. *Brain,* 1878, *1,* 304–330. Reprinted in J. Taylor (Ed.), *Selected writings of John Hughlings Jackson,* Vol. 2. London: Hodder & Stoughton, 1932. Pp. 155–330.

Kinsbourne, M., & Warrington, E. K. Jargon aphasia. *Neuropsychologie,* 1963, *1,* 27–38.

Liepmann, H. *Dres Anfsätze aus dem Apraxiegebiet.* Berlin: Karger, 1908.

Marie, P. La troisieme circonvolution frontale gauche ne joue aucun role special dans la fonction du langage. *Semaine Medical,* 1906, May 23. Reprinted in *Truvaux et memoires.* Vol. I. Paris: Masson, 1926.

McFie, J., & Piercy, M. F. The relation of laterality of lesion to performance on Weigl's sorting test. *Journal of Mental Science,* 1952, *98,* 299–305.

Meyers, R. Relation of "thinking" and language: an experimental approach using dysphasic patients. *Archives of Neurology and Psychiatry (Chicago)* 1948, *60,* 119–139.

Newcombe, F. *Missile wounds of the brain: A study of psychological deficits.* Oxford Neurological Monographs. London & New York: Oxford Univ. Press, 1969.

Paterson, A., & Zangwill, O. L. Disorders of visual space perception associated with lesions of the right cerebral hemisphere. *Brain,* 1944, *67,* 331–358.

Pick, A. Aphasie. In A. Bethe, G. von Bergman, G. Embden, & A. Ellinger (Eds.), *Handbuch der normalen und pathologiochen Physiologie.* Vol. 15, Part 2. Berlin: Springer, 1931. Pp. 1416–1524.

Premack, D. Language in chimpanzee? *Science,* 1971, *172,* 808–822.

Raven, J. C. *Progressive matrices.* London: H. K. Lewis, 1938.

Semmes, J., Weinstein, S., Ghent, L., & Teuber, H.-L. Correlates of impaired orientation in personal and extra-personal space. *Brain,* 1963, *86,* 747–772.

Smith, A. Speech and other functions after left (dominant) hemispherectomy. *Journal of Neurology, Neurosurgery, and Psychiatry*, 1966, *29*, 467—471.

Sokolov, A. N. *Inner speech and thought*. New York: Plenum, 1972.

Teuber, H.-L., & Weinstein, S. Ability to discover hidden figures after cerebral lesions. *AMA Archives of Neurology and Psychiatry*, 1956, *76*, 369—379.

van Woerkom, W. Über Störungen im Denken bei Aphasie Patienten. *Monatsschrift für Psychiatrie und Neurologie*, 1925, *59*, 256—322.

Vygotsky, L. S. *Thought and language*. (Edited and translated by E. Haufmann & G. Vaker) Cambridge, Mass.: MIT Press, 1962.

Warrington, E. K. Constructional apraxia. In P. J. Vinken & G. W. Bruyn (Eds.), *Handbook of clinical neurology*. Vol. 4. Amsterdam: North-Holland Publishing Co., Pp. 67—83.

Warrington, E. K., James, M., and Kinsbourne, M. Drawing disability in relation to laterality of cerebral lesion. *Brain*, 1966, *89*, 53—82.

Wechsler, D. *The measurement and appraisal of adult intelligence*. (4th ed.) London: Baillière, 1958.

Weinstein, S. Deficits concomitant with aphasia and lesions of either cerebral hemisphere. *Cortex*, 1964, *1*, 154—169.

Weinstein, S., Teuber, H.-L. Ghent, L., & Semmes, J. Complex visual performance after penetrating brain injury in man. *American Psychologist*, 1955, *10*, 408.

Weisenburg, T. M., & McBride, K. E. *Aphasia: A clinical and psychological study*. New York: Commonwealth Fund, 1935.

Zangwill, O. L. Intelligence in aphasia. In A. V. S. De Reuck & M. O'Connor (Eds.), *Disorders of language*. Ciba Foundation Symposium. London: Churchill, 1964. Pp. 261—274.

7. Minor Hemisphere Language and Cerebral Maturation

Marcel Kinsbourne

Language processes are predominantly represented in the left cerebral hemisphere in almost all adults. But after callosal section, the right hemisphere can decode speech, and after extensive left hemisphere damage, it can also in time assume a degree of control over speech production. Left-hemisphere dominance is progressively asserted over a right hemisphere which had substantial language potential in the first few years of language acquisition. After early destruction of the left hemisphere, the right can alone support virtually normal language development. But in the left hemisphere's presence, right hemispheric language potential dwindles over time, and the right hemisphere's ability to compensate for acquired aphasia following left hemisphere damage decreases to the adult level in the course of the first decade. It may be that the left hemisphere exerts increasingly effective transcallosal inhibition of right-sided, speech-decoding processes and competes successfully for control of language response mechanisms at brainstem level.

Almost all right-handed people and a majority of left-handers have language processes primarily represented in their left cerebral hemispheres. This inference has been made mainly by observing the effects of cerebral disease that is confined to one hemisphere; when such injury occurs on the left side, it often induces aphasic language disorder, but when it occurs on the right, aphasia rarely appears (Penfield & Roberts, 1959; Russell & Espir, 1961). More recently, this has been confirmed by the results of injection of amobarbital into the carotid artery. Most of the cerebral hemisphere on the injected side is transiently anesthetized. In almost all right-handers and a majority of left-handers, the patient becomes unable to speak after left-sided injection but not after right-sided injection (Milner,

Branch, & Rasmussen, 1964; Perria, Rosadini, & Rossi, 1961). Although the doctrine of left cerebral dominance for language (Broca, 1865) is generally accepted, there remains some uncertainty about the role of the right, subdominant hemisphere in normal adult language and in language development. Nor has it been firmly established what compensatory role the right hemisphere might play in language if the left is damaged in either the developing or the mature brain.

Different facets of language behavior can be selectively impaired by focal lesions in the mature and fully differentiated brain, so that adult patients can display a variety of different patterns of aphasic deficit. When children's developing brains are damaged, such differences in pattern of language deficit are less usual. This is partly because differentiation of brain function is as yet incomplete and partly because, when a child is beginning to acquire language, language processes interact, so that deficit in one process can obstruct full use of the rest. Nevertheless, the classical adult categorization of aphasia into comprehension (decoding) and production (encoding) deficits of language is definitely applicable to children (Kinsbourne & Peel-Floyd, 1965). We shall discuss the decoding and encoding processes separately because the minor hemisphere does not contribute equally to each process. First we characterize the end point, the minor hemisphere's participation in adult language, and then we consider how development brings this about.

It has been believed that the minor hemisphere does not take part in normal adult language behavior (although mild verbal deficit may follow right hemisphere lesions according to Archibald & Wepman, 1968; Eisenson, 1962; Swisher & Sarno, 1969). This conclusion has been based on the knowledge that language is left substantially unaffected by minor hemisphere damage, even when this amounts to right hemispherectomy (Smith, 1969). But that fact need not exclude the possibility that the right hemisphere participates in language in the intact brain, provided that its role can speedily be taken over by other structures when necessary. But this is difficult to prove. A number of behavioral indices of hemispheric involvement during normal language functioning have been developed (Kimura, 1967; Kinsbourne, 1970a, 1973), but these at present only indicate the side that is most involved and have not been refined enough to reflect the presence or degree of any participation by the other side of the brain. Because the left hemisphere is involved in the programming of all oral and manual speech output, verbal input must at some stage reach that hemisphere. It may be that the minor hemisphere normally decodes speech signals that reach it first (through the left ear and the left visual field) before passing the information on to the left hemisphere across the interconnecting commissure, the corpus callosum, but this is not known. That it can do so under abnormal circumstances is shown by neuropsychological studies.

The right hemisphere has been separated from the left by cutting the corpus callosum in certain epileptic patients (Bogen & Vogel, 1962). In such "split-brain" patients, it is found that spoken instructions given exclusively to the left ear or by briefly exposed printed instructions to the left visual field can be carried out correctly by the left hand but not by the right hand (Gazzaniga & Sperry, 1967). As the right hemisphere is the primary recipient of left-sided information and is in primary control of the left hand, it follows that it, unaided, must have decoded the verbal message so as to transform it into the requested hand-movement response. However, the subject cannot repeat the verbal message aloud or speak in response to it or to questions about it. The right hemisphere in callosectomized patients has little or no control over speech output (Butler & Norsell, 1968; Levy, Nebes, & Sperry, 1970). This demonstrates that it is possible to grasp the meaning of a verbal message (decode) without being able to encode the message into verbal motor output. In a language disorder called conduction aphasia (Wernicke, 1874), which is caused by left-sided focal brain damage, a similar independence of the ability to repeat from the ability to understand occurs. This independence has been experimentally verified in this syndrome (Kinsbourne, 1972). Lenneberg (1967) has shown that a child can easily comprehend language without any ability to speak. Thus the dissociation between comprehension and repetition in the disconnected right hemisphere is not unique to that hemisphere. Auditory feedback is involved in language acquisition but not in maintaining language once acquired. Motor-kinesthetic feedback is essential for neither the acquisition nor the maintenance of speech comprehension.

Is the mature right hemisphere unable to control speech because it lacks the requisite neural organization or because although it possesses encoding potential, the mature dominant left hemisphere competitively displaces it from control of the motor facilities that program the muscles of vocalization? Several sources of evidence support the latter interpretation.

Mere disconnection of right from left hemisphere suffices to reveal at once that the right hemisphere can *decode* speech to a fairly complex level of semantic and syntactic sophistication (Gordon, 1972); but it is necessary for the left hemisphere to be substantially reduced in function for a period of weeks before the right hemisphere gains a measure of control of speech *encoding* or output. One hemisphere can be suddenly temporarily inactivated in normal people by injecting sodium amobarbital into the carotid artery on that side (Wada & Rasmussen, 1960). It is found that while left-sided injection leaves the subject able to understand and carry out commands, he cannot speak for the 3 min during which the injection is effective (Perria *et al.*, 1961). Thus the right hemisphere, suddenly relieved of left-hemispheric competition, is unprepared at once to assume speech output control. But, after *permanent* surgical removal of the left hemisphere, speech is initially lost and then slowly re-established in the right hemisphere, although it remains subject to severe limitations (Hillier, 1954; Smith, 1966). The right-hemispheric speech strikingly shows the property speculatively attributed to it by Hughlings Jackson (1874) of being far more readily elicited in an emotional context than under the influence of the will alone. Presumably, emotional stimulation opens up to the right hemisphere output channels otherwise not under its control.

It is not essential for the whole left hemisphere to be removed; damage limited to the left language area can disinhibit the right hemisphere. Some right-handed patients who had been rendered aphasic by left-sided stroke were given intracarotid amobarbital. They showed no interruption of their aphasic speech when the injection was left-sided, but they totally stopped speaking after right-sided injection (Kinsbourne, 1971). It appears that aphasic speech does not, necessarily as has been generally assumed, represent the limited functioning of a damaged dominant language area. Rather, it may result from the unsophisticated compensatory efforts of the intact minor hemisphere. In other cases, we have found that aphasic speech does remain under left-sided control. These findings have since been confirmed (Czopf, 1972). It is not yet clear which type of dominant hemisphere damage switches in the right hemisphere and which does not; nor is it known how far recovery from aphasia based on right-hemispheric function may progress. If the preferred ear in dichotic listening can be assumed to be contralateral to the verbally dominant hemisphere, then there is evidence that, in aphasics, right hemisphere dominance develops and remains though language improves (Pettit, 1969). If isolated clinical case reports are to be believed, recovery based on right hemisphere verbal function may be virtually complete. Patients have been reported who, after recovering speech after left-sided disease causing aphasia, were again rendered aphasic, this time by lesions on the right side (Nielsen, 1964). It remains to be established whether it is typical for right-sided compensation in the adult to be complete, or whether recovery in such cases is usually mediated by resumed left-hemispheric functioning.

However, for our present purposes, the following salient findings can be relied on. The mature minor hemisphere has managed to develop speech decoding abilities that spring immediately into observable action when the left hemisphere is inactivated or excluded from transcallosal communication with the right. Thus the left cerebral dominance has not precluded the right hemisphere from some practice in decoding, in addition to maintaining its genetically preprogrammed decoding potential.

The situation is quite different as regards speaking. Substantial time has to pass after the occurrence of a lesion before the right hemisphere can assume even a limited degree of control over speech output. This makes it virtually certain that the right hemisphere plays no role in normal speaking and that it is precluded from such a role by neural arrangements that take time to reverse. This reversal could occur in one of two ways. Either speech output programs must be built up in the right hemisphere, or those programs take time to gain access to the brainstem output facility because they have to displace competing neural connections from the left. If the former process is the one that limits the rate of recovery, then speech therapy for at least some aphasics can be regarded as language education for the right hemisphere. If the latter process is crucial, then the situation might be analogous to that which occurs when one eye is deprived of patterned visual input for a long time early in life. The resulting visual defect, *amblyopia ex anopsia*, has been shown by Hubel and Wiesel (1965), working with kittens, to be set up by a process of synaptic disconnection. Certain neurons in the visual cortex normally receive synaptic connections from both eyes, and the disused synaptic terminals that emanate from the visually deprived eye are gradually displaced by those from the active eye. When patterned input is readmitted to the deprived eye, its vision improves only slowly; as a correlate of that improvement, synaptic terminals from the affected eye resume contact with the visual cortical cells. By analogy, the normally evolving dominance of the left hemisphere may be implemented by a progressive, genetically preprogrammed displacement of right-hemispheric connections from the speech output control neurons. Such connection would take time to re-establish when left-hemispheric influence is removed.

These considerations would lead us to predict that the left hemisphere is not fully dominant at the time of the origin of language, but that its dominance is established progressively. We shall suggest a possible mechanism for its establishment and consider the available evidence on the time course of this phenomenon.

A paradox in the adult aphasia literature will help us further develop our model of left-hemispheric ascendancy for language. The right hemisphere can decode speech, but left-hemisphere disease can cause severe receptive aphasia, in which the patient understands virtually nothing of what is said to him. Why does not the right hemisphere assume responsibility for language decoding in these patients as it does in split-brain patients? It must be because the left hemisphere continues to be involved in language processing and inhibits the decoding facility on the right. Even in split-brain subjects, if verbal messages are given simultaneously to both ears (Milner, Taylor, & Sperry, 1968; Sparks & Geschwind, 1968), the input to the left side is usually ignored or "neglected" (Kinsbourne, 1970b).

When there is verbal activity on the left, mental capacity seems to be pre-empted by that side, and the right hemisphere remains dormant. A similar phenomenon could account for receptive aphasia. The aphasic is still processing verbal input, or even trying to think in words, with his left hemisphere, and this either channels the available mental capacity to his imperfect left processor. Precisely because he is aphasic, it is harder for him to think in words than for a normal person. Therefore, any verbal processing he attempts will tend to create a great strain on the left hemisphere. We know that intentional verbal processes come from the left, and thus verbal processing in an aphasic's left hemisphere will use up even more of his mental capacity than it would in a normal person. Thus, an aphasic's left-hemispheric activity would exclude his right brain from language functioning even more than would a normal person's left-sided activity; in an aphasic this is especially troublesome because *his* left hemisphere is no longer verbally intact. *If* this effect is transcallosal, such a patient's ability to understand speech could be improved by callosal section. *If* the competition between the hemispheres takes place at the level of the brainstem, this maneuver would be ineffective.

We can now voice a further speculative expectation for language development: The competitive efficiency of the hemisphere dominant for control of language is self-aggrandizing, at a rate proportional to the degree of language use.

In young children, the developing functions of the cerebral hemispheres are embedded in complex, innate, lateral-orienting synergisms. The child turns his eyes and head, points his arm, swings one leg around, and, if standing, pivots on the other, opens his mouth, and vocalizes. The left hemisphere develops control over turning to the right, the right hemisphere over turning to the left. Left brain ascendancy is previewed in the strong tendency of newborns to make spontaneous head-turning movements to the right rather than to the left (Turkewitz, Gordon, & Birch, 1968). Reliable isolated right hand preference emerges later in that context, as the infant becomes able to differentiate out individual hand movement of the type customarily tested (Belmont & Birch, 1963). But it cannot be, as Gazzaniga (1971) has suggested, that dominance results from unilateral experience gained by the contralateral preferred hand, as according to this view, left-handers should have right hemisphere dominance for language, whereas in fact the majority are left dominant.

If one hemisphere is inactivated by early (prelanguage) disease, language development pursues a normal course, whether the lesioned hemisphere is the right or the left. Although one cannot be sure that language development in such individuals fully realizes its premorbid potential, it is clear that psychometrically, after either right or left hemispherectomy, language skills equally attain the normal range (Kohn & Dennis, 1974).

If the early damage is limited to only part of a hemisphere, the results are somewhat different. Annett, Lee, and Ounstead (1961) studied children with early hemispheric damage as judged by the location of isolated abnormal foci seen on the electroencephalogram. Both groups achieved substantial language development, but children with left-sided foci had significantly lower verbal aptitude than right-sided cases. Paradoxically, a partial lesion has here results in a measurable deficit, although total hemispheric removal does not. An explanation consistent with the type of mechanism we have been considering is that continuing control of language by the damaged left hemisphere results in imperfect language development, whereas complete left removal releases the full language potential of the still plastic hemisphere. As regards speech, the hemispheres differ not in their early potential but in their potency in competing for output control. Correspondingly, after left hemisphere damage in childhood, the language difficulty is relatively mild and evanescent as compared to the effects of comparably extensive lesions of the more mature brain. The literature on the effects of left-sided lesions suggests that the right hemisphere of children can compensate rather better than of adults for language disorder. The ultimate "adult" situation appears to be by puberty (Lenneberg, 1967). Up to then, the later the left-sided lesion occurs, the more severe and persistent is the language disorder. The right hemisphere, possibly through disuse, as well as diminishing plasticity, is progressively excluded from readiness to compensate should occasion arise.

The evolution of cerebral dominance can be tracked by studying normal children's ability to report different speech messages simultaneously presented to the two ears. Right-handers report messages to the right better than to the left ear under these dichotic conditions; this holds even for preschool children (Kimura,

1963) and is demonstrable as early as 3 years of age (Nagafuchi, 1970). Though according to one study, the effect becomes more salient with advancing years (Bryden, 1970), three others (Berlin, Lowe-Bell, Hughes, & Berlin, 1973; Geffner Hochberg, 1971; Kimura, 1963) find no developmental trend beyond age 5. It has two components: (1) an attentional bias to the right during verbal activity, which is due to general activation of the left hemisphere (Kinsbourne, 1970a, 1972), and (2) a processing advantage for right-ear presentation, which survives holding attention constant (insofar as this can be done by specific instruction as to where to attend: Bryden, 1971). In children, these components have not yet been disentangled, but for present purposes, the presence of cerebral dominance in children as young as 3 years of age is sufficiently demonstrated by the existing studies. Lefthanders, although as a group they also overall favor the right ear, do so less strikingly.

The dichotic listening technique yields further information when applied to children after early brain damage and hemispherectomy. Such subjects can report monaural messages presented through either ear (Kinsbourne 1975a), demonstrating that both contralateral and ipsilateral connections to the residual hemisphere are functional. With dichotic input, the response incorporates rather little of the ipsilateral message, particularly if the original lesion occurred in early childhood rather than perinatally (Netley, 1972). The remaining hemisphere is sufficiently plastic in its ability to program attention to either side for it to receive single messages from both locations. If the damage was very early, it can divide attention to some extent between both sides even when a contralateral message elicits its own natural contralateral attentional bias. So the earlier the lesion, not only the better is the compensation for speech production, but also the better is the right hemisphere's ability to distribute attention to verbal inputs over space or to attend selectively to one several of competing inputs (Kinsbourne 1975a).

Given that lateralization of language is so general and so characteristically human a development, what deleterious consequences might attend its failure to develop, as for instance in a minority of left-handers who appear to have bilateral language representation (Milner *et al.*, 1964)? Much has been predicted about the possible relationship of failure to lateralize language to developmental backwardness in learning to read (Orton, 1936), but it is not clear that most children with developmental reading backwardness in fact have bilateral language dominance. If some "dyslexic" children have bilateral language representation, it remains unclear which is cause and which is effect. No peripheral manipulations, such as changing children's hand preference, have been shown to influence a person's genetically preprogrammed pattern of cerebral dominance. Quite distinct from the question of how language processes are cerebrally distributed is the question of how mature they are at any one time. A case can be made for the view that a variety of patterns of reading unreadiness in grade-school children reflect immaturity in relevant processing by the left hemisphere (Kinsbourne, 1975b;

Kinsbourne & Warrington, 1963). But whether the extent to which there is language functioning on the right at all affects this is quite unknown.

Equally speculative is the possibility that some stutterers are experiencing a decision conflict at their speech output facility due to concurrent but imperfectly synchronized instruction from the language areas of both hemispheres. One study found four stutterers to have bilateral language representation. After excisions of part of one hemisphere on account of cerebral tumor or malformation, their language processes were found to be lateralized to the unoperated side only, and they no longer stuttered (Jones, 1966). Corroboration is needed for this intriguing claim.

In summary, whereas language representation in adults has been studied for over a century, almost all that is known about mechanisms of cerebral dominance in children is the product of work in about the last decade. We now know that language can originally be supported by either hemisphere but that the right hemisphere becomes less capable of compensatory language function as cerebral maturation proceeds. The right hemisphere, however, seems always to retain some such potential, particularly in the receptive sphere. Both hemispheres are equipped for language representation. Cerebral dominance involves active competition between hemispheres, which the left hemisphere is genetically destined to win. It may be not so much the cause as the result of the more advanced language specialization of one hemisphere than the other.

References

Annett, M., Lee, D., & Ounstead, C. Intellectual disabilities in relation to lateralized features in the EEG. In *Hemiplegic cerebral palsy in children and adults.* Little Club Clinics in Developmental Medicine. London: Heinemann, 1961.

Archibald, Y. M., & Wepman, J. M. Language disturbance and nonverbal cognitive performance in eight patients following injury to the right hemisphere. *Brain,* 1968, *91*, 117–130.

Belmont, L., & Birch, H. Lateral dominance and right-left awareness in normal children. *Child Development,* 1963, *34*, 257–270.

Berlin, C. I., Lowe-Bell, S. S., Hughes, L. F., & Berlin, H. L. Dichotic right ear advantage in males and females. *Proceedings, 84th Meeting of the Acoustical Society of America, Miami Beach,* 1973.

Bogen, J. E., & Vogel, P. J. Cerebral commissurotomy in man; preliminary case report. *Bulletin of the Los Angeles Neurological Society,* 1962, *27*, 169–172.

Broca, P. Sur la faculte du langage articule. *Bulletin de la Société de Anthropologie (Paris),* 1865, *6*, 493–494.

Bryden, M. P. Laterality effects in dichotic listening: relations with handedness and reading ability in children. *Neuropsychologia,* 1970, *8*, 443–450.

Bryden, M. P. Attentional strategies and short term memory in dichotic listening. *Cognitive Psychology,* 1971, *2*, 99–116.

Butler, S. R., & Norsell, U. Vocalization possibly indicated by the minor hemisphere. *Nature (London),* 1968, *220*, 793–794.

Czopf, J. Uber die Rolle der nicht dominanten Hemisphere in der Restitution der Sprache des Aphasischen. *Archives Psychiat. Nervenkr, 216,* 162–171, 1972.

Eisenson, J. Language and intellectual modifications associated with right cerebral damage. *Language and Speech*, 1962, 5, 49—53.

Gazzaniga, M. S. Changing hemispheric dominance by changing reward probability. *Experimental Neurology*, 1971, 33, 412—419.

Gazzaniga, M. S., & Sperry, R. W. Language after section of the cerebral commissures. *Brain*, 1967, 90, 131—148.

Geffner, D., & Hochberg, I. Ear laterality performance of children from low and middle socioeconomic levels on a verbal dichotic listening task. *Cortex*, 1971, 8, 401—409.

Gordon, H. W. Verbal and non-verbal cerebral processing in man for audition. Unpublished doctoral dissertation, California Institute of Technology, 1972.

Hillier, W. Total left hemispherectomy for malignant glioma. *Neurology*, 1954, 4, 718—721.

Hubel, D. H., & Wiesel, T. N. Binocular interaction in striate cortex of kittens reared with artificial squint. *Journal of Neurophysiology*, 1965, 28, 1041—1059.

Jackson, J. H. On the nature of the duality of the brain. *Brain*, 1874, 38, 80—103.

Jones, R. K. Observations on stammering after localized cerebral injury. *Journal of Neurology, Neurosurgery, and Psychiatry*, 1966, 29, 192—195.

Kimura, D. Speech lateralization in young children as determined by an auditory test. *Journal of Comparative and Physiological Psychology*, 1963, 56, 899—902.

Kimura, D. Functional asymmetry of the brain in dichotic listening. *Cortex*, 1967, 3, 163—178.

Kinsbourne, M. The cerebral basis of lateral asymmetries in attention. *Acta Psychologica*, 1970, 33, 193—201. (a)

Kinsbourne, M. A model for the mechanism of unilateral neglect of space. *Transactions of the American Neurological Association*, 1970, 95, 143—146. (b)

Kinsbourne, M. The minor cerebral hemisphere as a source of aphasic speech. *Archives of Neurology (Chicago)*, 1971, 25, 302—306.

Kinsbourne, M. Behavioral analysis of the repetition deficit in conduction aphasia. *Neurology*, 1972, 22, 1126—1132.

Kinsbourne, M. The control of attention by interaction between the cerebral hemispheres. In S. Kornblum (Ed.), *Attention and performance*. Vol. 4. New York: Academic Press, 1973.

Kinsbourne, M. The mechanism of hemispheric control of the lateral gradient of attention. In P. M. A. Rabbitt, & S. Dornic (Eds.), *Attention and Performance V*. London: Academic Press, 1975. (a)

Kinsbourne, M. Looking and listening strategies and beginning reading. In J. Gutherie (Ed.), *Aspects of reading acquisition*. Newark, Delaware: International Reading Association, 1975. (b)

Kinsbourne, M., & Peel-Floyd, C. Cue deprivation in relation to impaired language development. *Proceedings of the Congress Phoniat. Logoped., Vienna*, 1965.

Kinsbourne, M., & Warrington, E. K. Developmental factors in reading and writing backwardness. *British Journal of Psychology*, 1963, 54, 145—156.

Kohn, B., & Dennis, M. Patterns of hemispheric specialization after hemideconnection for infantile hemiplegia. In M. Kinsbourne & A. Smith (Eds.), *Hemispheric disconnection and cerebral function*. Springfield, Ill.: Thomas, 1974.

Lenneberg, E. *Biological foundations of language*. New York: Wiley, 1967.

Levy, J., Nebes, R. D., & Sperry, R. W. Expressive language in the surgically separated minor hemisphere. *Cortex*, 1970, 7, 49—58.

Milner, B., Branch, C., & Rasmussen, T. Observations on cerebral dominance. In Oldfield, R. C., & Marshall, J. M. (Eds.), *Language*. London: Penguin, 1964.

Milner, B., Taylor, L., & Sperry, R. W. Lateralized suppression of dichotically presented digits after commissural section in man. *Science*, 1968, 161, 184—186.

Nagafuchi, M. Development of dichotic and monaural hearing abilities in young children. *Acta Otolaryngolia*, 1970, 6, 409—414.

Netley, C. Dichotic listening performance of hemispherectomized patients. *Neuropsychologia*, 1972, 10, 233—240.

Nielsen, J. M. *Agnosia, apraxia, and aphasia*. New York: Harper (Hoeber), 1964.

Orton, S. T. *Reading, writing and speech problems in children.* New York: Norton, 1936.

Penfield, W., & Roberts, L. *Speech and brain mechanisms.* Princeton, N.J.: Princeton Univ. Press, 1959.

Perria, L., Rosadini, G., & Rossi, G. F. Determination of side of cerebral dominance with amobarbital. *Archives of Neurology (Chicago),* 1961, *4,* 173—181.

Pettit, J. M. Cerebral dominance and the process of language recovery in aphasia. Unpublished doctoral dissertation, Purdue University, 1969.

Russell, R., & Espir, M. *Traumatic aphasia.* London & New York: Oxford Univ. Press, 1961.

Smith, A. Speech and other functions after left (dominant) hemispherectomy. *Journal of Neurology, Neurosurgery, and Psychiatry,* 1966, *29,* 467—471.

Smith, A. Nondominant hemispherectomy. *Neurology,* 1969, *19,* 442—445.

Sparks, R., & Geschwind, N. Dichotic listening in man after section of neocortical commissures. *Cortex,* 1968, *4,* 3—16.

Swisher, L. P., & Sarno, M. T. Token Test scores of three matched patient groups: left brain-damaged with aphasia; right brain-damaged without aphasia; non brain-damaged. *Cortex,* 1969, *5,* 264—273.

Turkewitz, G., Gordon, B. W., & Birch, M. G. Head turning in the human neonate; effect of prandial condition and lateral preference. *Journal of Comparative and Physiological Psychology,* 1968, *59,* 189—192.

Wada, J., & Rasmussen, T. Intracarotid injection of sodium amytal for the lateralization of cerebral speech dominance: experimental and clinical observations. *Journal of Neurosurgery,* 1960, *17,* 266—282.

Wernicke, C. *Der aphasische Symptomenkomplex.* Breslau: Taschen, 1874.

8. The Relationship between Aphasia and Disturbances of Gesture and Perception[1]

Henry Hécaen

An attempt has been made to consider the relationship between disorders of language and disorders of gesture and perception, not generally, but according to the different aspects encountered clinically.

Among forms of apraxia deriving from left posterior cerebral lesions, which are, of course, the only lesions considered here, constructional apraxia and ideational apraxia are regarded as "programming" apraxias. Their frequent, but not invariable, association with language disturbances seems to point rather to a topographical proximity of the damaged areas than to a relationship of dependence. Ideomotor apraxia is regarded as the disturbance of a system of movements, relatively independent of the language system.

The notion of agnosia has been accepted, and the relationships between nonrecognition of objects, central color-blindness, and language disturbances are discussed. Without discounting the role of these relationships, a degree of independence is recognized between these two categories of disorder while not denying either the characteristics that aphasia can give to perceptual disorders or, conversely, the compensation that can be achieved through the mediation of language.

Apraxia

Following Dejerine, we shall define apraxia as a disturbance in the performance of gestural activity in a patient whose motor apparatus is intact (absence of para-

[1]This research was carried out with assistance of the GRANT Foundation.

117

lysis, ataxia, and choreoathetosis) and who fully grasps the act to be performed (no gnosic disturbances or global intellectual deficiencies). However, the deficits must not be thought of as absolutes.

To envisage the problem of impaired performance of certain acts and their association with language disturbances, we must first consider the clinical differentiations of apraxia. Evidence for this may be obtained by studying the laterality of lesions.

Ideomotor apraxia, described by Liepmann (1900) under the name of motor apraxia, affects only simple gestures, while the ideational level, necessary for complicated acts, remains untouched. The trouble rarely becomes apparent in spontaneous activities, and it is principally in the test situations that it comes to light, either in the execution of a movement in response to a verbal command, or in the imitation of gestures performed by the observer. There is often dissociation between the response to verbal commands and the imitative response, though the aphasia cannot be held responsible for this, since the observer's gesture is more frequently reproduced than the verbal command.

The simple gestures used to demonstrate this apraxia have been classified as follows: more or less symbolic expressive gestures, conventional symbolic gestures, gestures miming the use of an object without that object, and imitation of purposeless and meaningless gestures.

Ideational apraxia is characterized by impaired performance of a complex act, each element of which—in isolation—can be performed correctly. A disturbance in the performance of an action sequence, ideational apraxia cannot be due to the involvement of one specific segment of the body; it is a disturbance of the integration of activities of various different bodily segments.

The individual affected by ideational apraxia is incapable of working out the action required to achieve the goal in view, although the motoric capacities of all limbs are unimpaired. Patients with this disturbance cannot envision the required act as a whole; they have lost the ability to organize, temporally and spatially, the individual movements that constitute it.

The trouble is proportionately more evident as the action to be performed requires a more extensive succession of partial acts. In instances when, so to speak, no conscious plan need be conceived, the movement is performed perfectly— almost automatically, in fact. We must add that the extent of the disturbance varies with the patient's degree of concentration, as well as with the situational necessities that motivate the act.

The relationship between ideomotor and ideational apraxia is still ill defined. In fact, though it is evident that the former occurs most frequently in the absence of the latter, the inverse situation appears more questionable.

We should also emphasize the other clinical defects associated with these two disorders are similar, but that their frequency and intensity is greater in the case of ideational apraxia (aphasia, constructional apraxia, intellectual deterioration or confusion, sensory impairments, finger agnosia, optic agnosias).

For Liepmann (1900), in his initial study, there was only a simple difference of severity between these two disorders. Denny-Brown (1958) also tended to treat them as a common deficit due to a conceptual impairment: the loss of the propositional use of objects. However, in a later paper, Liepmann (1908) distinguished between ideomotor apraxia, as reflecting a dissociation between the sensorimotor constituents of the act and the control of their ideational concept, and ideational apraxia, reflecting a disorder of the ideatory concept. Since Liepmann the tendency has been to consider ideational apraxia as a special disorder of predominantly generalized psychological function, though Foix (1916) regarded it as independent from both ideomotor apraxia and global psychic impairment. Morlaas (1928) commented that the disorder did not have to do with execution but was a variety of agnosia (agnosia for the utilisation of objects). Though the subject could name the object and even give a verbal description of its use, he was unable to evoke the movements necessary to its utilisation. Zangwill (1960) agreed in part with this hypothesis but refused to completely exclude a deficit in execution. He argued that the constant association with ideomotor apraxia pointed to an impairment in dexterity.

Constructional apraxia, described by Poppelreuter and named by Kleist (1934) and Strauss (1924), represents the most frequent form of apraxia.

At the time of its recognition as a symptom by Kleist and by Strauss, constructional apraxia was associated with lesions of the left parietal zone. Since the research done by McFie, Piercy, and Zangwill (1950) and by Hécaen, de Ajuriaguerra, and Massonnet (1951), it has been established that these constructional disorders are also found when there are lesions of the right hemisphere, and that their frequency of occurrence and their severity are even greater in that case, whatever the ultimate reason may be.

Naturally the symptom complex within which constructional apraxia shows itself differs according to the hemispheric lesion that has produced it. With lesions of the left side, it is primarily language difficulties that are most frequently associated with constructional apraxia; with right cerebral lesions, it is sensory and spatial disorders. Although the issue is not yet settled, the indications are that there is a qualitative difference in the constructional performances of subjects according to the laterality of the lesion. Thus various authors concede some visuospatial disturbance as a basis for the apraxias due to right cerebral lesions, and some disturbance in execution of "programming" when the apraxias are due to left-side lesions.

Apraxia for dressing, the last of the main varieties of apraxia, occurs almost exclusively with right-side lesions.

Apart from these four main varieties of gestural impairment, there are a certain number of other varieties of apraxia, or disorders described as such, but we shall omit these because of their very close affinity to motor or psychomotor disorders.

Apraxia and Aphasia

The four main types of apraxia are associated with lesions located in the posterior hemispheric regions, and the hemispheric dominance factor is of very special

importance here. Lesions in the retro-Rolandic area of the left hemisphere determine bilateral ideomotor apraxia, ideational apraxia, and one aspect of constructional apraxia. These three clinical aspects have been regarded as conceptual
disorders, impairments of action, or impairments of action "programming."
Damage to the posterior function of this hemisphere (supramarginalis gyrus and
angular gyrus) seems to be a special factor in the mechanism of these disorders,
particularly in constructional apraxia. According to our anatomoclinical data,
frontal lesions can be discounted as causes of these three types of apraxia, whereas there is a statistically important link between the presence of constructional
apraxia and damage, isolated or not, to the parietal lobe. It seems, furthermore,
that for ideational apraxia more massive and more extensive lesions are required.

The problems of the connections between language disorders and disturbances of
gesture cannot, therefore, be presented in general terms, but only according to the
type of apraxia and, of course, only for the apraxias caused by left-side lesions.

As early as 1905, Liepmann was insistent on the connection between ideomotor
apraxia and aphasia, stressing the occurrence of language disturbances in 17 out of
24 cases of apraxia; be it noted, however, that most of these were cases of motor
aphasia. On the other hand, in 42 observations of left hemiplegia, there was no sign
of impaired gesture in the upper right limb.

Thus the role of left hemispheric lesions and the frequent association of impaired
performance of movement and language disorders was being asserted as far back as
that date. In this series, however, seven cases could already be noted in which
apraxia was not associated with aphasia.

Since then, the part played by left hemispheric lesions in producing ideomotor
apraxia has been confirmed by study of extensive series of cases (de Ajuriaguerra,
Hécaen, & Angelergues, 1960; de Renzi, Pieczulo, & Vignolo, 1968; Goodglass
& Kaplan, 1963). Controversy remains, however, and the discussion on the nature
of the relation between apraxia and aphasia depends on whether we believe that
this relationship is merely a matter of anatomic proximity of the underlying
structural correlates or whether we believe in a global disturbance of communication compromising both linguistic and paralinguistic behavior. This latter theory
has a remote origin in the conception of asymbolia upheld by Finkelnburg (1870),
who considered impaired performance of gesture to be only a part of the range of
disturbances in the ability to express or understand symbols. Finally, along with the
two preceding questions, that of the relationship between impaired performance
of gesture and general intellectual impairment had to be considered.

Goodglass and Kaplan (1963) attempted to find an answer to all three questions.
Twenty aphasic patients, and 19 subjects having suffered cerebral lesions but
showing no aphasia, were submitted to a battery of quantified gesture tests. The
two groups were paired as regards age and intellectual efficiency. The results of this
study allow the following conclusions. While gestural defect is more severe in the
aphasic group, there is no clear-cut relation between the intensity of the defect
and the gravity of the aphasia. The essential impairment in the aphasic patients,
in comparison with the control groups, is evidenced above all on the higher

standard of their imitative performances, which implies a formulation impairment, compared to their performances in response to verbal commands. Furthermore, if we consider only those subjects in the control group affected by right hemispheric lesions, we find an indisputable gestural superiority. It follows from all these results, according to Goodglass and Kaplan, that impaired gestural capacity can be considered as a praxic disorder arising from left hemispheric damage, and not as an aspect of a central communication impairment.

If we now consider ideational apraxia in its relationship with language and intellectual disorders, our analysis (de Ajuriaguerra *et al.*, 1960) shows a very high frequency of association of these disorders with impaired gestural performance, since out of 11 cases observed, 10 evinced aphasic disorders and 9 a state of confusion or intellectual deterioration.

De Renzi *et al.* (1968) studied the ability of patients to handle objects presented to them; one group of their subjects had unilateral lesions, the other group served as control. They noted that impairment in the utilization of objects occurred in 34% of the aphasic patients and in 6% of subjects affected by left hemispheric lesions without aphasia, but there was no impairment in any of the patients suffering from right hemispheric damage. Furthermore, the ideational apraxia scores showed a high level of correlation with the scores for a verbal comprehension test, whereas the degree of correlation with the scores for "intelligence" tests and ideomotor apraxia tests was relatively low. These results are interesting. First, the formal relationship between ideational apraxia and a left hemispheric lesion locus is confirmed. Second, a point to note is the frequency of these impairments in the utilization of objects upon more detailed testing. Last—and most important— the association between aphasia assessed in terms of verbal comprehension deficiency and deficiency in the handling of objects emerges clearly from these results. It was in the cases of global aphasia and severe Wernicke's aphasia that ideational apraxia was most often noted. This inability to associate the appropriate movement with the object presented, which de Renzi and his associates (1968) relate to the difficulty they had already noted among aphasic patients of associating drawings with corresponding colors or sounds, seems to them to denote a common underlying disorder. The basic disorder would seem to consist of an inability to associate the different aspects of the same concept.

De Renzi *et al.* (1968) consider that this deficiency, like that affecting abstract thinking or verbal memory, is probably inherent in aphasia. But they do not entirely reject the hypothesis that the link between these disorders and language impairment may depend on anatomical proximity of lesions. Their study also stresses the independence of ideational apraxia and ideomotor apraxia.

However, on examining the gestures required of patients by these Italian authors, it emerges that their test battery does not include descriptive actions simulating the handling of objects; they are either conventional symbolic or expressive gestures. One might therefore suspect that the pathological dissociations are between the disorders of expressive gesture and the disorders of descriptive gesture (showing the handling of an object, with or without the actual object). Indeed, that was the conclusion which I reached from systematic analysis of the performances of my own apraxic patients.

Turning now to constructive apraxia consequent to left hemispheric lesions, in the writer's series of patients it occurs with ideomotor apraxia in 72.34% of the cases only, whereas it is always found with ideational apraxia. This difference may prove important, since some authors (Hécaen & Assal, 1970; Warrington, James, & Kinsbourne, 1966) regard constructive apraxia following a left hemispheric lesion as a disturbance in the programming of acts, and this deficiency is evident in ideational apraxia. The ability to program sequences of acts would thus be more easily disturbed in a constructive activity than in the manipulation of concrete objects, the recourse to less abstract strategies can be envisaged by the patient if he does not suffer from more diffuse lesions. We must stress that we have observed that the impairment of constructive activity consequent on left hemispheric lesions can be overcome if the patient is provided with elements that eliminate the need for preliminary organization of the task. Further, the link between aphasia and constructive apraxia cannot be considered as absolute. In one of my series studied earlier, language troubles were present in only 71.95% of the cases of constructive apraxia following left hemispheric lesions. It is also easy to cite cases of severe sensory aphasia, either of the comprehension impairment or of the verbal deafness type, which are not accompanied by constructive apraxia. These observations are arguments for merely an indirect association between praxic disturbances and language disturbances. In apraxia, the basic disorder consists of a difficulty of programming; it is caused by damage to a specific area of the dominant hemisphere (supramarginalis gyrus and angular gyrus), with "a degree of fragility" intervening to account for the differences of frequency in the appearance of constructive apraxia and ideational apraxia. The extensive lesions needed to produce ideational apraxia would also explain the high frequency of its association with aphasia, an association which, in fact, would depend only on the proximity of the programming activity area to the areas controlling linguistic activity. This programming disorder may also be revealed in linguistic performances when both areas are damaged, but it is not clearly distinguishable in an aphasia in which the temporal damage is minimal.

As regards ideomotor apraxia, its locus is more difficult to specify. Its association with aphasia is certainly remarkable, but even Liepmann could envisage a link between the two only on anatomical grounds; the results of the study by Goodglass and Kaplan (1963) rule out the possibility of lumping together gestural disorders and language disorders as elements in a general disturbance of communication.

It is therefore necessary to define these gestural modalities and the nature of the disturbances affecting them before it is possible to understand the different types of relations they have with disorders of linguistic activities. A "naive" description of movements, allowing for the dissociations effected by pathology, permits of an initial classification into actions performed with or without objects, and of a third modality, the ability to make graphic and constructional actions. In the first category we shall put the highly codified gestures, replacing language, such as the gesture language of deaf-mutes, the artificial sign languages, the gestures accompanying the spoken language, conventional symbolic gestures (the sign of the cross, military salute, etc.), more or less conventionalized expressive gestures (threatening, pleading, etc.), and finally, descriptive movements relating to activity on the body or simulating the use of objects. The disturbances of these different groups of actions represent ideomotor apraxia in its classical definition. Among the actions for the manipulation of actual objects, a distinction will be made between those that have no direct connection with the body (ideational apraxia) and those performed essentially by reference to the body (apraxia for dressing).

If we seek to define the relationship between language and the various types of action, it becomes possible to exclude the actions operating on the body and a certain type of praxic activity (visuospatial), since pathology has taught us that disturbances of these activities appear only following lesions of the right cerebral hemisphere. To return to our inventory, we shall try to apply a classification based on a logical division of signs, such as that proposed by Peirce (1932, p. 129) and revived by Jakobson (1964), with the addition of the temporal dimension (successivity, simultaneity):

	Sign quality	*Temporal quality*
1. Symbolic gestures	Codified system, language substitute	Successivity
	Conventional symbols	Simultaneity— in most instances
2. Expressive iconic gestures		Simultaneity
3. Indexical gestures		
a. Actions representing the utilization of objects	i. Simple ii. In sequence	Simultaneity Successivity
b. Actual handling of objects	i. Simple ii. In sequence	Simultaneity Successivity

Lastly, another plane of dissociation also warrants acceptance, namely that of response according to the stimulus considered: action in response to a verbal command, action in imitation of the action of the observer (optical), reproduction of action in which the subject has first been physically guided (kinesthetic), descriptive actions in response to the visual or auditory presentation of the object.

It is therefore not surprising that pathology does not offer us rigorous distinctions between the different types of action. In addition to this, all too often our clinical data are not sufficiently precise; we have only the results of more or less rapid observation, and not of proper experimentation with systematic use of control groups.

Thus the kind of classification proposed (Hécaen, 1972) makes it possible to form a picture of the differing role of linguistic activity according to the type of action response. The connection would probably be nil with the sensory—motor apraxias, such as unilateral kinetic apraxia or melokinetic apraxia, which still are very close to the disorders of sensory—motor coordination, and nil also in the somatospatial apraxias (visuoconstructive disorders, apraxia for dressing), in which only the integration of the spatial qualities of the sense messages is impaired.

In the other varieties of gestural capacity, we cannot but expect a relative independence vis-à-vis linguistic activity; as much, however, for anatomical as for genetic reasons, the intervention of linguistic factors cannot be totally excluded.

The analysis by Piaget (1960) on the development of the systems of coordinated movements as functions of either some result (goal) or some intention leads to the recognition of the developmental stages (sensory—motor coordination stage, intermediary stage with the appearance of the symbolic function, stage of representations with a twofold aspect [symbolic and operative]) corresponding to the three main groups of gestural disorders, which I and my colleagues attempted to describe (de Ajuriaguerra *et al.*, 1960). In our last group, which we would now be more inclined to call programming apraxia, the disorders appear to indicate damage to at least two different gestural abilities. The first subgroup concerns disorders of "gesture language," in the sense of a system of coding characteristic of particular sociocultural levels, but not formally conventionalized; it could correspond to Piaget's figurative level and include the ideomotor apraxias with impairment of symbolic and expressive actions (symbolic icons). The second subgroup is represented by the disorder of the propositional use of objects (Denny-Brown, 1958) or of the programming of sequential actions, and corresponds finally to the operative level. Ideational apraxia (impairment of actual handling of objects) evidences disturbance at the level of concrete operations, whereas ideomotor apraxia, which affects actions descriptive of the use of objects, shows a disorder situated at an intermediary level between the foregoing and a level of more complex structuring and interiorization, where damage would result in constructive apraxia of the programming process.

It may thus be satisfactory to distinguish a gestural "language," depending essentially on the sociocultural standards of a given society, from a programming activity (and we have seen that pathology gives some support to this conception); and, at the same time, to consider that both involve only indirect relations with linguistic activity. However, such distinctions cannot be absolute; Zangwill's observations show that movements simulating the handling of objects may be preserved, whereas actual handling of objects may be impaired. Again, given the sequential nature of certain expressive or symbolic actions and the need for some kind of programming for the execution of these movements, it is possible that they may be disordered by a lesion affecting the area controlling programming, whereas other nonsequential actions remain unaffected.

Despite these reservations, it seems possible by methodical examination of the pathological actions to subject a hypothesis of this kind to verification and then to study more specifically the relationships between each type of gestural activity and the various aspects of verbal performance. But even if it were successfully shown that none of these gestural disorders has a direct and necessary connection with language, the question would still arise as to whether the systems of abstract rules and transformations postulated for the linguistic activity do not also apply to these codified systems whose original or derived character vis-à-vis the system of language cannot be assumed a priori.

It would also remain to be settled how far these different gestural codes are arbitrary in nature, and whether they can be considered as being made up of discrete elements. The attempts to establish a kinetics, by seeking analogies with the linguistic system, do not seem, at first glance, to be particularly satisfactory.

Agnosias

The relationships between perceptual and linguistic disorders present in many ways a similar appearance to the language-disorder—praxic-disorder relationships, in the sense that the existence of language disorder cannot be excluded in many instances of agnosia; but here, again, the association is not invariable. Further, a certain number of recognition disorders are determined by right hemispheric lesions and consequently have no relationship, at least directly, with language disorders.

Without going into detailed discussion of the nature of these perception disorders, a brief examination will be made of the links between language disorders and visual agnosias—the latter limited to agnosias of objects and colors, since spatial and physiognomic agnosias appear to derive from right hemispheric lesions.

Despite criticisms of the notion of agnosia, it seems possible to accept this term in order to define the disorders of the ability to "recognize" objects, persons, or spatial data, in patients in whom nothing appears to be wrong with elementary sensory capacities or intellectual functioning—or, at least, not enough to account for the nonrecognition.

Evidence for the existence of such disorders includes the selectivity of the impairments as regards external data, the diversity of the symptomatic associations presented by these different types of visual agnosia, and, finally, the difference of laterality, if not lesional localization, that they present.

The problem of the links between language and high-level perceptual disorders will therefore be centered essentially on object agnosia and color agnosia, whose derivation from left hemispheric lesions seems confirmed.

Agnosia of objects is an extremely rare pathological state. I have observed it only four times in a series of 415 hemispheric lesions (Hécaen & Angelergues, 1963), while de Renzi, Scotti, and Spinnler (1969) noted it in only one case among 124 patients affected by unilateral cerebral lesions.

In the majority of the observations reported, language disturbances and intellectual deficiency are manifest, and the lesions established are, in general, bilateral or even diffuse. As a consequence, in the majority of these cases no special selectivity is observable in the disturbance of visual recognition—objects, images (realistic or otherwise), faces, even spatial data, cease to be identified.

As long ago as 1914, von Stauffenberg, after reviewing the published clinico-pathological cases, was able to demonstrate the importance of left occipital lesions; here, the isolated forms of the disturbance were indeed observed (von Stauffenberg, 1914). This was true of the most conclusive case study within the writer's experience (Hécaen & deAjuriaguerra, 1956). The patient, after a left occipital lobectomy, was unable to identify visually the most familiar objects, but exhibited no disturbance in the handling of spatial data and could recognize persons known to him before or after his illness, perfectly well, both in face-to-face encounters and from small amateur snapshots. On the other hand, he could not distinguish any color, and he exhibited global alexia. Although language difficulties were, in the immediate postoperative stage, fairly marked (paraphasia, slight difficulty in comprehension), they disappeared almost completely with the exception of the alexia (which remained total) and of some slight graphic trouble. Aphasia could not account for the disturbance in recognition, since the patient was capable of naming the object if, instead of being presented visually, it was given to him to touch or if its characteristic sound was made. Occasionally the object could not be designated in terms of the nonvisual modalities, but paraphrased or schematized, the patient showed that he recognized it, which he was unable to do when the object was presented visually. At a second stage, when spontaneous speech was fluent and verbal comprehension excellent, visual identification often became possible, more often, in fact, for images than for objects (when the score was 2 recognized objects out of 10). But the increase in the time taken for recognition was very marked, since the process consisted of the successive identification of the parts of the object presented (which often resulted in wrong identifications).

With another of the writer's patients (a victim of carbon monoxide poisoning), there was also object-recognition disturbance, but to a much lesser degree. The characteristics of the disorders were, however, very similar to those observed in the first case. There was no disturbance in oral or written language, and no impairment of the visual field.

There is no question, but that, as Teuber emphasized in 1968, the majority of published reports of visual agnosia fail to satisfy the conditions necessary for us to know definitely whether there is an absence of a subtle change in the reception of sensory input or an absence of naming disorder such that we can distinguish an optic agnosia corresponding to a normal perception deprived of its signification.

In opposition to this scepticism, as expressed by Teuber, are more recent findings. De Renzi and coll. (1969) have demonstrated, in a large series of unilateral hemispheric lesions, the presence of mild association deficits with lesion of the left hemisphere and apperceptive deficits with right-sided lesions. Moreover, new and more completely studied observations of object agnosia have been reported, such as those of Taylor and Warrington (1971), and above all by Rubens and Benson (1971), Lhermitte, Chedru, and Chain (1973), and Albert *et al.* (1975).

In 1974, Hécaen *et al.* also reported a particularly pure case of this type. In effect, the patient presented a relatively mild defect of recognition limited to the visual sphere. The disorder was selective and concerned only objects, pictures of realistic figuration, colors, and graphic symbols, while forms, faces, and spatial material were well discriminated. There was no intellectual deterioration; visual acuity was normal and oral language was unimpaired. The difficulty in writing was minimal except for a complete inability to copy. Special testing confirmed that the disorder of naming or designation to verbal command was limited to visual stimuli, while the ability to match and discriminate forms was, in this patient, largely conserved. Last and most importantly, these investigations employing tasks as little verbal as possible, have enabled the demonstration that the perceptual deficit in this patient concerned the apprehension of the signification and/or the category to which the object belonged. Isolated elements, forms, colors, and even letters were handled relatively well, but they could no longer be brought together in a meaningful whole.

Thus, the most recent findings indicate that it is only in the most exceptional case that a perception is deprived of its meaning: The patient is no longer able to determine the inadequacy of an object to a context, to apprehend its unity under diverse appearances, and perhaps above all, to realize that two objects of different form belong to the same category.

Impairment of the visual recognition of objects can, thus, occur without any direct relationship to language disturbance. Furthermore, it cannot be maintained that it always depends on the inability of visual information to reach the language centers since, on one hand, in one of our patients, there was no hemianopsia and no problem of color recognition or alexia, and on the other, it has been recently demonstrated that patients are able to name geometric forms but fail on tests where they are required only to match two objects or two object pictures of the same category but of different form.

It does not seem likely that this implies the exclusion of language in all sensory identification, but only that the disturbance, at a certain level, is governed by other factors and represents an impairment independent of language disorders.

Naturally, it is difficult to exclude the role of a disorder of verbal mediation in the deficit of association or categorization. However, apart from the total absence of aphasia in our last patient (Hécaen *et al.*, 1974), the results of certain tests tend to indicate a compensatory role of language. Thus, on the test of association of pictures of homonymous objects, our patient made fewer errors than on other association tests. The patients of Rubens and Benson (1971), and of Taylor and Warrington

(1971), seem to have been equally aided by recourse to verbal mediation. We should also note that De Renzi *et al.* (1969) have not observed a correlation between the results on tests of naming and association: Patients with severe naming-deficits achieve high scores on the association test.

Color agnosia is a term used to cover several different aspects of color-identification disturbance. Besides deficiency in color perception as a sequel to cortical blindness, which may even be limited to one-half of the visual field and aphasia for color names, there seems to be a true color agnosia. It seems to be characterized by retention of color perception, on the one hand—assessed by tests such as those of Ishihara, Pollack, or Rayleygt—and, on the other, by an inability to pick out the other shades of a particular color, to designate and to name the colors (even though there is no aphasia), and to evoke the specific colors of particular things (cherries, the sky, lemons, etc.).

Any breakdown of color-identification disturbances on the basis of these characteristics proves difficult in the clinic, where one finds that the kinds of disturbances can occur in association. In the event of dissociation, the different aspects of the syndrome do not fit the classical descriptions.

It was long ago suggested (Wilbrand, 1887) that color-identification disturbance might, in fact, come from a language disturbance limited to the domain of colors (amnesic color-blindness). Lewandowski (1908) records a very different case from Wilbrand's: the disturbance consisted of "a separation between the idea of the color and the idea of the object," and it could not be explained by a language disturbance. This patient had suddenly exhibited an aphasia with alexia, acalculia, and right hemianopsia. He was unable to name the colors but could differentiate between them, appreciating that the colors shown to him were different, and consistently matching the two identical samples in a very large number of colored strands of wool. He was also unable to indicate verbally or to designate among color samples the color of an object named verbally. He was, however, able to recognize, in a range of colored images, the one which was colored inadequately.

According to Sittig (1921), a distinction must be made between patients whose color sense is impaired (color blindness) and those in whom it is spared. When the patient can no longer name or understand the names of colors, the correct term is color amnesia, but if the patient is also incapable of classifying color samples correctly, that is, grouping the different shades of the same basic color, then the term is color agnosia, combined to a varying extent with a disorder of an aphasic type.

True color aphasia occurs in those cases in which the patient—who is not otherwise aphasic and who does not show any perceptual deficiency—cannot name or designate colors in response to a verbal command. Gelb and Goldstein (1924) take the view that this aphasia of names of colors means only impairment of the categorical attitude in regard to colors; for these patients, colors cease to be conceived independently of the objects with which they are concretely connected.

Geschwind and Fusillo (1966) have described an alexic patient who was perfectly capable of naming objects, photographs, and drawings, but whose naming of colors was regularly incorrect. He could, however, match colors and group shades correctly according to basic color independently of their brightness or saturation, and his colorimetric tests were normal. The lesion of the corpus callosum present in this subject, according to Geschwind and Fusillo, by disconnecting the right visual area—the only receiver of visual information because of right hemianopsia caused by left occipital damage—precluded the association between verbalization and color, while, on the other hand, the associations restricted to one sensory modality were still possible. Thus the tasks consisting of naming the color of an object named verbally (auditory association) or associating a color with a drawing of an object of that color (visual association) were performed quite correctly by the patient.

As regards retention of the ability to name objects, this would seem to be explained by the fact that objects, unlike words and colors, arouse somaesthetic associations at the level of the parietal lobe. According to Geschwind, the misnamings of colors by these patients are in fact genuine confabulations due to the absence of control by the language area over the visual activities, now confined, through the lesion, to the right occipital lobe. (Certain patterns of verbal behavior on the part of the patients dealt with by Gazzaniga and Sperry [1967] who had undergone a surgical section of the corpus callosum provide arguments in favor of such an interpretation.)

This explanation cannot, however, be extended to all the cases encountered, even when the verbal aspect of the disorder is predominant. The patient reported on by Kinsbourne and Warrington (1964), for instance (with normal scores for color perception tests at the visuosensory level and a normal field of vision), had a severe disturbance both in naming colors and in pointing them out on command. He was also incapable, in nearly every case, of giving the correct name of the color corresponding to an object when the name of the object was given to him verbally, and he was unable to fill in drawings with the right colors. He was able to recognize his mistakes, however. Likewise, in tests of ability to learn names of colors and objects or figures, there was potent failure, as was also true of a test of association of colored blocks with nonverbal material. On the other hand, this patient could grasp verbal associations that did not include the names of colors. In the view of these authors, the presence in this case of color-recognition disturbances may be secondary to disturbances of verbal color evocation. The deficiency would appear to consist essentially of an inability to match up color names with the rest of the information.

In a case fairly similar to that cited by Kinsbourne and Warrington, Stengel (1948), despite the predominance of color-naming disturbance, diagnosed a disturbance in color recognition on the grounds that there was no language disorder and that the patient had difficulty in classifying colored samples.

This discussion of a few isolated observations clearly shows that several factors play a part in these disturbances of color identification. Apart from the elementary sensory factor—which may occur independently in the sequelae of cortical blindness but which is perhaps not always absent in the other color-recognition disturbances—the part played by linguistic and amnestic factors must be defined before a truly cognitive disorder is admitted.

De Renzi and Spinnler (1967) tackled these problems by submitting a control group and a group of subjects suffering from lesions in one cerebral hemisphere to a test battery designed to measure both color perception and color naming, along with the ability to fill in drawings with colors; this last task calls for both color discrimination and the ability to recall the color of the object.

Failure at the perceptive level was principally a characteristic of the subjects with lesions in the right cerebral hemisphere, whereas failure in the verbal tests went with lesions in the left hemisphere. In the coloring test, the aphasic group showed the most severe impairment.

De Renzi and Spinnler conclude that deficient nonverbal association between objects and colors, although concomitant with aphasia, comes from a general associative disturbance that is specific to lesions in the left hemisphere.

The presence in their series of four cases showing very low scores in color naming, without there being any particular drop in the scores for image naming, suggests to them the real existence of a color-naming aphasia. As they did not conversely discover any disturbance in color recognition where there was no perceptive or verbal disturbance, de Renzi and Spinnler consider the existence of color agnosia highly unlikely.

Following an investigation of the color-vision disturbances in 42 patients with posterior cortical lesions, Lhermitte, Chain, Aron, Leblanc, and Souty (1969) reach completely contrary conclusions. The examination of their patients comprised a chromatic discrimination test of the Ishihara type, a color sorting test, the Farnsworth-100-Hue test, verbal identification tests, and nonverbal tests of recognition and evocation of object colors. Only patients with probable bilateral posterior lesions showed disturbances in chromatic vision as explored by the discrimination and sorting tests, whereas in two other groups, the failures in the Farnsworth test were only of the tritanopic or dyschromatoptic type. In one of these two groups, failure in the Farnsworth test was unaccompanied by other failures; in the other, both the verbal identification test and the nonverbal color recognition and evocation tests revealed a considerable degree of error.

Impairment of chromatic vision is therefore present in all three groups: in the group with lesions in both hemispheres, it reflects a global elementary sensory disturbance; in the other two groups it is specifically blue—yellow color-blindness, or else it reflects a loss in chromatic discrimination evidenced only in an organizing activity.

As regards the disturbances in the designation, naming, recognition, and evocation of colors, these cannot be directly attributed to a language disturbance, since the failures occur whether the task is verbal or not and since the patients' verbal errors are preponderantly in terms of two parameters linked to the quality of chroma, namely the blue—yellow axis and the degree of saturation.

In the view of Lhermitte and his associates, what these subjects have lost is the knowledge of color as a specific attribute of the object. The subject is color agnostic in the sense that he sees colors but does not recognize them, the agnosia being then considered as a regression of the acquisition of relationships between colors and objects.

There seems to be general agreement to attribute impairments of color recognition, whatever their supposed character, to lesions of the left hemisphere. Only de Renzi and his associates have observed a greater frequency of disturbances in color perception where the lesions are in the right hemisphere, especially if the field of vision is affected.

There are, then, definite divergences of opinion as to whether color agnosia really exists; accepted by Lhermitte and his associates, it is denied by De Renzi and his associates. Thus, the writer feels that the conclusions of the latter authorities should not be accepted without reservation. The fact is that, although the study of extensive series of observed cases chosen with reference solely to lesional lateralization is of certain interest, it also presents limitations, particularly because of our imprecise knowledge of the sites of the lesions; nor can we rule out the possibility of associations of impairments due to simple anatomical proximity. Moreover, if we examine the cases of so-called color agnosia one by one, we cannot help being struck at once—despite a certain similarity that exists between them—by the particularities of the impairment in each case. Not one case seems to correspond to the classical types defined as central color blindness, color aphasia, color agnosia, or amnesia regarding the specific attributes of colors.

May we not then suspect disturbances of different basic functions affecting a specific function, and accordingly giving the deficiency a special character in each instance? The sole possibility of verifying the hypothesis then consists of clinico-pathological observation, comprising at once the examination of the diverse performances and a precise anatomical study of the lesions. If we take the example of an amnesic aphasia limited to the names of colors and without other language disturbance, we must follow Gelb and Goldstein (1920) in looking for a disturbance of a fundamental function operating, for anatomical or other reasons, only in the domain of color, while presenting certain characteristics that approximate it in its mechanisms to verbal evocation disturbance in general.

Similarly, the disturbance of color–object association (which has its parallel in the domain of disturbance of the association of sounds with corresponding objects), instead of being conceived as inherent in the presence of aphasia, might also be envisaged as signifying the impairment of a precise area involving a fundamental function but finding expression in this or that domain according to the extent of the lesion. To call this disorder amnesic may therefore appear rather arbitrary, and it seems to the writer to be just as valid to call it agnostic, since it is the significance of the color that is lost.

We are thus brought back to the question of the connections between language and color recognition. By way of conclusion, let us take a look at the studies made on normal subjects on the relation between color naming, color recognition, and color discrimination.

Lenneberg (1961) reviews the prior experiments and, on the basis of new data, shows that shade discrimination is not linked to naming habits when the task is simple and does not call for much effort of memory. Conversely, lexical habits come into play when the mnestic task is greater. Thus, it is conceivable that in a color recognition task, our habit of structuring colored material semantically can supply anchor points on a continuum; but "codability" (Brown & Lenneberg, 1954) is probably only one of the ways in which linguistic categorization enters into color recognition since, conversely, codability as a nuisance factor in color discrimination tests may be kept at a minimum or can be controlled experimentally (Burnham & Clark, 1955).

It is also noted that color naming remains very stable, in spite of great variations in the conditions of intensity and the lengths of exposure; certain modifications of color naming can, however, be obtained, more particularly by changes in luminosity (Luria, 1967).

These results reveal both the role of language and its limitations in the question of color recognition. It is at least logical to think that linguistic disturbance has a different incidence, depending on the type and relative difficulty of the discrimination task. We can thus envisage a series of disturbances in color recognition ranging from those impairments in which linguistic disturbances are the essential factor to those in which their role is reduced to a minimum; in the latter case, it is even possible that the pathological language impairment actually facilitates nonverbal color recognition by blocking the normally occurring language interference.

References

Albert, M. L., Reches A. & Silverberg, R.: Associative visual agnosia without alexia. *Neurology*, in press.

Brown, R. W., & Lenneberg, E. H. A study in language and cognition. *Journal of Abnormal and Social Psychology*, 1954, *49*, 454—462.

Burnham, R. W., & Clark, J. R. A test of hue memory. *Journal of Applied Psychology*, 1955, *15*, 73—86.

de Ajuriaguerra, J., Hécaen, H., & Angelergues, R. Les apraxies: Variétés cliniques et latéralisation lésionnelle. *Revue Neurologique*, 1960, *102*, 566—594.

Denny-Brown, D. The nature of apraxia. *Journal of Nervous and Mental Disease*, 1958, *126*, 9—33.

De Renzi, E., Pieczulo A., & Vignolo, L. A. Ideational apraxia: a quantitative study. *Neuropsychologia*, 1968, *6*, 41—52.

de Renzi, E., Scotti, G., & Spinnler, H. Perceptual and associative disorders of visual recognition: relationship to the side of the cerebral lesion. *Neurology*, 1967, *19*, 634—642.

de Renzi, E., & Spinnler, H. Impaired performance on color tasks in patients with hemispheric damage. *Cortex*, 1967, *3*, 194—216.

Finkelnburg, F. C. Niederrheinische Gesellschaft Sitzung vom 21 Marz 1870, Bonn-Berlin. *Berliner Klinische Wochenschrift*, 1870, *7*, 449—450, 460—462.

Foix, C. Contribution à l'étude de l'apraxie idéomotrice. *Revie Neurologique*, 1916, *1*, 285—298.

Gazzaniga, M. S., & Sperry, R. W. Language after section of the cerebral commissures. *Brain*, 1967, *90*, 131—148.

Gelb, A., & Goldstein, K. *Psychologische Analysen hirnpathologischer Fälle.* Leipzig: Barth, 1920.

Gelb, A., & Goldstein, K. Über Farbenamnesie. *Psychologische Forschung*, 1924, *6*, 127—186.

Geschwind, N., & Fusillo, M. Color naming defects in association with alexia. *Archives of Neurology (Chicago)*, 1966, *15*, 137—146.

Goodglass, H., & Kaplan, E. Disturbance of gesture and pantomime in aphasia. *Brain*, 1963, *86*, 703—720.

Hécaen, H. *Introduction à la neuropsychologie (Langage, geste et perception)*. Paris: Larousse, 1972.

Hécaen, H., & Angelergues, R. *La cécité psychique*. Paris: Masson, 1963.

Hécaen, H., & Assal, G. A comparison of constructive deficits following right and left hemispheric lesions. *Neuropsychologia*, 1970, *8*, 289—304.

Hécaen, H., & de Ajuriaguerra, J. Agnosie visuelle pour les objets inanimés par lésion unilatérale gauche. *Revue Neurologique*, 1956, *94*, 222—233.

Hécaen, H., de Ajuriaguerra, J., & Massonnet, J. Les troubles visuoconstructifs par lésions pariéto-occipitales droites. Rôle des perturbations vestibulaires. *L'Encéphale*, 1951, *1*, 122—179.

Hécaen H., Goldblum M. C., Masure M. C., & Ramier A. M. Une nouvelle observation d'agnosie d'objet. Déficit de l'association ou de la catégorisation, spécifique de la modalité visuelle? *Neuropsychologia*, 1974, *12*, 447—464.

Jakobson, R. On visual and auditory signs. *Phonetica*, 1964, *11*, 216—220.

Kinsbourne, M., & Warrington, E. K. Observations on colour agnosia. *Journal of Neurology, Neurosurgery, and Psychiatry*, 1964, *27*, 296—299.

Kleist, K. *Gehirnpathologie*. Leipzig: Barth, 1934.

Lenneberg, E. H. Color naming, color recognition, color discrimination: a reappraisal. *Perceptual and Motor Skills*, 1961, *12*, 275—382.

Lewandowski, M. Über Abspaltung des Farbensinnes. *Monatschrift für Psychiatrie und Neurologie*, 1908, *23*, 488.

Lhermitte, F., Chain, F., Aron, D., Leblanc, M., & Souty, O. Les troubles de la vision des couleurs dans les lésions postérieures du cerveau. *Revue Neurologique*, 1969, *121*, 5—29.

Lhermitte F., Chedru, F., & Chain F. A propos d'un cas d'agnosie visuelle. Revue Neurologique 1973, *128*, 301—322.

Liepmann, H. Das Krankheitsbild der Apraxie (motorischen Asymbolie). *Monatsschrift für Psychiatrie und Neurologie*, 1900, *8*, 15—44, 102, 182—197.

Liepmann, H. *Drei Aufsätze aus dem Apraxiegebiet*. Vol. 1. Berlin: Karger, 1908.

Luria, S. L. Color-name as a function of stimulus-intensity and duration. *American Journal of Psychology*, 1967, *80*, 14—27.

McFie, J., Piercy, M. F., & Zangwill, O. L. Visual spatial agnosia associated with lesions of the right cerebral hemisphere. *Brain*, 1950, *73*, 167—190.

Morlaas, J. *Contribution à l'étude de l'apraxie*. (Thèse.) Paris: Legrand, 1928.

Peirce, C. S. Speculative grammar. In *Collected papers*. Vol. 2. Cambridge, Mass.: Harvard Univ. Press, 1932. Cited by Jakobson (1964).

Piaget, J. Les praxies chez l'enfant. *Revue Neurologique*, 1960, *102*, 551—565.

Rubens, A. B. & Benson D. F. Associative visual agnosia. *Archives of Neurology*, 1971, *24*, 305—316.

Sittig, O. Störungen im Verhalten gegenüber Farben bei Aphasischen. *Monatsschrift für Psychiatrie und Neurologie*, 1921, *49*, 49—63.

Stengel, L. The syndrome of visual alexia with color agnosia. *Journal of Mental Science*, 1948, *94*, 46—58.

Strauss, H. Über konstruktive Apraxie. *Monatsschrift für Psychiatrie und Neurologie*, 1924, *56*, 65—124.

Stauffenberg, W. von. Über Seelenblindheit. *Arbeiten Hirnanatom.*, 1914, *8*, 1—212.

Taylor A. & Warrington E. K. Visual agnosia: A single case report. *Cortex*, 1971, 7, 152—161.

Teuber H. L. Alteration of perception and memory in man. In L. Weiskrantz (Ed.), *Analysis of behavior change*. New York: Harper & Row, 1968. pp. 268—375.

Warrington, E. K. James, M., & Kinsbourne, M. Drawing disability in relation to laterality of cerebral lesion. *Brain*, 1966, *89*, 53—82.

Wilbrand, H. *Die Seelenblindheit als Herderscheinungen und ihre Beziehungen zur homonymen Hemianopsie, zur Alexie, und Agraphie*. Wiesbaden: Bergmann, 1887.

Zangwill, O. L. Le problème de l'apraxie idéatoire. *Revue Neurologique*, 1960, *102*, 595—603.

II. Deafness and Blindness

A careful study of language development in the deaf and in the blind is indispensable for a proper understanding of the nature of language and of the true prerequisites for a knowledge of language. Most important of all is the realization that man can acquire a knowledge of language in the absence of either hearing or sight; this clearly demonstrates that the essential nature of language is quite dissociable from specific sense modalities (and, as will be shown in the next section, from articulatory skills as well). Thus it has little to do with sensory association mechanisms. These observations are merely preliminaries to the present section. The chapters included here deal with more specific points, most of them of a fairly practical nature. Thus Fry makes the important point that the handicap of a hearing deficit may be overcome by proper management of the small child. Of special interest here is the empirical fact that optimal results of auditory education of the deaf can be obtained only if the child's exposure to sounds occurs within a fairly limited age range. Abberton and Fourcin present an important new prosthetic instrument that materially aids in articulation training of the congenitally deaf. The chapter by Furth and Youniss emphasizes once more that the language lag of the congenitally deaf does not cause a lag in cognitive development, thus showing that language is not a prerequisite for cognition (as is so commonly assumed), although cognition does seem to be a prerequisite for language acquisition. The last chapter in this section, by Fraiberg and Adelson, is of special interest in that it presents some entirely new discoveries that are of considerable psychological interest: although congenitally blind children appear to learn all the essentials of language without undue difficulty, they seem to suffer a particular cognitive cut-back in their ego development, that is, their appreciation of the relation between self and not-self; this, in turn, is reflected in certain semantic difficulties, particularly the semantics of the pronoun system.

9. Phonological Aspects of Language Acquisition in the Hearing and the Deaf

D. B. Fry

The phonological system is basic to any language in the sense that it is composed of the smallest functional units and that these form a closed set. The normal child has acquired the complete system by the age of 4−5. In the process of acquisition, reception precedes production; the child learns to distinguish between sounds and to recognize them before he learns to make them. The system is built up and expanded step by step, but always works as a whole. The brain organizes incoming acoustic information and evolves effective cues for making differentiations demanded by the system.

Children with impaired hearing can learn to operate successfully with speech; their success is a function of amount of exposure to audible speech much more than of their degree of hearing loss. Three important requirements are early diagnosis of hearing loss, the provision of suitable hearing aids, and the maximum help to the child's parents. Given these conditions, the deaf child will acquire the phonological system and will also learn to produce speech that is readily intelligible to ordinary people.

Introduction

Acquiring one's mother tongue is basically a process of accumulating in the brain a very large store of information about a particular language system. A good deal is known about many of the natural languages of the world, enough certainly to indicate that language systems have common features. Two in particular occur and recur; the first is that the systems comprise several levels, forming a hierarchical structure in which each level operates with its own linguistic units. Thus the English system embodies four operational levels, those of the phoneme, the morpheme, the word, and the sentence. The second feature is that a language is a self-consistent and interlocking system such that the function of each of the units that make up the system is specified by its relation to all the other units. To say that an individual has acquired the English language implies that he has stored in his brain the complete inventory of phonemic units operating in English, the knowledge of the rules that govern the combining of phonemes into morphemes (the grammatical units of the language), an extensive dictionary of words, together with a knowledge of the rules governing the combining of morphemes into words and of the rules governing sentence structure, that is, of the ways in which words may be combined to form sentences.

Whenever we take in or send out a spoken message, the brain circuits that act as the stores of all this information and those that give access to it come into play. In the reception of speech, decoding proceeds from the level of the phonemic units, the phonological level, upward through the morpheme and word levels until the complete sentence is reconstituted and the listener takes in what it means. The decoding process is possible only because the sequence of units on all four levels is very much constrained by the language system and by the situation in which the message is sent. At any point in a spoken message there are severe restrictions on what may come next; not every phoneme in the inventory is equally probable in the next position in the phoneme string, and some, indeed, are quite impossible from the point of view of the language system; similarly the succeeding morpheme or word at any point is very largely determined by what has preceded it, and as the message continues the constraints at each level become stronger and stronger. Although as ordinary language users we are generally unaware of the effects of these constraints, we carry the requisite information in our brains and compute their strength at the various levels all the time we are processing speech. Because of the hierarchical nature of the language system, there is continuous interaction between the linguistic levels of operation, from the point of view of constraints as from all other points of view. Knowledge of the form of these interactions and of their effects in a given situation is again an important part of the information held in the brain of the language user.

The encoding of speech, the generating of a message, involves sequences of operations broadly in the reverse order. When sending out speech we do not often plan a whole sentence before embarking on an utterance, but we do begin with some key ideas and a provisional plan for the structure of the sentence. On this basis the brain writes the program necessary at each level, for the syntactic structure of the sentence, for the selection of the consequent function and content words, for the morpheme sequence, and for the phoneme string. These programs are subject to the constraints of the language and the situation in the same way as is the decoding process; indeed the latter to a great extent reflects the constraints that shaped the encoding.

It has been stressed that a language is a system which works as a whole, "un système où tout se tient," as de Saussure expressed it. This chapter will concentrate upon the phonemic or phonological level of language operation, but it is important to bear in mind that the phonological level implies the existence of the higher levels and works in conjunction with them. There are some senses, however, in which the phonemic level may justifiably be looked upon as basic, as a level that can be considered somewhat apart from the others. The phonemes are the smallest functional units in the system, and they are the units that are directly correlated with the sensory and motor events of speech. On the transmission side, the nerve and muscle actions and the consequent sound waves of speech are the direct result of the phoneme program; on the reception side, the phoneme string is the first formulation of the information borne by the sound waves, middle-ear movements, and nerve impulses upon which the brain can perform the essentially linguistic processes of decoding.

A further important characteristic of the phonological level lies in the fact that the phoneme inventory for a given language is a closed set. The English phonological system comprises (in round numbers) 40 phonemic units. By the time the English-speaking child is about $4\frac{1}{2}$- to 5-years old, he is operating with the whole phonemic system, and he will make no additions to it for the rest of his life. He will always be adding to his stock of morphemes and words, but each fresh word will be a new arrangement of items from the phoneme inventory, just as each new word he learns to read will be a rearrangement of letters of the alphabet. In a rather specific sense, therefore, the phonological system is the basis of the language, since it consists of a closed set of small units that combine together to form the higher order units of the language. Moreover we may reasonably speak of the acquisition of the phonological system and discuss the ways in which it comes about, since there is a point in the child's development at which one can say that he has acquired the complete system.

So far we have been concerned only with those parts of the speech communication process that are carried on by the brain. This emphasis is very necessary because the fact is all too often overlooked that functioning with speech is much more brain work than anything else, a fact that will be doubly important when we come to consider the situation of the child who is deaf. However, the message that is generated in the speaker's brain and later decoded in the listener's brain goes through a number of transformations in the course of its transmission. On the speaker's side, the phoneme program is implemented through a continuous flow of operating instructions in the shape of nerve impulses transmitted to the very complex muscle systems used in speaking—the breathing muscles, the laryngeal muscles, and those of the head and neck required for articulation. The highly complicated speech movements generate sound waves, which are radiated around the speaker, and some of this acoustic energy serves to set up movements in the peripheral mechanisms of the listener's ear. The effect of these movements is transmitted in the form of nerve impulses to the listener's brain, where the information forms the input to the phonemic level of the decoding process. Hence the form in which speech information is publicly available, as it were, is that of sound waves.

Two important facts about these sound waves, from the point of view of language acquisition, are that they occur in certain sequences and in certain situations. It is this patterning in both the sounds and the situations in which they recur that makes it possible for the human being to acquire a whole language system. The brain is *par excellence* a device for detecting and remembering patterns, particularly through the auditory and visual modes. When a child learns his mother tongue, his brain is exploiting this capacity to the full—and perhaps more successfully and completely than it will do in any other context for the rest of its life. It is through continual exposure to speech stimuli in situations to which the speech is highly relevant that the child acquires the elements of the language system. Provided he is so exposed, his brain will abstract from the sensory events the features on which it builds, first of all, the phonological system. If the child is deprived of the stimuli, for whatever reason, his brain will fail to evolve a workable system.

The Priority of Speech Reception

This brings us to one of the cardinal facts about language acquisition, one that is particularly important with reference to the acquisition of the phonemic system; that is that in speech and language learning, reception always precedes production. Any new element in the language system is first of all detected and recognized on repetition before it plays any part in the speech produced by the person concerned. We can all confirm this from ordinary adult experience as language users. Each of us has stored in his brain a comparatively large dictionary of words, perhaps some tens of thousands, any one of which we should recognize if we heard it. Among these is a very much smaller number, only about 4000–5000 or less, which we would ever utter ourselves in speech; in every case these are words that we first learned to recognize. In the last 10 or 15 years, for example, many English-speaking adults have learned to recognize, through hearing them on the radio or television, words such as "astronaut," "module," and so forth; only when the word had become thoroughly familiar in reception did they venture to add it to the stock of words they themselves would use in conversation. Similarly in the early stages of language acquisition, the child learns to detect and recognize an element, whether it be a sound, a grammatical form, or a word, before he introduces the element into his own speech productions.

This principle plays a major role in the acquisition of the phonemic system of a language, as it does at other levels of language. Many cases are known, and a particularly striking one is described in Chapter 13 (Lenneberg & Lenneberg, Vol. 2, 1975), in which a person can function with a language system, can take in and understand spoken messages perfectly normally, even though he is incapable of producing speech himself. In such a case the person has acquired the phonemic system and is operating with it purely on the basis of reception and recognition. We must say, therefore, that the phonological system has been acquired as soon as it is fully operative in speech reception—in the case of the young child who is acquiring his native language, this will mean when he can make all the discriminations called for in the complete phonemic system and does not make errors at the phonemic level in reception. This stage is reached some considerable time before the child is capable of making all the necessary distinctions in his own speech productions, and this fact has led to a good deal of confusion in discussions of the child's acquisition of the phonological system. This is not to say that there is not considerable interaction between speech reception and speech production, especially in the learning stages; in the normal child the producing of speech sounds contributes materially to the stabilizing of phonemic distinctions. However, this does not alter the fact that phonemic differences have to be noticed and recognized before they can be effective in speech production and that the primary function of the phonological system is to make possible the decoding of speech signals.

A related fact is that, although there are undoubtedly brain circuits that are specific to speech reception or to speech production, the great store of linguistic information in the brain is required for both purposes and in the normal case is applied in the two processes.

The Phonological System

We must now look more closely at the nature of the phonological system before considering the way in which it may be acquired. The function of phonemes within a language system is to signal differences between one word and another (or one morpheme and another). In a list of English words like *heed, hid, head, had,* each one a three-phoneme sequence, it is a change in the middle phoneme that signals that we are dealing with four different items in the language; similarly in *tin, sin, win,* a change in the first phoneme, and in *wig, with, wing,* a change in the third signals a change of word. All the 40-odd phonemes that make up the English phonological system have this differentiating function; each one exists simply as an item distinct from all the others. The interdependence of all the members in such a system is evident; a reduction of the total number of phonemes to 35 or an increase to 45 would change the relationship of every phoneme to every other phoneme in the system. Hence the phonemic system is essentially a system of relationships.

Since speech is transmitted from speaker to listener and the brain of each deals with the message in phonemic terms, these relationships must be reflected in one form or another at the various stages in speech communication. This means that there are features in the patterns of nerve impulses, of muscle actions, of sound waves, and of middle-ear movements that are correlated with the phonemic differences embodied in the message. Concentrating attention for the moment on the sound waves, we can say that the speaker in encoding the message makes sure that the sounds are so structured as to reflect the relationship between successive phonemes in the string, while the listener is concerned to process the information contained in the sound waves in such a way as to enable him to reconstruct the phoneme string. For this purpose he relies, on the one hand, on his knowledge of the constraints of the language, and on the other, on the use of features in the sound waves, now usually referred to as "acoustic cues," which past experience has shown to be reliable signals of the differences between phonemes.

An important difference has to be noted, however, between the system of relations that constitutes the phonemic system and the set of acoustic cues made use of in decoding. It is not a situation in which a single and invariable cue is associated with the occurrence of a given phoneme, in such a way that the presence of the cue signals with certainty the occurrence of that phoneme in the string while its absence indicates that the phoneme does not figure in the string. There is a considerable range of acoustic cues that the brain can fasten on and that it uses in various combinations in deciding which phoneme is the most probable at any point. This can be illustrated by looking at just one part of the English phoneme system, the fricatives /s, ʃ, f, θ/, and /z, ʒ, v, ð/. The sounds that signal the occurrence of any one of these phonemes contain a marked noise component, so that when the brain picks up this cue in an English sequence, it tends to look for the phonemic solution within this group. If the sound also has a noticeable amount of low frequency energy with some periodicity, this cue will place the phoneme among the second group of four, the voiced fricatives. However there are other cues that may replace or supplement this cue for the voiced group; if the noise is preceded by a relatively long vowel sound or if there is onset of periodicity before the noise is switched off, the solution will be found within the voiced group. Other cues operate to distinguish sounds within each set of four. If the noise component is of relatively high intensity, then the solution lies within the first pair in each case, if of low intensity, then in the second pair. Various frequency cues provide further resolution within the whole group of phonemes. If the noise energy begins relatively low in the frequency range, in the region of 2000 Hz, the phoneme is likely to be /ʃ/ or /ʒ/; if the noise energy is concentrated in the region around 4000 Hz, *s* or *z*; if it is restricted to higher frequencies, from 6000 Hz upward, it will be /f, v, θ/ or /ð/; the distinction between /f/ and /θ/ will rest upon differences in the adjacent periodic sounds, in particular on rapid changes in the frequency of the second and third formants of the associated vowels.

This complex system of acoustic cues refers to only a restricted part of the English phonemic system. In dealing with the whole inventory, the brain uses something vastly more complicated still, but the example is enough to show that there is no question of one phoneme, one acoustic marker; there are always a number of cues available, and the selection used for a given phonemic decision will depend on the conditions of communication, the context, and also on the individual concerned, for there is no compelling reason why different language users should use cues in the same way, even within the same language. The important part of the operation is making the right phonemic decisions, that is, decoding the speech without error; provided the listener does this, he is free to proceed with whatever cues he pleases or can make use of. As we shall see later on, this principle has a great bearing on the case of the deaf person.

Acquisition of the Phonological System by Hearing Children

SPEECH RECEPTION

We can now turn to the question of the acquisition of the phonological system and consider how it is that the normally hearing child builds up the system and learns to use it. It has already been emphasized that reception precedes production; we shall be concerned, first of all, with the system as a set of units used in the process of recognition, before we discuss the interactions between listening and speaking in the learning phase. The first important point here is that acquiring the phonemic system is a process of building up the system. The adult listener to English operates with 40 phonemic categories; his brain has, as it were, a framework of 40 pigeonholes into which incoming sounds are sorted in the act of recognition. Since any unit in the system, any phoneme, has only a differentiating function, the very framework of categories is a result of the number of distinctions that need to be made. The child who is beginning to acquire the phonological system cannot start out with the complete framework of 40 categories, most of them as yet unused, for the system of distinctions must work as a whole. He begins with a very small framework of two or three categories and expands this as the need to differentiate among more and more phonemes arises.

In order to follow some of the steps in this process, we must first consider how it is that the child embarks on the acquisition of language. In the prelinguistic stages, the baby hears the sounds of speech continually, but they remain undifferentiated for him—that is to say, they constitute noise from his point of view. Fairly soon there are various events, people, and objects in his surroundings that take his attention and become particularly important for him. In the great majority of cases the mother is the earliest focus of attention, since she is the source of many pleasant experiences like feeding, bathing, dressing, and so on. As a consequence, the speech sequence that so frequently accompanies her appearance is quite commonly the first to stand out from the noise and to be recognized by the young child. We naturally have to depend on various behavioral signs for evidence that the baby does recognize the sequence, but these are readily noticeable, at least to mothers, in the form of smiles or movements of one sort or another. The moment the child consistently associates the sequence /mama/ with the person, he has begun his acquisition of his native language, and it is important to notice that it is the demands and interest of the situation, in short the "meaning," that come first and entail the act of differentiation and recognition.

With this first step the child has begun his construction of the phonological system and effectively has his first two phonemic categories, although he cannot as yet do anything with them. There can be little doubt that /mama/ is recognized as a whole, but even so the child has already registered an important feature of the phonemic system, which is that time sequence is significant. He hears and remembers the reduplicated syllables as /mama/; they never turn up, for example, as /amam/. In this sense he has a phonemic system consisting of two units, /m/ and /a/.

Very shortly a second person may assume great importance in his baby world, and the speech sequence associated with this person will come to be recognized. The child can consistently associate /mama/ with his mother and /dada/ with his father only by distinguishing /da/ from /ma/ or /d/ from /m/. Here again it is the pressure of the situation that imposes the need for a further phonemic distinction and obliges the child's brain to find a basis for the differentiation. Like the adult with his complete phonemic system, he must do this on the basis of acoustic information coming in, and hence his task is to find acoustic cues that will work consistently in the particular situation. We know little as yet about the ways in which acoustic cues are developed during language acquisition, but we do know something of the interactions between the phonemic system and the use of cues. In particular, we know that if in a given language a certain distinction has no linguistic function, as is the case, for example, with /s/ and /ʃ/ in Dutch, or /n/ and /ŋ/ in Spanish, then the users of that language are incapable of noting any difference between the two sounds. This means that in the course of language acquisition we develop the capacity to notice acoustic cues necessary for making linguistically important distinctions, but not cues for differences lying within phonemic categories. What evidence there is (Liberman, Harris, Eimas, Lisker, & Bastian, 1961; Liberman, Harris, Hoffman, & Griffith, 1957) certainly favors this view and not the opposite one, which would hold that the child begins with the ability to make many more distinctions between sounds than the language calls for and has to learn to disregard many of the differences. The need for the differentiation, brought about by the social situation, is the primary factor; it is rather that linguistic oppositions evoke the cues than that language makes use of differences that are inherently easily perceived.

The young child, then, needs to distinguish /da/ from /ma/, and his brain will find the means of doing so. His system now includes three items, one "vowel," /a/, and two consonants, /m/ and /d/. In his use of cues all that is demanded is that they suffice for these differentiations; they can therefore be a very restricted set. The difference in intensity between /a/ and /m/ of about 8 dB would form an adequate cue for this distinction, and the interrupted nature of /d/ in contrast to the continuous character of /m/ and /a/ would function satisfactorily for the remaining distinctions. Although we do not as yet know how the child operates at this early stage, there can be no doubt that these acoustic cues would be enough for the functioning of this small system.

The importance of the interlocking nature of the phonological system becomes clear when we consider how it develops. Let us suppose that the next sequence that the child recognizes consistently is /baba/ or /nana/. Again the addition comes about only because a new feature of the environment takes on a particular degree of interest. Not uncommonly this is one of the grandparents, who is referred to by one or the other of these sequences. The increase in the number of phonemic units from three to four means that the whole system is changed, because all the items have to be distinguished from one another. If the new phoneme is /b/, then a cue must be evolved that will distinguish it not only from /a/ and /m/, but also from /d/.

The interrupted character of /d/ is shared by /b/, so that some fresh cue has to be found. This may well lie in the second formant transition, which has been shown to play an important part in adults' processing of speech and also to be perceptible to very young children. The same cue would serve equally well if the required distinction were between /n/ and /m/ instead of /b/ and /d/, but would in this case be applied to splitting the class of continuants (nasals) and not the stops.

These hypothetical examples serve to illustrate the kind of process that is going on during the acquisition of the phonological system. It is not necessary, and indeed is scarcely possible, to follow out the complete process. There is undoubtedly much individual variation among children, in this as in every other aspect of language development and use, and we have, unfortunately, very little firm information about the reception and recognition of speech in young children. The main features of the process are clear, however: In the early stages, a child will learn to recognize a speech item only if it is associated with something in his world that concerns and interests him, and he learns it through the consistent repetition of the association. His phonemic system works as a complete whole at every stage and includes only the phonemic units required for recognizing the items he has learned. In order to differentiate these units from one another his brain evolves acoustic cues, of which the only requirement is that they work effectively; provided this condition is met, it can make use of any cue that it likes. While there is a small number of units, there will be few cues, and they may be of a gross kind—simply, the cue may be one which, if used with reference to the adult phonemic system, would characterize a whole class of units. For example, in the child's three-unit system /d/ might be distinguished by its interrupted character, but in the adult system this cue would specify a subset of ten units in English, the six stops and four affricates. As the child learns to recognize more and more items, he expands his phonological system, and every addition to this system means additional cues. As we have seen, the new cue is often needed to split an existing class, so that a complicated cue system is soon built up, but it is a self-evolving system.

The normally hearing child will usually be capable of all the differentiations called for on the reception side by the time he is three to four years old (though there is, of course, great individual variation). He achieves this because he is all the time surrounded by the sounds of speech and because they are associated with the events of his daily life. If he is deprived of this experience, for any reason, he will not develop the capacity for taking in speech and will not acquire the phonological system, but provided the stimuli are continually supplied, the brain will evolve the means of processing them. At a certain stage in normal children an interesting and important shift of emphasis takes place. At first the person, the object, the event—the "thing itself"—has to be interesting enough to trigger the acquisition of some language item, but when the phonological system is in a fairly advanced stage, then for most children language activity per se becomes actually more interesting than many of the things it represents. This is the stage at which the small child spends a great part of his time asking questions, often repeating the same question many times on one occasion. Most adults, including parents, misread this activity as betraying a consuming interest in the subject of the question, but it generally means that the child is now interested in the linguistic information rather than the thing itself and is eager to confirm that, for instance, the word is *bicycle* rather than that the thing is a bicycle. It is by triggering many repetitions of an item that the child is able to expand his phonemic system and add to his grammatical and lexical information. As always, he does this through reception first, and it is noticeable that, when in the questioning phase, children will not often speak back spontaneously the answer they are given, though they are often pressed to do so by the adult concerned, who seems to feel the need for some overt reward and is not aware that he is making a vital contribution to the child's acquisition of his language.

SPEECH PRODUCTION

By such means then the child eventually expands his phonemic system to the point where it coincides with that of adult speakers, and we have to say that this point is reached when the child can consistently employ the whole set of 40-odd phonemes, in English, when decoding speech. So far we have said little about speech production except to note that it is always preceded by reception and recognition and that it is possible for complete recognition to develop even in cases where speech production is impossible. In all normal conditions, however, there is a great deal of interaction between speech reception and speech production, and parts of the two processes certainly call for the use of common circuits in the brain. At the same time, recognizing sounds and making them are not the same thing; it is clear that a speaker, whether a child or an adult, may fail to make a consistent difference between two sounds in producing them and yet be well aware, on the reception side, of the distinction between them and not make errors in recognizing them. Among adult speakers of English, for example, there is the occasional case of the person with a lisp who produces only one sound to represent the two phonemes /s/ and /θ/, and similarly for the voiced sounds. It is clear however that he has no difficulty in decoding words containing any of these four sounds and does not confuse them in reception.

In the case of the young child, when a difference between, say, /t/ and /k/ is consistently made in speech production, we can be sure that these two units are already functioning in the child's phonological system and that by this time the distinction is quite stable. On the other hand, we cannot say during the time when he is still articulating /t/ for both /t/ and /k/, that his system is lacking the unit /k/; this could be demonstrated only on the basis of his reception of speech. This fact is often overlooked even by those professionally concerned in the study of children's acquisition of language—understandably enough, since the child's own speech is the most obvious behavioral evidence we have of his progress in language development. The fact remains that there is a time lag between learning to recognize the difference between sounds and learning to reproduce that difference. At present our knowledge about the child's acquisition of the phonemic system on the reception side is very incomplete, much more so than our knowledge of the production side. It appears that among English-speaking children, for example, though there are great individual variations in the rate at which different sounds are acquired, there is some uniformity in the order in which they are learned, particularly in the case of consonants. The first ones, as was suggested earlier on, are /m, d, b/ and /n/, and to these are added fairly soon /t/ and /p/. Rather later on /k, g, w/ and /y/ appear, and it is only very considerably later that the child produces the fricatives, the affricates, and /l/ and /r/ (Lewis, 1936; Morley, 1957).

The interaction between reception and production is perhaps most apparent in the later stages of the acquisition of the phonological system, where it affects particularly the distribution of sounds. The sequence of events is essentially that the child first learns to recognize the difference between two sounds, then learns to reproduce this difference, and finally learns in what words and sequences the sounds are to be used. A particularly striking example in English often occurs with the affricate sounds in *chain* and *train*. The first step is that the child learns to distinguish /tʃ/ from /tr/ and knows which of the two words has been said. Some time later the words will appear in his own speech, but he will produce the same sound at the beginning of the two words, making them both sound like *chain*. At a considerably later stage he will succeed in producing distinctly different sounds in the two cases, and he will of course have added many more words to his vocabulary by this time. As a consequence he will very probably become uncertain about the distribution of the two sounds, especially of the new sound /tr/, which he has more recently learned to make, and one may hear productions such as *treeks* instead of *cheeks* and *trocolate* instead of *chocolate*. These errors in distribution are, of course, soon corrected through repeated hearings and utterances of the words in question.

An important point has still to be made with reference to the normal child's acquisition of the phonological system; this concerns the part played by the speech models with which he is provided. We have already stressed that the basis for the development lies in the auditory speech stimuli that reach the child. The major factor in the forming of his phonemic system will therefore be his principal speech model, in the normal case his mother. The phoneme system represented in her speech will be basically the one learned by the child, since he hears more speech from her than from anyone else in the early stages. This effect is very much reinforced by the fact that the child's pronunciation is the result of imitation of his mother's speech; in other words his "accent" will resemble hers, at least throughout the early years of his life. It is clear, therefore, that auditory sensations play a vital role in the acquisition of the phonological system, and we must now see what in this respect is the situation of the child born with a hearing loss.

Acquisition of the Phonological System in Cases of Hearing Impairment

From all that has been said so far about the case of the hearing child it will be clear that learning to take in speech and to produce it is essentially a matter of brain work. The basis of the phonological system is the brain's organization of the acoustic information that comes into the receiving apparatus, rather than the character of the sound waves themselves. This is a fact of the greatest importance for our understanding of the situation of the child born with a hearing loss, since a deficiency in the ear does not imply a deficiency in the brain. A deaf child has (or is as likely as the hearing child to have) intact the vital component for language learning, the brain. Given this condition, the important factor, as we have seen, is continual exposure to the sounds of speech. Cases have been reported from time to time over the years off "wild" boys and girls who, despite the possession of normal hearing, have not developed speech simply because they never heard any; it is evident that amount of exposure to speech stimuli takes priority over the condition of the actual hearing.

This has been borne out repeatedly by experience with deaf children. Again and again children have been found with a comparatively mild degree of hearing loss, for instance losses not exceeding 50 dB in either ear, whose ability to use speech is very poor indeed. On the other hand, there are many instances of children with very considerable losses of hearing, of the order of 80—100 dB, who have learned to take in speech through their hearing and have also learned to produce speech that is readily intelligible to the ordinary listener (Whetnall & Fry, 1971). In other words, whether a child is going to learn to talk and understand speech depends much more on the amount of exposure to speech stimuli than it does on the degree of hearing loss.

Naturally it is not easy to understand why this should be the case. The common assumption is that "deafness" is a very specific condition, which simply prevents sound from affecting the person afflicted with it, so that there would seem to be little chance of such a person's being exposed to speech stimuli. This is very far from being the true state of affairs. Any ear may exhibit something less than normal sensitivity for sounds of certain frequencies, and it is this fact that is expressed by saying that the ear shows a hearing loss of so many decibels. A hearing loss of 80 dB at 2000 Hz implies that a pure tone of 2000 Hz will become just audible to that ear provided its intensity is raised to 80 dB above the normal threshold. The loss of sensitivity generally varies from frequency to frequency in one ear, it usually varies between the two ears in one individual and certainly varies from person to person. It is in fact very rarely that one comes across an individual who cannot respond to sound at all, no matter what the stimulus frequency or intensity, and a majority of children who are discovered to have a hearing loss do have some usable hearing. The methods of measuring hearing loss that are commonly used aim at establishing the organic condition of the hearing mechanism, but none of them is independent of learning on the part of the subject; a person who has never been in the habit of using his hearing and then learns to do so will show a distinct improvement in hearing as indicated by a pure-tone threshold audiogram. This is one reason, among many, why it is no use predicting solely from a pure-tone audiogram whether a child is going to succeed in using speech or not.

In order for hearing to be used, sounds must of course be audible; where there is a hearing loss, the first requirement is for hearing-aids of a suitable type and power to bring as many sounds as possible within the range of sensitivity of the ears concerned. The whole question of the relationships between hearing aids and types of hearing loss is very complex and cannot be treated here, but two general points must be made. The first is that, as far as the development of speech and language is concerned, a hearing aid is useless unless it makes speech stimuli very audible to the child most of the time. The child must hear speech loud enough and often enough for his brain to work on the information, and hence an aid that delivers too little power, in view of the hearing loss, will be of very little avail. The second point is that there is quite a body of evidence that shows that for language acquisition binaural hearing is a marked advantage. As normally hearing people, we use our two ears in order to orient ourselves in the world of sound and, most particularly, to direct our attention to one source of sound rather than another. This factor is likely to be of even greater importance during the learning period, especially for the child who in any case has defective hearing; it is therefore wise, wherever possible, to provide the child with two hearing aids so that he may have the advantage of a binaural system (Whetnall, 1964).

PRELINGUISTIC DEVELOPMENT OF THE DEAF CHILD

It will be useful to follow in general terms the development of a child who is born with a serious loss of hearing in order to see where this is liable to diverge from that of the normal child and to consider how it is possible for him to achieve effective use of speech and language.

During the first months of life there are few obvious signs of difference between the hearing baby and the one with a hearing loss. The deaf baby cries with discomfort in the first weeks and months and soon begins to express pleasure by cooing and gurgling; in both cases the sounds are not distinguishably different from those uttered by a hearing child. His development continues into the babbling stage, at about the age of 6 months, again without noticeable differences. Deaf babies begin to babble at the normal time, and the sounds they make have no special character (Lenneberg, 1966).

The babbling period is of vital importance for the development of speech, and it is significant for several reasons that deaf children should babble spontaneously. In the normal baby, two very significant processes are taking place during this period. First, the child is exploring many of the possibilities of the speech mechanism. He discovers how to control breathing for speech, how to break up the regular rhythm used for inhalation and exhalation in quiet breathing and to replace it by the quick intake and the slow, controlled expiration that speech demands. He finds out that the larynx mechanism can be switched on and off and that there is a whole range of articulatory movements possible in the pharynx, the mouth, and the nose. All this activity is prelinguistic, but it is essential experience as a basis for the later learning of sounds by imitation and for the translating of the phonological system into terms of articulation.

An even more important aspect of the babbling activity lies in the fact that it establishes in the brain the links between motor actions and auditory impressions during speech. In normal conditions of speech production, we rely on the combination of auditory and kinesthetic feedback for the control of our speech movements. It is during the babbling period that the circuits are set up in the brain that make this control possible. The baby learns that a certain kind of movement or combination of movements will result in a particular kind of sound; that a movement repeated will produce the "same" sound. Through many hours of this activity he sets up the mechanism and accumulates a capital of information that will serve him for the remainder of his speaking life.

There can be little doubt that a major motive force behind the child's persistent and repeated babbling is the pleasure he derives from the sounds he is making. Even if in the early stages the balance may be tilted somewhat in the direction of pleasure from movement, the effect of the sounds themselves soon becomes apparent. The babbling of the deaf baby is therefore doubly significant, because it makes it highly probable that, despite the hearing loss, such a baby does get some auditory stimulation from the sounds he makes and is capable of developing the brain mechanisms through which kinesthetic and auditory information are related. If this were not the case, we should expect that the deaf baby's babbling would be markedly different in sound from the hearing baby's and also that the activity itself would fade within a fairly short time. All the evidence is in the contrary direction, which would argue, as indeed we know on other grounds, that the necessary control circuits for speech can be established in the brain of a child with a hearing loss.

Up to this point, therefore, the development in the normally hearing and the deaf baby run parallel, but there is a stage at which their paths will diverge unless some special measures are taken. Babbling, in its earlier manifestations, is very much a spontaneous activity; it tends to take place when the baby is alone in his crib, particularly on waking and before going to sleep. Later on, a development takes place that is of the utmost importance for speech—the baby's babbling activity begins to be triggered by the sound of a human voice. If someone speaks directly to the child or if he simply overhears people talking, he will now start to babble. The character of the babbling remains the same as before; he makes no attempt to imitate the sounds he hears, but these sounds act as a trigger. At this moment the capacity for hearing external sounds becomes a critical factor; in a child with a hearing loss, babbling is liable to fade at this point. It is indeed frequently reported of deaf babies that they began to babble in the normal way, but that after a time the activity ceased. The coincidence of two developments is often responsible for this fading of babbling. The first is the trigger mechanism we have already noted; the second is the mobility that the child begins to achieve at about the same time. It is just at this stage that the baby begins to crawl and so gets further away from his mother, who is the most common source of speech sounds. In the normally hearing child this has no effect on babbling because these sounds are still highly audible, but the situation will be very different for a child with a hearing loss. Up to this point he will generally have spent a good deal of time in his mother's arms or on her lap, and her voice may well have been perceptible to him. A few feet of space between him and his mother will in many cases be enough to place the sounds below his threshold; the vital stimulus for the continuing of speech development is missing and the babbling fades.

This breakdown in the process of speech development is not inevitable. If external sounds are made audible to the child it will not occur. There are many reported cases in which mothers have achieved this by continually speaking into the child's meatus and of course it can be done more effectively through the providing of hearing aids. It is obviously important that the presence of a hearing loss should be diagnosed at the earliest possible moment and certainly by the age of 8–10 months when the baby is likely to begin to crawl. In clinical experience, the best results in speech and language development have been obtained when this condition is fulfilled, but this does not mean that no progress is possible if diagnosis takes place later. It is significant that cases are reported in which a baby's babbling has faded and the activity has started again after an interval when hearing aids were provided and the sounds of speech were made audible for the child. This is a good indication of the importance of the babbling stage for speech.

SPEECH RECEPTION IN THE DEAF CHILD

Given that the child's hearing loss is diagnosed very early and that he is given suitable hearing aids, there still remains the question as to how he can achieve anything like normal functioning with speech and language. Since, as we have seen, reception precedes production, we shall look at the question first with reference to reception, that is, to the acquiring of the phonological system. The answer here lies in what has been said about the operation of acoustic cues and their relation to the system. The acoustic information reaching the brain of the child with a hearing loss, even when he has been fitted with hearing aids, is certainly going to differ in character and in total amount from that supplied to the hearing child's brain. If spoken language were a medium very different from what it really is, and if we could understand speech only when presented with "mint copies" of a very restricted and closely specified set of acoustic stimuli, then this defect in the deaf child would make any operation with speech out of the question (and, incidentally, it would be virtually impossible for even two normally hearing adults to speak to each other). We have already seen that spoken language is not like this. In any spoken message, we receive very much more acoustic information than we need for decoding the message; what we have to draw out of this information is just enough in the way of acoustic cues to implement the distinctions carried by the phonological system.

The child with a hearing loss, provided speech is made audible enough to him, sets about developing the phonemic system in the same way as the hearing child. He has in the early stages to make only a very few differentiations, and his brain forges its own cues for doing this out of the acoustic information supplied to it.

As the system is expanded, it evolves the further cues needed at each stage, again from the acoustic information it has. What makes the process hard for most of us to understand is our natural conviction that the only way of distinguishing between two sounds is the way in which we do it ourselves, ignorant though we may be as to what this way is. In the visual world we can perhaps just about accept the parallel situation of the color-blind person and conceive of his differentiating between certain colors on the basis of their monochromatic tone or of his coping with red and green traffic lights, on the basis of their different spatial positions. The same principle holds in the auditory sphere; if distinctions have to be made, the brain finds a basis for making them in the available information.

Among the cues that have been shown experimentally to be effective for hearing people, there is in any case a proportion that can work equally well for those with a hearing loss. For example, the short silence or interruption that acts as a cue for the whole class of stop consonants can be used by the deaf child as well as by the hearing; the whole range of formant cues on which vowel differentiation is based are available, since they are carried by the high intensity stretches of the speech wave, so that speech which is audible necessarily carries this information. Similarly the various cues that depend on formant transitions, the second formant transitions as cues to place of articulation, the rate of transition for distinguishing semivowels from other classses of consonant, the onset of the first formant as a cue for voicing—all these are types of cue that can remain operative in the presence of even a considerable hearing loss. In addition, hearing people make use of a variety of frequency cues, some of which appear to depend upon the transmission of energy in the higher frequencies, which are generally most affected by hearing defects. However, acoustic analysis shows that all the noises that constitute the fricative consonants are in fact wide spectrum sounds. Even though they may all show spectral peaks in the higher frequency bands, they also show differences in the lower ranges, and it is these differences that provide a cue basis for the deaf child's discrimination of the sounds.

All of this does not mean that there will be no noticeable difference between the progress of a hearing child and a deaf child in acquiring the phonological system. The latter will progress more slowly, and will be more liable to errors and over a longer period. He will also need more specific help from his mother than the hearing child, who generally goes through the successive stages without anyone's being aware of the fact. The mother has to pay a great deal more attention to her task and see that the child is continually supplied with audible speech stimuli related to his everyday life and its events. This is not an easy matter, since all too easily the attitude may develop that the child is deaf and that therefore it is of no use to talk to him. The truth is quite the opposite; because he has a hearing loss, he needs to hear even more speech than the hearing child, not less. His progress therefore depends to a very great extent upon the efforts of the mother, upon her understanding of what the nature of the task is and upon her application in carrying it out. The very many cases in which deaf children have successfully acquired the phonemic system and developed a normal use of language are the result of the mother's success in playing her part, combined with the advantages of early diagnosis and the provision of suitable hearing aids.

SPEECH PRODUCTION IN THE DEAF CHILD

In the large majority of such cases, the child not only learns to operate the phonological system in reception, he also learns to produce speech which, in the best case, is scarcely distinguishable from that of a normal child. That this is possible has been demonstrated by many hundreds of children, many of them now adults, in various centers in different parts of the world. If indeed there were only one such case, we should still be faced with the task of explaining how such a thing is possible, and it must be admitted that an explanation is not easy. The problem can be stated specifically in the following way. The production of speech sounds is the fruit of imitation; the procedure is that the child first becomes familiar with a sound of a certain type, which is stored as an acoustic pattern in his brain. He next tries to produce a sound with his own vocal tract that will provide a good match with this stored pattern. The auditory impression of his own sound reaches his brain through the auditory feedback loop, and it is this impression that is matched with the stored model. His first attempts do not afford a very close match, so he improves the match by repetition over a long period in which the judgment of his own ear and brain is supplemented by feedback from his listeners, especially his mother. Through this process of convergence, he eventually produces a sound that is an adequate match and is accepted by a range of listeners. In ways that are as yet little understood, this operation of pattern-matching disregards certain dimensions of difference, such as the differences between a child's and an adult's fundamental frequencies and formant frequencies.

In the case of the deaf child, it is certain that the pattern represented by the model is distorted in comparison with that perceived by a normally hearing person. However, the auditory impression of his own production will also be distorted and in the same way, so that if he succeeds in making these two patterns coincide, he has the basis of a satisfactory reproduction of the model. We can readily see that if the degree of distortion is not very great, this may be sufficient to explain a measure of the deaf child's success in producing acceptable speech. In the overwhelming majority of instances, the effect of deafness is to introduce a marked deficiency in high frequency information. The matching of auditory feedback from his own production with the incoming model would lead the deaf child to considerable success in the case of vowel sounds, semivowels, nasals, and /l/ and r sounds, as well as in the all-important matters of timing, rhythm and intonation, and voice quality, for in all these cases the patterning in the low frequency end of the spectrum plays a predominant part. There can be little doubt that this accounts for the very "natural" impression made by the speech of many deaf children who have been auditorily trained and have acquired speech through their hearing.

There remains, however, one further fact to be explained, which is that the speech of such children often embodies articulatory distinctions that one would expect to depend on something other than low frequency information. To take a concrete, if hypothetical, example, if a child's hearing is such that he receives practically no information relating to frequencies above, say, 1500 Hz, we should expect that he would be incapable of producing in his own speech distinctively different sounds to represent the phonemes /s/ and /ʃ/, or that if he did so, they would not be very readily distinguishable by ordinary listeners. We have seen that, on the reception side, he could learn to differentiate them as incoming sounds on the grounds of differences that undoubtedly exist in the range below 1500 Hz. By monitoring his own productions to match the incoming model he would also produce different sounds, but in fact the process seems to go much further than this, since such children learn to make sounds remarkably like those of hearing speakers. The properties and characteristics of the articulatory mechanism and the vocal tract are such that in generating a close match for [ʃ], for example, in the range below 1500 Hz, the speaker in fact articulates a sound with higher noise components lying in a range where he gets virtually no auditory feedback; these are, as it were, a by-product of the articulatory action necessary to make a match at all.

Not all children with a hearing loss produce speech that is close to normal speech, and not all of those who do are equally successful with all sounds. The effect of very weak or nonexistent feedback in the higher frequency range is often apparent, but there are enough cases in which the speech is almost normal to make it necessary to seek some such explanation as has been given here. To take a very rough parallel in the visual world, it is somewhat as though one looked at a figure through a distorting lens and then, still looking through the lens, tried to make a faithful copy of the figure. A really successful attempt would be a figure which would also constitute a faithful copy when the lens was removed and both patterns were seen undistorted.

In conclusion it may be well to emphasize once again that it is the amount of exposure to audible speech that will determine the success of a deaf child in learning to receive and send out speech much more than the degree of his organic hearing-loss. Give the three requirements that have been mentioned—early diagnosis, early provision of hearing aids, and the maximum of help to the parents of the child, especially the mother—it is only a very small proportion of children with a hearing loss who cannot learn to operate with spoken language.

References

Fry, D. B. Acoustic cues in the speech of the hearing and the deaf. *Proceedings of the Royal Society of Medicine*, 1973, 66, 959–969.

Lenneberg, E. H. The natural history of language. In F. Smith & G. A. Miller (Eds.), In *The genesis of language*. Cambridge, Mass.: MIT Press, 1966. Pp. 219–252.

Lewis, M. M. *Infant speech*. London: Routledge & Kegan Paul, 1936.

Liberman, A. M., Harris, K. S., Eimas, P., Lisker, L., & Bastian, J. An effect of learning on speech perception: the discrimination of durations of silence with and without phonemic significance. *Language and Speech*, 1961, *4*, 175—195.

Liberman, A. M., Harris, K. S., Hoffman, H. S., & Griffith, B. C. The discrimination of speech sounds within and across phoneme boundaries. *Journal of Experimental Psychology*, 1957, *54*, 358—368.

Morley, M. E. *The development and disorders of speech in childhood*. London: Livingstone, 1957.

Whetnall, E. Binaural hearing. *Journal of Laryngology and Otology*, 1964, *78*, 1079—1089.

Whetnall, E., & Fry, D. B. *The deaf child*. London: Heinemann, 1971.

10. Visual Feedback and the Acquisition of Intonation[1]

Evelyn Abberton / A. J. Fourcin

Rhythm and intonation are basic to the normal development of speaking ability in children. Like other speech skills, they cannot be properly developed unless speech feedback paths are available. An auditory path is ordinarily crucial to this development, but its replacement may prove possible by the use of a visual presentation. This section describes a method that derives its information from a direct monitoring of vocal fold vibration and gives some examples of its application to the teaching of rhythm and intonation to the profoundly deaf.

Abnormalities of Deaf Speech

In normal speech, timing and intonation play a vital role. They convey grammatical, semantic, and emotional information, and the intelligibility of speech depends greatly on their appropriate use. The normal child begins to develop control of the patterning of intonation in what will be his native language during the babbling stage before he has begun to acquire selective control of articulation (Weir, 1966). Intonation is not a superficial attribute of speech; normally it is the basis on which all else is built.

Without sufficient auditory feedback, intonation and rhythm, like other speech skills, are abnormal. Deaf people who have been taught to speak talk more or less

[1]The first work on teaching using the visual display derived from the output of the laryngograph was supported by a Research Grant from the Department of Education and Science. The illustrations were made possible by a current award to A. J. Fourcin from the Science Research Council.

157

on a monotone or use pitch in a random, uncontrolled manner. Either the pitch range employed is too narrow, or it is extremely wide with excursions into falsetto. Some speakers use high-pitched falsetto as their usual voice quality, whereas others have the appropriate register but a voice quality that is rough and tense. In addition, their breathing and speaking are often uncoordinated.

The speech of such people, particularly those with a severe hearing loss, lacks the essential framework of rhythm and intonation patterning, even if articulatory positions for vowels and consonants have been learned (John & Howarth, 1965). The impression is of a string of segments individually conceived and produced; this is often intelligible only with familiarity and concentration.

In principle, this difficulty can be reduced if an alternative speech feedback pathway can be employed. Either or both of the senses of touch and vision can most readily be utilized. Tactile displays of some degree of complexity have been developed as visual substitution systems for the blind (White, Saunders, Scadden, Bach-y-Rita, & Collins, 1970), and the theoretical neurophysiological basis of this sensory replacement has been discussed by Bach-y-Rita (1967). Tactile speech-analyzing aids for the deaf (Kringlebotn, 1968; Pickett, 1968) also exist, but important difficulties arise from the limited frequency-analyzing capacity of the skin and the spatial spread of masking. Much work has been done, however, in developing displays of visual correlates of acoustic patterns to help the deaf and hard of hearing in both the reception and production of speech (Pickett, 1968). Teaching with a display of this type will be effective only if it results in the establishing of effective speech motor activity. The student will acquire this from learning the motor actions he must employ in order to produce the same visual pattern with his own speech as is presented by the teacher. The student can acquire this in an error-correcting feedback situation. A visual pattern derived from the speech of a teacher, when copied by a student, requires the use of the right motor activity. It is the way of arriving at this motor activity that is subsequently retained.

Design Requirements and Operation of a Visual Feedback System

A visual display of intonation information could, then, in principle, help to solve many of the problems of the deaf speaker in timing and pitch control. If such a display is to be useful, however, the following factors must determine its design:

1. The physical signal it presents to the student must be clear and must correspond in a simple way to the normal experience of pitch changes.
2. The display must be substantially instantaneous and not associated with time lag, which would interfere with visual control of the articulators.
3. Pattern proportions must be similar for speakers with different pitch ranges.
4. The patterns must not be transient: the ear can deal with successive rapid stimuli and provide a satisfactory basis for their recall, but visual memory of

transient events is inadequate. The display must thus be stored, to supplement the user's visual memory, and must not be overloaded with information.

5. Since the teaching method depends on pattern matching, the facility must provide for both stimulus and response to be displayed together for comparison. The device should be usable by a teacher and student working together, or by a student alone.

6. The apparatus must be inexpensive, and reliable and simple to use.

The major physical correlate of intonation in speech is fundamental frequency; over the years numbers of displays have been produced in different countries whose aim is to show the changing patterns of fundamental frequency for teaching purposes. The general impression gained from the literature is that such displays can, indeed, be helpful in teaching control of pitch register and intonation. Pronovost (1967), Risberg (1968), and Mártóny (1968) describe work in this area; more recently, Boothroyd and Decker (1970), Boothroyd (1971), James (1971), and Anderson (1971) have reported on new visual displays of fundamental frequency for teaching both normal and deaf students. None of these displays, however, fulfills all of the requirements listed above. Some are very costly, some not reliable, and all involve complex processing of speech to extract the fundamental frequency, always with some delay in presentation of the visual pattern. The use of a larynx microphone does not increase reliability, because its output is largely dependent on the shape of the vocal tract as well as on the vibration of the vocal folds.

Our own work in this area has utilized a completely new approach to the problem of obtaining the physical correlate of intonation for purposes of a visual display. The display we are using (Fourcin & Abberton, 1971) is derived from the output of the laryngograph, a device developed in the Department of Phonetics and Linguistics at University College London, which is based on the principle of Fabre's (1957) glottograph. The laryngograph responds to changes only in electrical impedance produced by the vibrating vocal folds, by means of two electrodes superficially applied on each side of the speaker's larynx. It is unaffected by acoustic noise from the speaker or his surroundings, and allows continuous and instantaneous monitoring of vocal fold activity during ordinary speech. The waveform of the output of the laryngograph is devoid of the complexities of the acoustic speech signal and gives information about vocal fold closure and, to some extent, associated voice quality. The laryngograph waveform, Lx, can be used in two ways for teaching purposes: directly, and as the basis of a display of fundamental frequency. If Lx is displayed on an oscilloscope screen, a deaf speaker can see whether he is producing voice at all (the instrument will not respond to whispering) or voice in the correct register; falsetto and creaky voice, for example, have distinctly different waveforms from normal voice (see Fig. 10—1).

This facility can help a deaf speaker to overcome voice breaks and can show how the fundamental frequency of the voice changes during speech. (It is worth noting that if the electrodes are placed across the nose, nasal vibration can be independently detected, a waveform being obtained for nasal and nasalised sounds

(a)

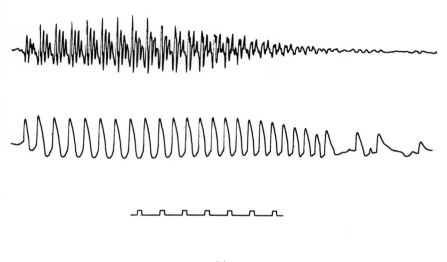

(b)

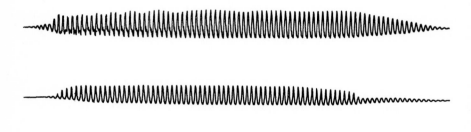

Figure 10–1. *Speech and Lx Waveforms.* (a) The top trace is for the acoustic pressure waveform corresponding to *Oh!* spoken by a normal adult male. The lower waveform shows the corresponding simultaneously recorded laryngograph response. The increase in speech fundamental frequency, *Fx*, is clearly shown in both the speech and *Lx* waveforms at the beginning of the utterance: at the end, the vowel transition and the reduction in speech intensity make the *Fx* variation difficult to follow in the speech; it is easily seen in *Lx*, however. *Lx* also shows a final abrupt change in voice quality to creaky voice, which can be heard but, normally, hardly seen in the pressure waveform. (b) The top trace is again the acoustic pressure waveform and the lower trace is the corresponding *Lx* from the same speaker as in (a). This time, however, he was speaking in a falsetto register.

In the *Lx* waveforms the positive-going direction corresponds to vocal fold closure. In normal voice and in creaky voice the rapid closing phase of the vibratory cycle and the slower opening phase are clear. In normal, chest, voice the pattern is regularly repeated, but in creaky voice there is considerable variation in the length of the open phase. In falsetto the waveform is of smaller amplitude and is sinusoidal in shape. The lowest trace in (a) and (b) is a time marker and shows 10 msec intervals.

but not for oral ones.) For intonation and rhythm work, however, another, non-transient, display is provided on the screen of a storage oscilloscope, which has time on the horizontal axis and a logarithmic vertical frequency scale. The display, which is also produced instantaneously, is obtained by measuring each period of the Lx waveform and deriving the negative of its logarithm. This gives not only the overall fundamental frequency contour of an utterance, but shows variation in excitation from moment to moment (see Fig. 10–2). The logarithmic frequency scale is used to normalize pattern proportions for speakers with different pitch ranges, a vital factor in a teaching method that depends on pattern matching. A logarithmic scale corresponds to our perception of these patterns more closely than does a linear scale.

Using the electrodes, the student can attempt to copy in the lower half of the screen a model contour in the upper half. The model may be provided live from the teacher, or from tape, or could take the form of a photograph or drawing of the contour to be practiced. As the student responds, he has immediate correcting of reinforcing visual feedback. The pattern is built up from left to right (corresponding to our reading and writing habits) as it is spoken. Thus continuous correction is possible; the student does not have to wait until his utterance is complete and presented in its entirety before he can compare it with the model. In practical teaching situations it is important to have this synchrony and form of presentation.

A dynamic visual display of this kind allows effective crossmodal transfer and learning of new laryngeal gestures.[2] When the display is no longer present, the deaf speaker can monitor his output kinaesthetically. We have concentrated on teaching correct rhythm and intonation patterns for short, useful utterances, at no time asking the student to do exercises in pitch sustention or movement that are not speechlike. Immediate improvement in timing results once the speaker can see that the length of trace for his utterance does not correspond to the model trace. Not only can the overall length be adjusted, but, just as importantly, control of the internal temporal syllabic composition of the utterance can be learned. Since duration and fundamental frequency are major physical correlates of what we perceive as linguistic stress in English (Fry, 1958), the display can be used to teach the basic concepts of nuclear tone and contrastive stress (see Fig. 10–3). We hope to investigate whether an additional indication of intensity (by a relative brightening or broadening of portions of the trace) would give any more useful information. A separate display for intensity, however, would certainly only distract the learner. Falling intonation patterns are fairly easily acquired. Rises are more difficult to achieve, sometimes because of faulty breathing. However, a motivated learner can learn to produce both these basic patterns (and even combine them) and use them in appropriate linguistic contexts.

The display has also contributed to segmental control. Since the laryngograph only gives an output for voiced sounds, the display can be used to correct the

[2]Crossmodal transfer takes place in the case of normally hearing students learning a foreign language. In the case of the profoundly deaf, the process is essentially that of sensory substitution.

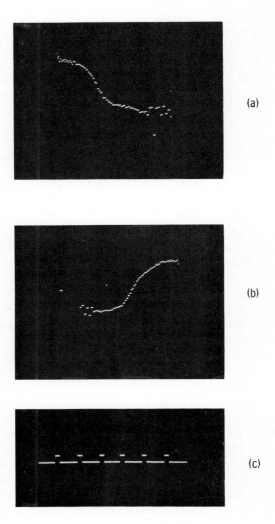

(a)

(b)

(c)

Figure 10–2. *Normal fundamental frequency traces.* (a) This trace represents *Oh* spoken with a falling intonation pattern. At the beginning and end of the pattern the broken lines represent larynx periods of very different lengths producing the auditory effect of creaky voice or vocal fry. This effect, which is more noticeable in the lower *Fx* range, is visible because the *Fx* display responds on a period-by-period basis to *Lx* variations. (b) This trace represents *Oh?* spoken with a rising intonation pattern. Creaky voice is again visible in the lower portion of the speaker's range where it is characteristic of much English speech. (c) This is a time marker showing 0.1 sec intervals.

These traces show the fundamental frequency variation throughout the course of a fully voiced utterance. The subject is a man speaking British English. The *Fx* frequency scale has not been shown, since only the overall shape is of importance to the deaf learner; the logarithmic frequency scale used for the display essentially normalizes pattern proportions for speakers with different pitch ranges.

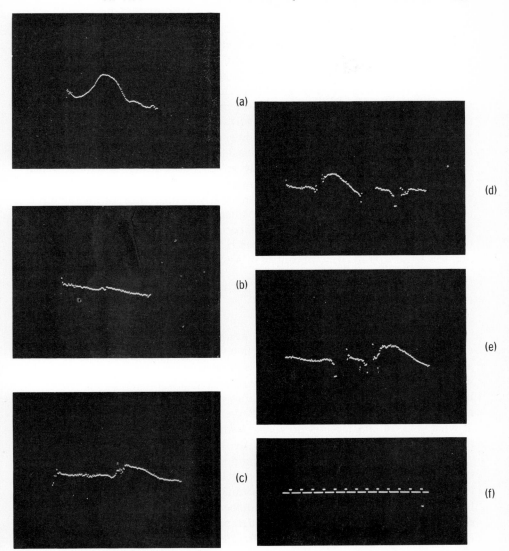

Figure 10–3. *Fundamental frequency traces from a deaf speaker.* Traces (a), (b), and (c) represent the greeting, *How are you?* (a) is from a normal speaker putting nuclear stress (most prominence) on *are*. (b) is from a congenitally profoundly deaf man with orthodox training in speech skills, and characteristically flat intonation. (c) is the same deaf man's output after 5 weekly half-hour practice sessions with the *Fx* display, and the pattern in (a) as model.

The normal speaker has a larger range than the deaf speaker. Nevertheless, the narrower fall produced by him is perceptually satisfactory because it is in the lower half of his range. Falls produced in the upper half of the range (from high- to midlevel) are not acceptable.

Traces (d) and (e) were produced by the same deaf speaker after five lessons. They represent *Can I come with you?* and show his manipulation of contrastive stress. In (d) the falling nucleus is on *I* and in (e) it is on *you.* Trace (f) is a time marker showing 0.1 sec intervals.

inappropriate use of phonetically voiced or voiceless segments in an utterance. Time relationships are important components in the linguistic voiced—voiceless distinction, which in English is not always signalled by the simple presence or absence of phonetic voicing. Perceptually significant differences in the durations of vowels, nasals, and laterals preceding linguistically voiced or voiceless consonants can be more easily appreciated by the profoundly deaf when they have simple visual correlates. Pairs such as *built—build* can thus be kept distinct in a natural English way, instead of the member that ends in a linguistically voiced consonant appearing to the listener as a disyllabic word (in this case, *builder*), which can result if the final consonant is fully voiced phonetically. Listening to deaf speech is rather like listening to normal speech under adverse conditions. In such conditions, natural time relationships are of great importance for intelligibility, both at the level of individual sounds (Miller, 1956) and of sentence structure. It is also significant that as the deaf speaker becomes accustomed to producing more natural time and pitch patterns in his speech, his voice quality becomes smoother and less tense, and his general control of segments also improves.

Conclusion

We have described how a particular processing device that directly monitors one crucial component of speech can be used in several important ways to help the deaf acquire more natural speech. Because it is simple and reliable to use, and relatively inexpensive, we believe it may be able to make a substantial contribution in teaching and therapy. So far we have been mainly concerned with remedial work with adults, but a project is now in progress (Parker, 1974) to ascertain in what way and at what stage of language development children may best be able to benefit from the sort of information it provides.

The display we have described is the product of basic research in speech perception and production. More displays of speech information will become available as fundamental work progresses. Vocal tract information such as vowel quality will be presented visually (Lindblom & Sundberg, 1971). Electronic aids will not diminish the role of teachers or speech therapists, however. On the contrary, their effectiveness will be increased, but greater demands will be made of them as the effective use of speech processing devices in teaching and therapy depends on the teachers having a thorough knowledge of the phonetic bases of the linguistic structures of their language.

References

Anderson, F. The speech visualizer. The South African Inventions Development Corporation. Mimeographed description, 1971.
Bach-y-Rita, P. Sensory plasticity. *Acta Neurologica Scandinavica* 1967, *43*, 417—426.
Boothroyd, A. An experiment on the learning of pitch control by profoundly deaf children. SARP 5.

Clarence V. Hudgins Diagnostic and Research Center, Clarke School for the Deaf, 1971.

Boothroyd, A., & Decker, M. Concept and control of fundamental voice frequency in the deaf. SARP 4. Clarence V. Hudgins Diagnostic and Research Center, Clarke School for the Deaf, 1970.

Fabre, P. Un procédé électrique percutané d'inscription de l'accolement glottique au cours de la phonation: glottographie de haute fréquence. Premiers résultats. *Bulletin de l'Académie Nationale de Médecine, Paris*, 1957, *141*, 66—99.

Fourcin, A. J., & Abberton, E. First applications of a new laryngograph. *Medical and Biological Illustration*, 1971, *21*, 172—182. (Reprinted: *Volta Review*), 1972, 74, (No. 3), 161—176.

Fry, D. B. Experiments in the perception of stress. *Language and Speech*, 1958, *1*, 126—152.

James, E. Unpublished doctoral dissertation, University of Aix, Aix, 1971.

John, J. E. J., & Howarth, J. N. The effect of time distortions on the intelligibility of deaf children's speech. *Language and Speech*, 1965, *8*, 127—134.

Kringlebotn, M. Experiments with some vibrotactile and visual aids for the deaf. *Proceedings of the Conference on Speech-Analyzing Aids for the Deaf. American Annals of the Deaf*, 1968, *113*, 311—317.

Lindblom, B. E. F., & Sundberg, J. A quantitative theory of cardinal vowels and the teaching of pronunciation. In G. E. Perren & J. L. M. Trim (Eds.), *Applications of linguistics*. London & New York: Cambridge Univ. Press, 1971.

Mártóny, J. On the correction of the voice pitch level for severely hard of hearing subjects. *Proceedings of the Conference on Speech-Analyzing Aids for the Deaf. American Annals of the Deaf*, 1968, *113*, 195—202.

Miller, G. A. The perception of speech. In M. Halle, *et al.* (Ed.), *To honor Roman Jacobson*. The Hague: Mouton, 1956. Pp. 353—359.

Parker, Ann. The laryngograph. *Hearing*, 1974 Volume *29*, (No. 9), pp. 256—261.

Pickett, J. M. Recent research on speech-analyzing aids for the deaf. *IEEE Transactions on Audio and Electroacoustics*, 1968, *AU—16*, No. 2, 227—234.

Pronovost, W. Developments in visual dispalys of speech information. *Volta Review*, 1967, *69*, 365—373.

Risberg, A. Visual aids for speech correction. *Proceedings of the Conference on Speech-Analyzing Aids for the Deaf. American Annals of the Deaf*, 1968, *113*, 178—194.

Weir, R. H. Some questions on the child's learning of phonology. In F. Smith & G. A. Miller (Eds.), *The genesis of language*. Cambridge, Mass.: MIT Press, 1966.

White, B. W., Saunders, F. A., Scadden, L., Bach-y-Rita P., & Collins, C. C. Seeing with the skin. *Perception and Psychophysics*, 1970, 7, 23—27.

11. Congenital Deafness and the Development of Thinking[1]

Hans Furth / James Youniss

Congenital deafness is characterized as a life situation of a child growing up without being immersed in society's language. With proper methodological precautions, one can consider research with deaf children as strong evidence for a development of thinking that is not tied to linguistic knowledge. Deaf persons without a language frequently perform similarly to hearing persons with language who live in an intellectually undemanding environment. In agreement with Piaget's theory, no specific symbolic system or medium is a prerequisite for the development of preoperatory to formal thinking.

The Linguistic Background of Deaf Children

If one approaches the study of the intellectual development of the child profoundly deaf before the onset of speech, it is imperative to sketch at least in rough outline the life situation of such a child. It is understood that no "typical" deaf child ever exists. The factors to be mentioned in the following two or three paragraphs are typical in the sense that they describe important aspects in the life of the great majority of deaf children.

Most deaf children are born to hearing parents and are kept away from the adult deaf community until close to the age when they leave school and enter the world of work. In any case, the "sign language" that is used in the American deaf com-

[1]Prepared with partial support of SRS grant No. 14-P-55084, United States Department of Health, Education, and Welfare.

munity is frequently not a native language in the sense that deaf children are exposed to it during infancy. Most deaf children get to know the sign language during their teens through informal contact with deaf peers or adults. Even where there is some residual hearing, these children cannot acquire knowledge of society's language through the ear. They sometimes start formal instruction in speech as early as 3 years; by age 6 nearly all attend special schools for deaf children. The main focus in these schools, almost the only focus, one could say, at least until the quite recent past, is the teaching of language.

It is important to distinguish knowledge of language from skill in speech or speech reading, as well as from reading or writing. Fingerspelling is a skill similar to reading and writing except that the fingers form individual letters in the air instead of symbols on paper. All of these linguistic forms belong to English, whereas sign language is a codified gesture language different from English and also from spontaneous or home-made gestures. Keeping these distinctions in mind, the following statements summarize the actual condition of deaf children. Good speech reading is an extremely rare event, worthy of publicity, as is any exceptional talent. Good speech is also very rare. Good reading and writing—if one uses achievement tests indicating at least a fifth-grade reading level—is found in between 10 and 20% of deaf adults. Fingerspelling has only recently found a general use in education. Most young deaf children use gestures and pantomime at home for purposes of communication and gradually and informally pick up the American Sign Language as they have contact with deaf adults.

This, then, is the linguistic background of deaf children. Since the great majority of them never succeed in being at home in English even after many years of schooling, and since they acquire proficiency in sign language only at a relatively advanced age, it is plain that one deals here with children who, at least during the years of intellectual development, are without a language in the sense of a conventional linguistic system. This statement does not deny that deaf children produce gestural or imaginal symbols—of course, they do this spontaneously—or that they may succeed in learning English labels for objects and events or some English phrases. But what they lack is the transmission of a ready-made, complete, and all-embracing symbol system such as the language of a social group. In this respect they are uniquely different from any other group of people, and their intellectual development has to be considered in the light of this special condition, namely, the lack of an available language.

Intellectual Development of the Deaf

It is instructive to recall briefly that historically deafness was always linked to dumbness in the pejorative sense. And even in modern times, the stereotype of stupidity was only taken away when deaf persons were able to prove to society that they could learn speech. In other words, the link *speech—intelligence, speechlessness—stupidity*, seems still as strong as ever. The main difference could be that today the opportunities for fostering an exceptional talent are greater, and success is more widely broadcast than before. Scholars would hardly insist on external speech as a prerequisite of adequate intelligence, but many theories of intellectual development would readily find a crucial role for language. These theories would consider that the internalized language of society gives the child an "inner language" that lies at the base of further intellectual development. It is our contention that deaf children do not have this kind of inner language, which comes from internalization of an externally transmitted language, and that a scientific demonstration of the essential adequacy of their intellectual development seriously undermines the basis of these theories.

In order to observe indicants of intellectual development[2] in deaf children, it is of course necessary to make use of procedures that do not in themselves require linguistic knowledge; otherwise one merely demonstrates that their knowledge of English is indeed poor. A second critical question concerns the use of hearing controls. In comparison to a selected sample of hearing children, a sample of deaf children may have a higher incidence of neurological impairment, a greater degree of test anxiety, and a more heterogeneous socioeconomic background, quite apart from uncontrolled factors due to the child's and other persons' attitude towards and management of deafness. Considering all these points, one may indeed despair of ever setting up an adequate comparative research design.

Fortunately, this problem becomes crucial only when small statistical differences have to be given a reasonable explanation. When differences are so glaring that there is practically no overlap between the hearing and deaf sample, one may be justified in attributing the differences to an overall condition, present in one sample but not in the other. When there are no differences, one need only make sure that the hearing group was not sampled in a systematically biased fashion—a rather unlikely situation—and that the task itself was intellectually and developmentally meaningful, for example, that younger children perform at a lower level and older children at a higher level. If these two conditions are satisfied, one need not be overly concerned about the admitted heterogeneity of influences bearing on deaf children's performance and can conclude that the common factor of linguistic deficiency did not seriously affect performance on the experimental task.

There remains then the third possibility of finding small mean differences that are statistically significant and require a reasonable explanation. This much should be clear by now. If one hypothesizes the crucial importance of language and one further finds that in many studies deaf children perform as well as hearing controls, one cannot selectively cite studies in which deaf children perform statistically more poorly as confirmation of the initial hypothesis. On the contrary, even one relevant study of no difference is a serious counterindication for this linguistic hypothesis. Moreover, relatively small, even though significant, differences cannot be easily

---

[2]We would like to make it clear that this review is concerned with the development of logical structures (in Piaget's sense) and not with the acquisition of factual knowledge in which deaf persons are often found to be deficient.

reconciled with a supposedly necessary contribution of language. Because statistical differences do not exclude a large area of overlap, such a result would mean that most deaf children without language would still perform as well as or even better than many children with language.

Prior to 1960, the psychological literature characterized deaf people's thinking as if it resulted from a blend of brain injury and mild mental illness (cf. Myklebust, 1960). Commonly used descriptive terms were "perceptually bound," "concrete," "figure-ground confused," "suspicious," "perseverative," and "rigid." By the 1970s these characterizations have changed so that, in general, thinking in deaf children and adults can be said to be comparable to thinking in normal, hearing language users. This dramatic shift over a relatively short time can be attributed to three major factors. First, a break from the confines of strict behaviorism allowed for the possibility that thinking might be viewed apart from a mechanistic inner-language framework. Second, this philosophical liberalization encouraged psychologists to take seriously other theoretical perspectives on thinking, which, unlike the internalized language model, did not a priori rule out an adequate intellectual development for persons without language. Third, a considerable amount of research was done in this fresh milieu and data were accumulated that empirically established important points of comparability between deaf and hearing individuals.

Much of this research has been reviewed by Furth (1964, 1971), who summarized the results of 84 studies, the subjects of which ranged from preschool age to middle adulthood. Although a numerical ratio in itself is useless for a meaningful interpretation, it may be of interest to mention that the two reviews list 62 points of similar performance between the deaf and the hearing subjects, versus 44 points of difference, the latter mostly in the form of a slight but statistically significant inferiority. Since these differences are evenly spread throughout various problem areas and are not limited to narrowly defined specific tasks or age levels, it is obvious that one's theoretical perspective will always be the main determiner of the interpretation of such data. However, one is justified in making the following supposition: The same theoretical considerations that explain the slight statistical inferiority in some tasks must also make sense concerning the substantial amount of overlap and particularly the over 60 tasks in which no differences at all were observed.

How can one explain the fact that young deaf children, from age 3 to age 9, perform similarly to hearing children on simple tasks of discovery, shift, and transfer of rules (Blank & Bridges, 1966; Pufall & Furth, 1966; Weigl & Metze, 1968, Youniss, 1964)...? Success on these tasks has been traditionally related to strategies of using verbal mediators. With hearing children one may be inclined to attribute to society's language the determining factor for the presence of mediating strategies. But the performance of deaf children throws a different light on the role of these symbolic mediators. If symbols are required to succeed on the task, then for the source of these symbols one must look not to an external language that supplies them as ready-made working entities, but to the developing intelligence of the child who produces them as they are needed. Success on these tasks may very well involve the coding of certain rules in a symbolic medium, whether verbal, visual, or gestural. The remarkable fact is that children without linguistic skills do seem to make use of whatever symbolic instruments are required in the service of thinking. This illustrates strikingly that symbols are basically produced by the thinking person and used according to his available thinking skills. No radical distinction between verbal and other symbols is indicated. That is, just as the existence and the use of private symbols by deaf children argues for an internal source, similarly the use of verbal symbols by hearing children must be subordinate to the thinking of the children, even though the existence of the symbols derives from an external source. In this perspective, no symbols in themselves, verbal or otherwise, can explain thinking.

We studied somewhat older deaf children at the "concrete operatory" level. By definition, in concrete operations children apply operative schemes, which comprise a self-consistent logical system, to physical objects or events (perceived or imagined). A viewpoint that considers a linguistic system as the basis of the schemes would put the deaf child at a distinct disadvantage.

Since deaf children cannot easily be interviewed and asked to offer adequate justifications for their performance, we designed tasks where a given event was being transformed radically from its perceptible starting point. In these situations the figurative aspect of the perceptual situation or of the symbolic medium did not directly facilitate operative understanding. Moreover, the design of the tasks required the child to display his operatory skill across logically equivalent but physically varying situations. It can be presumed that the child who succeeds in one situation and, further, maintains this success across varying situations is effectively subordinating figurative variations to stable operative structures. At the same time, mixed performance is also instructive, since it can show which situational variations produce decrements, hence which strategies of reasoning the child is employing. The experimental procedure also included a correction phase and retest. Thus it allowed for a qualitative comparison between deaf and hearing subjects, rather than merely yielding a gross pass—fail quantitative evaluation.

Our work on children's anticipatory visual imagery, patterned after the mental image studies of Piaget and Inhelder (1966), illustrates the procedure. After an initial response to a visually presented object, the child was asked to imagine seven figurative transformations of the object. When the child had completed this request, he was exposed to correction by presentation of four rotated positions. Finally the child made a second attempt at indicating all eight positions.

Four imagery problems were studied in two experiments. For *horizontality* the child was shown colored liquid in a square bottle and asked to draw the liquid on a paper showing the bottle's outline. Next, the bottle was covered with a sock and rotated to the right 45°, 90°, 135°, and so on, up to 235°. Each time the child was to draw the liquid on a paper on which an outline of the bottle was shown in the specific rotated position. For *shadow projection*, a rod was presented between an artist's easel and a light source. When the light source was removed, the rod was rotated in the vertical plane 30°, 60°, then 90°, and in the horizontal plane 30°, 60°, and 90°. Each time the child was to draw a line on the artist's pad to represent the projected shadow.

Results from these two problems, more fully described in Robertson and Youniss (1969), were quite systematic: (1) children of ages 11 and 12 were better than children of age, 8 and 9; (2) the performance of deaf children was indistinguishable from that of their hearing peers; and (3) performance differences within age groups were systematically related to the physical dimensions of transformation. The figurative-perceptual component strongly influenced the operative component of the child's performance, and this influence was similar in hearing and in deaf subjects.

This pattern of results was replicated on two other imagery problems (Youniss & Robertson, 1970). For *perspective*, the child was seated before a three-object scene on a table top. As the experimenter moved from the child's perspective (0°) around to 45° left, the child had to select the photograph representing the experimenter's perspective. As in previous problems, all children did worse with greater angular transformations, the younger more than the older children. Here also, with one exception, the deaf were remarkably similar to hearing children. The younger deaf children were qualitatively similar but quantitavely inferior, particularly in not benefitting from corrective input. For *rotation*, a child had to indicate the relative position of two squares as one was rotated in 45° steps around the other fixed square. The performances of the two samples were substantially similar.

A first consideration shows that hearing and deaf groups had the same systematic error source and broke out of this pattern to achieve full operativity at about the same age. Once an object was removed from view and rotations were performed by the experimenter, the child was of course free to imagine that the object had taken any one of several possible positions. Nonetheless, the typical error source for *perspective* was the "egocentric" choice, the child's own perspective; for *rotation*, it was imagining the movable square in a diagonal rather than a vertical or horizontal position. With *horizontality*, subjects failed predominantly by imagining the water level to be parallel with the base of the bottle, and many children who were correct on other positions made this "parallel" error with the bottle in a diagonal orientation.

Second, detailed analyses of results indicated that performances varied systematically as a function of the figurative input. The systematic changes observed in the hearing samples applied also to the deaf samples. Third, there was the expected improvement with increasing age: Children with more developed concrete operations could maintain operative control over a wider range of figurative situations. These three considerations taken together show more than a gross similarity between deaf and hearing children on tasks that Piaget considers characteristic of the latter part of the concrete operatory stage.

In another experiment, deaf and hearing youngsters, ages 11—15 were evaluated on probability concepts (Ross, 1966). There were some slight differences favoring hearing children at the younger ages. But the most remarkable fact was the qualitative communality of probability behavior in several aspects: sensitivity to different ratios in odds, sure-thing predictions that were mainly determined by keeping track of the changing ratios, sex differences favoring boys, inappropriate alternation tendencies. On all these counts these two groups, with radically different linguistic experiences, were indistinguishable. As a consequence of such studies one is justified in concluding that the development of operative structures up to this stage proceeds substantially along normally expected lines, largely unaffected by the absence of language.

Deaf children were found to lag behind hearing controls on a number of discovery studies. One of these studies (Furth & Youniss, 1965) dealt with logical concepts of affirmation, negation, conjunction, and disjunction. Deaf adolescents, 16-years old, were still far behind 10-year-old hearing youngsters in discovering the logical meaning of symbols. The procedure required matching of written symbolic expressions against drawings of an instance. Subsequently this discovery task was administered as a task of comprehension and use. After clearly demonstrating the meaning of the basic symbols and some preliminary practice to insure comprehension of the instructions—which is always a problem with deaf persons—a transfer task was presented with a complex set of potentially confusing instances. On this task of symbol use the same deaf adolescents who had failed on symbol discovery performed very similarly to a group of hearing adults.

This result so far indicates an interesting distinction between two types of cognitive tasks. Possible reasons for deaf children's failure on discovery tasks can be advanced from points mentioned in the introduction. A subsequent investigation delved more deeply into underlying causes for those occasional failures. We tested a sample of hearing adolescents from a rural environment and discovered a performance pattern almost identical to the deaf sample: failure on symbol discovery, success on symbol use. A number of other studies also reported similarities in terms of relatively low performance levels with hearing youngsters from a cognitively impoverished environment. This was particularly notable in tasks of conservation of liquid (Furth, 1966) and more complex logical symbols (Youniss, Furth & Ross, 1971). All these facts confirm a general hypothesis that links the slightly retarded performance level of deaf children to a general deficiency in experience rather than to the specific lack of language. The implication of this hypothesis points to a misplaced emphasis in the early education of deaf and of many hearing youngsters, namely the traditional stress on language and reading and an almost total neglect of intellectually challenging activities of which elementary school children are psychologically most in need (Furth, 1970, 1973).

Moreover, the conservation task well illustrates the need for a critical and cautious interpretation of isolated failures. As reported in greater detail in Furth (1973), Oléron and Herren (1961) and Furth (1966) found 0% success for deaf children below age 11, but a change in procedure resulted in 25% success. This same modification produced 67% success in 11-year-old deaf children, whereas Oléron and Herren (1961) reported only 20% and Furth (1966) 45% success for 12- to 14 years, and in this respect make more sense than the 5—10 years retardation implied by the earlier studies. Agreement with this interpretation and the hypothesis of an experiential deficiency is given by conservation experiments with hearing rural children who also showed a 2-year lag.

These remarks form a fitting introduction to our final topic—the deaf person's functioning on formal propositional reasoning. Piaget (1972) suggests that formal thinking is particularly sensitive to the prevailing intellectual atmosphere and may only become manifest on the basis of a specialized interest and commitment. Since we were interested primarily in "average" deaf adults, we selected for our investigation not the few who were scholastically successful, but those adolescents who after many years of schooling still had a reading level below grade four. Thus proficiency in English could not be taken seriously as a contributing factor in success.

In our most recent investigation, patterned after two others published elsewhere (Furth & Youniss, 1969, 1971), we selected 10 deaf adolescents. After 5 weeks' training in the use of logical symbols, 6 of our deaf subjects gave an almost errorless performance that included comprehension of negated conjunction and disjunction, conjunction and disjunction of two negations, and implication. Two of these six "logicians" were exceedingly poor in English, not able to reach a reading level of third grade. Additionally, we observed that neither of these two young men could use the sign language at the level required to comprehend a formal lecture. A follow-up testing with changed symbols 1 year later indicated that after a 40-min warm-up session, 4 of the 6 deaf adolescents made from 0—5 errors on 48 conjunctive and disjunctive problems. Here, as on other tasks, there is every reason to believe that our attempts to elicit formal reasoning and communication were a new type of experience for these deaf persons. Under such conditions hearing persons would probably have similar difficulties. These deaf adolescents were also tested on a number of other tasks that relate to formal thinking, such as complex probability and permutations. On the permutation task it was particularly instructive to observe how seven adolescents literally discovered an adequate combinatorial method as they worked on the task under the eyes of the experimenter.

From evidence reported in Furth and Youniss (1971) and in the literature, one can gather that regarding formal operations, deaf people are again in a position not unlike hearing people from an impoverished social environment. Language as such does not seem to be the crucial issue. If culture and life habits do not generally foster attitudes of curiosity and intelligent initiative, formal thinking is not as likely to occur as in a more favorable environment. Our experimental results would, at least, indicate that absence of language is no absolute barrier to the manifestation of some forms of formal operations. The findings of social scientists who surveyed the personal and social life in the deaf community (Furth, 1973) provide corroborating evidence for the presence of adequate intellectual and personality structures in the average deaf adult.

A word should finally be said about attempts to investigate the coding mechanism of deaf persons. Although some interesting possibilities have been investigated in color coding (Lantz & Lenneberg, 1966), letter coding (Conrad, 1970), and word coding (Youniss, Feil & Furth, 1965), no really far-reaching differences have yet been observed on this intriguing question of "What do deaf persons think *in?*" In any case, from the available evidence and our theoretical perspective we hold that the person's thinking mechanisms determine the value of a particular symbol. What counts is not the figurative medium of symbols, but the available thinking mechanisms and the manner in which the person uses the symbols in the service of these mechanisms.

In conclusion, it seems that notwithstanding the tremendous importance of the linguistic medium for the adult mind and human society in general, its absence in the developing individual does not in itself lead to serious intellectual short-comings. The spontaneous production of symbolic instruments is indeed the most striking aspect of the intellectual development of deaf children; it powerfully illustrates the subordinate role of all symbols in the developing structures of thinking. Occasional failures in comparison with hearing controls can reasonably be attributed to a general experiential deficiency that many deaf children share with hearing children from cognitively impoverished backgrounds. In this sense, deaf children's linguistic deficiencies contribute, at most, indirectly to a slight retardation; otherwise, up to and including the period of concrete operations, intellectual progress is remarkably normal both in gross performance levels and in detailed aspects of intellectual functioning.

The impact of early linguistic deficiency on the formal thinking of deaf adults is hard to evaluate, if only because its prevalence and rate in differing hearing populations is not well documented. In contrast to earlier stages, formal thinking focuses on aspects of reality that can be articulated only in a linguistic system; it is also more sensitive to the challenges and interests of the environment. On both counts deaf adults may be at a disadvantage in comparison with selected hearing persons. However, the evidence now available demonstrates that with no adequate knowledge of the language of society and only limited use of a gestural language, some individual deaf adolescents can function on a formal level.

References

Blank, M., & Bridger, W. H. Conceptual cross-modal transfer in deaf and hearing children. *Child Development,* 1966, *37,* 29—38.

Conrad, R. Short-term memory processes in the deaf. *British Journal of Psychology,* 1970, *61,* 179—194.

Furth, H. G. Research with the deaf: Implications for language and cognition. *Psychological Bulletin,* 1964, *62,* 145—164.

Furth, H. G. *Thinking without language: Psychological implications of deafness.* New York: Free Press, 1966.

Furth, H. G. *Piaget for teachers.* Englewood Cliffs, N.J.: Prentice-Hall, 1970.

Furth, H. G. Linguistic deficiency and thinking: Research with deaf subjects 1964—1969. *Psychological Bulletin,* 1971, *76,* 58—72.

Furth, H. G. *Deafness and learning: A psychosocial approach.* Belmont, Calif.: Wadsworth, 1973.

Furth, H. G., & Youniss, J. The influence of language and experience on discovery and use of logical symbols. *British Journal of Pscyhology,* 1965, *56,* 381—390.

Furth, H. G. , & Youniss, J. Thinking in deaf adolescents: Language and formal operations. *Journal of Communication Disorders,* 1969, *2,* 195—202.

Furth, H. G., & Youniss, J. Formal operations and language: A comparison of deaf and hearing adolescents. *International Journal of Psychology*, 1971, *6*, 49—64.

Lantz, D., & Lenneberg, E. H. Verbal communication and color memory in the deaf and hearing. *Child Development*, 1966, *37*, 765—780.

Myklebust, H. R. *The psychology of deafness: Sensory deprivation, learning and adjustment*. New York: Grune & Stratton, 1966.

Oléron, P., & Herren, H. L'acquisition des conservations et le langage: Etude comparative sur des enfants sourds et entendants. *Enfance*, 1961, *14*, 203—219.

Piaget, J. Intellectual evolution from adolescence to adulthood. *Human Development*, 1972, *15*, 1—12.

Piaget, J., & Inhelder, B. *L'image mentale chez l'enfant*. Paris: Presses Universitaires de France, 1966.

Pufall, P., & Furth, H. G. Double alternation behavior as a function of age and language. *Child Development*, 1966, *37*, 653—662.

Robertson, A., & Youniss, J. Anticipatory visual imagery in deaf and hearing children. *Child Development*, 1969, *40*, 123—135.

Ross, B. M. Probability concepts in deaf and hearing children. *Child Development*, 1966, *37*, 917—928.

Weigl, E., & Metze, E. Experimentelle Untersuchungen zum Problem des nicht sprachgebundenen begrifflichen Denkens. *Schweizerische Zeitschrift für Psychologie*, 1968, *27*, 1—17.

Youniss, J. Concept transfer as a function of shifts, age, and deafness. *Child Development*, 1964, *35*, 695—700.

Youniss, J., Feil. R. N., & Furth, H. G. Discrimination of verbal material as a function of intrapair similarity in deaf and hearing subjects. *Journal of Educational Psychology*, 1965, *56*, 184—190.

Youniss, J., Furth, H. G., & Ross, B. M. Logical symbol use in deaf and hearing children and adolescents. *Developmental Psychology*, 1971, *5*, 511—517.

Youniss, J., & Robertson, A. Projective visual imagery as a function of age and deafness. *Child Development*, 1970, *41*, 215—225.

12. Self-Representation in Language and Play: Observations of Blind Children

Selma Fraiberg / Edna Adelson

In longitudinal studies of children blind from birth we observed striking delays in the acquisition of *I* as a stable pronoun, in spite of adequacy in early language development. Similar delays in the use of imaginative play by these same children suggest that the acquisition of personal pronouns is closely united with the capacity for symbolic representation of the self and that vision normally plays a central facilitating role in each of these achievements. One case is presented to demonstrate how a form of the self is externalized and the self as object reconstituted.

Introduction

Among children blind from birth there is typically a delay in the acquisition of *I* as a stable pronoun. The meaning of this characteristic has been necessarily obscured because of the heterogeneous population usually designated as "blind," one that includes children with damage to other systems, as well as children with minimal vision and those blinded postnatally.

In our longitudinal studies[1] of the early ego development of blind children, we have followed 10 children, blind from birth. The children in this sample are, to the best of our knowledge, free of any other sensory or motor handicap and are neurologically intact. Babies admitted to the research program were totally blind or had

[1]The research program was supported by the National Institutes of Child Health and Development (Grant # HDO1-444). The intervention program was supported by the Office of Education (Grant # OEG-0-9-322108-246(032)).

light perception only. A concurrent guidance program was provided for all babies in this group.

Our group is advantaged, then, within a blind population by the intactness of other systems and by a guidance program that has facilitated development. They are disadvantaged in comparison with the general population of blind children by their total or near total blindness and blindness from birth. Both the selection process and the guidance program have enabled us to examine the developmental characteristics of blind infants and young children under the most favorable circumstances.[2]

All of the children in this group were followed by means of biweekly home visits from the first year through age $2\frac{1}{2}$. Four of the older children were available for continued study through the age of 5 years. The opportunity for continued study of these children was fortunate. In this advantaged group of blind children, we saw delays in the achievement of *I* as a stable pronoun and a concomitant delay in the representation of the self in imaginative play. As we analyzed the descriptive protocols and reviewed the videotape samples, we began to achieve some insight into the interlocking components of self-representation in language and play and to follow the extraordinary problems for the blind child in constructing an image of self and a concept of an objective self.

In this essay we propose to examine the relationship between the blind child's acquisition of *I* as a correct grammatical form and the correlates of *I* in representation of the self in play. We have selected one of the four older children, Kathie, as the subject of detailed study.

I/Me Usage in Four Blind Children

The four blind children who were available for continued study to the age of 5 years included three who were in the upper half of our group on most measures and one who placed in the lower half of the group.

Jackie, who consistently ranked in the lower half of our group, had not achieved *I* when last seen at 5 years of age. At $2\frac{1}{2}$ years of age his language achievements placed him in the lowest rank in our group of 10. The failure to achieve *I* was also a measure of his impaired ego development. Jackie presented a picture of a disordered personality with frequent regression to echolalic speech. We include this brief description of Jackie, who had no *I* at age 5, because he fairly represents the large number of ineducable blind children who do not achieve *I* or *me* even at school age or later. In Jackie's case, and others known to us, there was no evidence of neurological impairment, and one can fairly consider an alternative explanation for this form of deviant ego development: that blindness imposes extraordinary

---

[2]For two reports of the findings see Fraiberg (1968) and Fraiberg (1975). The intervention program is described in Fraiberg, Smith, and Adelson (1969) and Fraiberg (1971a).

impediments in the development of a self-image and the construction of a coherent sense of self.

The remaining three children in the older group all achieved *I*. Kathie, Paul, and Karen ranked in the upper half of our group on nearly all measures. Their language achievements at age $2-2\frac{1}{2}$ (judged by vocabulary, two-word combinations, and the use of words to make needs known) fell within the sighted age range. A syncretic *I* (*Iwanna*) appeared in their language records in this same age range, which again does not distinguish them from sighted children.

From this developmental picture in the language area, we would have predicted an unremarkable course, leading within a few months to a stable concept of *I* and versatility in the use of *I*. We were not prepared for our findings. The ages for the achievement of the nonsyncretic *I* for these three children were as follows: Karen, 2 years 11 months; Paul, 3 years 5 months; Kathie, 4 years 10 months.

The differentiation of a *syncretic I* from a *nonsyncretic I* follows Zazzo's usage (Zazzo, 1948). The syncretic *I* typically appears in the 2-year old's vocabulary embedded in verb forms of need or want. In the course of weeks or months *I* is gradually disengaged from this early set and is used inventively in new combinations. The two levels of *I* represent two levels of self-representation. The achievement of the nonsyncretic *I* requires a high level of inference on the part of the child in which he demonstrates his capacity to represent himself as an *I* in a universe of *I* s. (*I am an* **I** *to me; you are an* **I** *to you; he is an* **I** *to him,* etc.)

We credited the children with the achievement of a nonsyncretic *I* when these criteria were met: (1) *I* used inventively in new combinations (disengaged from set phrases); (2) *I* employed with versatility in discourse (management of *I* and *you* with rare or no confusion or reversals). It is of some interest that although these criteria were met by the three children at the ages given above, both Paul and Kathie had occasional lapses in *I—you* usage for many months afterward.

While the achievement of stable *I* usage impresses us as markedly delayed in these blind children, comparisons with sighted children cannot be fairly made through the use of any existing measures. There are no normative data for the achievement of the nonsyncretic *I* in sighted children. Gesell, who offers the only developmental scale that includes personal pronoun usage, does not discriminate between the syncretic and the nonsyncretic *I* (Gesell & Amatruda, 1947). He scores pronoun usage on two levels: at 24 months he credits the child with the pronouns *I, me,* and *you*—"not necessarily correctly"; at 30 months the child receives credit when he "refers to self by pronoun rather than name. May confuse 'I' and 'me.'" Gesell accepted parent reports for his language items, and his scoring, as cited, does not discriminate for our purposes the cognitive values of I.[3]

In the absence of comparative measures in standard developmental tests for sighted children, we cannot pursue some of the problems of apparent difference

[3]The primary source of data for our research group was naturalistic observation in the home, recorded as objective narrative description and documented on film or videotape. Parent report was a secondary source and will be indicated when used.

between the range for achievement of a stable *I* in three otherwise healthy and adequate blind children and that of sighted children. Yet the differences, on any level of comparison we can borrow, impose themselves upon us. If three blind children demonstrate language competence at the age of $2-2\frac{1}{2}$ years that can be objectively rated as normal for sighted children, if the syncretic *I* appears as a grammatical form in the range for sighted children, how can we explain a developmental course that detours in the middle of the third year and comes back on the sighted child's route in the fourth or fifth years? Were the apparently "very late" achievers of *I* (Kathie and Paul) cognitively impaired? Was Karen, the earliest achiever of *I*, the smartest in the group? Here again, all expectations and reasonable predictions come undone as strangely as the blind child's pronoun usage. At age $2\frac{1}{2}$ Kathie and Paul were among 3 highest ranking children in our group of 10 both in language achievements and in overall developmental achievements. Kathie's good intelligence will speak for itself in the history we present later. Paul, at 5 years, had a command of language and a capacity for abstract thinking that impressed us as superior even by sighted child standards. Karen, the "first achiever" of *I* was a very adequate blind child; her language and cognitive capacities at 5 years were good, but they did not equal those of Kathie and Paul. We are not able to explain this puzzle.

While we watched the protracted struggle with pronoun usage, another piece of the puzzle was emerging from the patterns of play we had observed and recorded.

At the age when sighted children begin to *imitate* domestic life in doll play (approximately 2 years), we find no such examples for the blind children in our group. If we tried to elicit such play—*Let's give the dolly her bottle, Let's put her to bed*—we got no response, not even mechanical compliance. In some instances there were other infants in the house being mothered, or other children in the family playing with dolls. Models were available but were not used.

Again, at age $2\frac{1}{2}$, when sighted children begin to *represent* themselves and their world in play, endowing the doll with a personality and an imaginary life, our blind children could neither represent themselves or other personalities nor invent in play.

Between the ages of 3 and $4\frac{1}{2}$ years we began to see imaginative play emerge in the records of Karen, Paul, and Kathie. In each case the emergence of representational play had correspondence with the emergence of the self-reference pronouns *me* and *I*. The data invited close scrutiny. They suggested that the acquisition of personal pronouns was closely united with the capacity for symbolic representation of the self, and that vision normally plays a central facilitating role in each of these achievements.

After we worked our way through this thicket we discovered that René Zazzo had arrived there by another route in his study of a sighted child. His observations on Jean-Fabien, which will be summarized in the last section of this paper, were most welcome; they provide another framework in which to place our detailed observations of Kathie as she pursued an elusive *I* between the ages of 2 and 5.

Kathie's Progress

Kathie has been followed by us since she was 9 months of age; she is now 6-years old. She is totally blind. Kathie was 3 months premature. The diagnosis, retrolental fibroplasia, was made at 5 months of age. She is a healthy, very bright child with no other sensory defects and is neurologically intact.

Kathie is the youngest of five siblings. Her parents have shown extraordinary ability to empathize with a blind child's experience, and every help that parents and our staff specialists could give has been available to promote the fullest use of her good capacities.[4]

Now, at 6 years of age, she has excellent command of language; she is inventive in imaginative play; she is well behaved but also mischievous and fun-loving. She is in the first grade in a classroom for sighted children and holds her own. She has considerable appetite for new experience. She enjoys cooperative play. She is independent in dressing and feeding. She is fully responsible for her own safety in outdoor play.

The story of Kathie's language and representational intelligence followed a different route from that of the sighted child. In the absence of pictorial memory, there were delays in the evolving forms of mental representation, the concepts of time and causality, self-representation, and the construction of a world of permanent objects. Yet, a simple vocabulary count and identification of word and thing or an analysis of phrase and sentence patterns would not have distinguished her speech at the age of 2 years from that of sighted children. It was between the ages of 2 years and 4 years that the study of Kathie's speech and play gave us a slow-motion picture of the relationship of language to other cognitive processes and thus provided the means for identifying those elements in self-object representation that are dependent upon a coherent and intact sensorimotor organization.

OBSERVATIONS AT 2 YEARS OF AGE

When Kathie was 2 years, 1 month old, she became the subject of a linguistic study conducted by Eric Lenneberg with our staff. Speech samples were obtained in home visits and Dr. Lenneberg and Nancy Stein of our staff worked out a dictionary: "What does Kathie *mean* when she *says*. . .?" Following a 3-month study, Dr. Lenneberg felt that Kathie's language competence compared favorably with that of the sighted child of the same age. Her vocabulary at that time was well within the range for sighted children. She correctly identified members of her family and a number of people outside of the family. She identified by touch or sound and named all the objects in her home with which she had contact. She quickly learned

---

[4]For the story of this family see Ulrich, S., *Elizabeth*, (Introduction by S. Fraiberg, Commentary by E. Adelson), Ann Arbor: University of Michigan Press, 1972.

the names of novel objects brought by us. She had four- or five-word phrases in which present tense verb forms were embedded, but not yet used inventively in new combinations.

She could express her wishes in phrases. Here are a few samples: *Wanna hear a record, Wanna go walkie, Wanna go lie down, Wanna hear music, Want to feel, . . . What's that?* (confronted with a novel object).

She had a range of useful words for the expression of affective experience. *Feels good! Tastes good.* And the dictionary records that she used the words *damn* and *shit* when she was angry.

She employed parental admonitions to inhibit forbidden actions. *Don't put your finger in your eye,* she said to herself, imitating her mother's voice when she pressed her eye, and sometimes succeeded in inhibiting the act. *Hot!* she said, to warn herself when near the stove.

There were examples of generalization in our records. At Christmas time, when we brought her a toy-sized Christmas tree, she explored its plastic bristles thoughtfully and said, *Feels like a brush!* She could identify a chair and name it, and generalize from chair to chair.

We heard pronoun reversal and pronoun confusion in nearly all the speech samples we have from this period. When she touched the hair of one of the observers, she said, *My hair,* using the wrong pronoun. *Want me carry you?* she said to her mother when she meant that she wanted her mother to carry her. The pronoun *I* was rarely used and, typically, appeared as a syncretic form *Ahwonna* or as an *I, you* reversal. However, at this early age, 2 years, the pronoun reversals and the unstable use of *I* do not distinguish Kathie from *sighted* children.

In Dr. Lenneberg's unpublished notes he records one item that puzzled him. "All attempts to make her listen to short stories (while sitting on laps and being quiet) have failed." In a summary statement he draws attention to the disinterest in stories as being one factor that points to "a somewhat different language beginning from that found in sighted children." As it turns out (in retrospect), this puzzle was already one of the clues to certain incapacities in symbolic representation that were later to be of considerable interest in our study of blind children.

Dr. Lenneberg moved to Cornell and had no opportunity to follow Kathie's language development beyond the age of 2 years, 3 months. When we now report further developments in Kathie's language history, we will find much that interests us from a developmental point of view, but we will also miss much that Dr. Lenneberg would have brought us from linguistics.

OBSERVATIONS AT 3 YEARS OF AGE

Between the ages of $2\frac{1}{2}$ and 3 years, we became aware that Kathie's language and her capacity to represent showed marked deviations from those of the sighted child. In both our detailed home observations and in the reports of her mother, it was very clear that Kathie could not represent herself through a doll or toy. She could not recreate or invent a situation in play. She could not attend to a story or answer questions regarding a story or tell a story herself. She could not spontaneously report an experience. And still, between the ages of 3 and 4, she continued to confuse and reverse pronouns, and the concept of *I* had not emerged as a stable grammatical form.

To illustrate the problem, we shall present some of our own observations of Kathie at the age of 3. In a later section, we will bring in observations at 4 years of age.

When Kathie was 3 years, 23 days, we arranged for her to visit us in our nursery. The nursery visits had been a special treat for Kathie in preceding months. Since we already knew from home observations that Kathie could not invent in play or represent herself in play, we sketched an observational plan and procedures that would tell us more precisely where the incapacities lay and what her limits might be.

We worked out a group of experimental play situations that would permit us to compare a blind child's capacity to represent herself in play with that of a sighted child. We were satisfied that the "pretend" games we had in mind could be played with any sighted child between the ages of 18 months and 2 years, giving much leeway for 3-year-old Kathie.

In order not to strain Kathie's tolerance, we moved freely between structured play periods and unstructured "free play intervals." In the 1-hr observational period that was recorded verbatim and documented on 16 mm film, the structured portions of the observation totalled 20 min. This gave us a balance between the two modes of observation, which favored the spontaneous productions and would permit us to fairly assess Kathie's play capacities and language. Kathie's mother was present throughout.

When we now present material from this play session, it is important to keep in mind that we already knew Kathie's play incapacities from naturalistic observations in her home, and that the purpose of the structured play observations was to get more precise information regarding the level of symbolic representation available to this bright, 3-year-old blind child. When S.F. pursued certain elements in play, though it was clear that Kathie could not follow her, it was because we needed the negative demonstration as much as the positive demonstration, both for this period of observation and for our projected retest at 4 years.

S. F. was not a familiar person to Kathie and gave her a good deal of time to greet old friends at the Project, to get accustomed to a new voice, and to begin some verbal exchanges. When Kathie seemed at ease and came close to S. F. at the work table, S. F. hinted that there was something on it. Kathie came over, sniffed, and said, pleasantly surprised, *Play dough.* S. F. waited to see what Kathie would do. She squeezed it, handled it, put it down. When it was evident that she would not invent with the play dough, S. F. suggested they make a cookie and guided Kathie's hands with the cookie cutter. Kathie was interested but did not extend the possibilities. Later, to test her notions of "pretend," S. F. asked, "Can *I* have a bite of the cookie, Kathie?" Kathie, clearly confused but amiable, said, **You** *have a bite!* and put it in *her own* mouth. Kathie said, reflectively, *This cookie different.*

Because of the confusion in *me* and *you* elicited in this sequence, we used a later occasion to test facial analogies. S. F. asked, "Where is *my* mouth, Kathie? There was no response to *my mouth*, but Kathie's hand moved to *her own* mouth. S. F.: "Where is *my* nose?" She made no effort. (Neither E. A. nor Kathie's mother had been able to get Kathie to name parts on their faces correctly if they used the pronoun *my*, i.e., in the question *Where is* **my** *nose?* If Kathie's mother asked, *Where is Mommy's nose?* she could "respond correctly.")

Knowing how much Kathie lover her own bath at home, we had sketched out a sequence for doll play. There was a basin of water, a doll, a towel. S. F. brought over one of our dolls and suggested giving the dolly a bath. (We knew, however, that Kathie had no interest in her dolls at home.) S. F. introduced the doll to Kathie, who gave it a few cursory touches and was clearly not interested. S. F. tried to elicit interest. "Where is the *dolly's* mouth?" —no answer. "Where is the *dolly's* nose?" —no answer. We were unable to get a demonstration when we played this game with other blind children of Kathie's age. Clearly, Kathie could not endow the doll with human characteristics either.

Kathie made it clear she did not want to give that baby a bath, but we were not prepared for the bath that took place within a few moments. As soon as Kathie touched the water, she herself stepped into the tiny tub, giving S. F. only a second to remove her new red shoes. She curled up in the tiny tub, legs folded up, and made joyful screeches. Then followed a series of little chants and songs, her own bathtub songs at home.

After several minutes of splashing and singing, S. F. decided to take a chance on reintroducing the doll. She suggested washing the dolly's hair (guiding Kathie's hands to the doll's hair.) She even went through a performance in which, representing the doll, she squealed protests and said, *No, no, I don't want a shampoo.* Kathie did not pick up the game, but now she did something else.

As Kathie squatted in the tub, pushing herself up and down in the water, she began to carry on a dialogue in two voices: *Swimming in the water Mama look at that! Whee, whee Can you feel it? Okay, you stay in the water. Okay, you sit down in the water.* Very clearly, one voice in this speech belonged to Kathie and one voice to her mother, bathing Kathie.

Before drawing inferences from this last anecdote, let us give a second set of very similar observations.

Later in the session, Kathie was walking around the room when she discovered the sink in the nursery. We did not tell her what it was. She climbed in and examined the sides and faucets with her fingers. One of us said, "What is *it*?" and, after a moment, she said, firmly, *It's a sink!* Kathie curled up inside it. She was unmistakably pretending that the sink was a bed and said, in a mother's intonation, *Night-night, have good sleep, night-night. Go sleep in the sink.* She closed her eyes, then opened them mischievously, and went through the whole routine again, with some variation. *Right here. You be a good girl!* Once S. F. tried to extend the game by saying, "Good morning *Kathie!*" Kathie, not to be distracted, said, *See you in the morning, good night. Then go in pool.* (Echo phrases—apparently her schedule for summer.)

Obviously, then, Kathie could "pretend" when she herself was the subject. Could she pretend now with a doll? It was doubtful, but S. F. brought over the doll for an experimental demonstration. She said, "The *dolly* wants to go to sleep. Let's put the *dolly* to bed." She gave the doll to Kathie. Without any ceremony Kathie dropped the doll over the side of the sink and pursued her own game.

In these last two examples (and others we have from this and other sessions), it is very clear that Kathie had a form of "pretend" in which she could take herself as object and play "subject and object" in a game. But she could not yet move beyond to the further objectivation (actually *projection*) that would permit the doll to represent Kathie, while Kathie herself represented her mother to that doll.

Note, too, how important it is for her to get *into* the basin, to put herself *into* the sink for "pretend." Where a sighted child would be able to *imagine* herself in the basin, the sink, and so forth, and then also to *imagine* her doll as herself in the basin and the sink, Kathie is still obliged "to go through the motions," to transpose through action that which would be transposed through vision. We must re- member, of course, that sighted children in nursery school also enjoy fitting them- selves into the doll bed or the doll carriage, but by this age they can move flexibly between such egocentric play to representational play, sometimes placing the doll, sometimes themselves, in the bed and the carriage.

Along with these failures in self-representation, we see throughout this session, even in this condensed form, that *I* and *you* are not yet used correctly, which ties in with observations in which subject and object pronouns are confused in com- prehension as in following the directions for the game "Where's *my* nose? Where's *your* nose?" The pronouns do not yet define subject and object, which may indicate the level of Kathie's conceptual development; she cannot yet see herself as an object to others. She is indisputably *Kathie* to herself and to others, and her mother is *Mommy*, but she cannot assimilate the semantic ambiguity in which she is a *you* to others and they are a *you* to her. The same ambiguity bedevils her in comprehending *me* and *my* usage in the "Where's *my* nose? Where's *your* nose?" game. Yet she could correctly identify facial parts by pointing if the questioner used the form "Where is *Mommy's* nose? Where is *Mrs. Adelson's* nose? Where is *Kathie's* nose?"

From the protocols of this session and home visits during this period we do not yet have an example of *me* usage in self-reference. Typically, when Kathie wanted something she would say, *Give it to her!* in the echo form.

The first example of *me* in self-reference (not echo or reversal) occurs at 3 years, 6 months, and the context happens to catch exactly a transition point. Kathie's mother called her in the midst of play. Kathie was clearly annoyed at the interrup- tion. She roared at her mother, *You leave her alone!* Then, shortly afterwards, *Leave* **me** *alone!*

The question should be raised of whether Kathie's performance in the nursery would have been more fairly tested if the play sequences had been undertaken by one of her old friends on the staff, or her mother. To test this possibility, we invited Kathie and her parents to another play session 4 months later and recorded the visit on videotape. This time E.A., a familiar person, took over some of the play sequences, and we also involved the mother in a "Where's *my* nose? Where's *your* nose?" game. Even under these most favorable circumstances, the limits of Kathie's performance remained the same.

Now we would like to suggest that the observations on subject and object in play and the problem of expressing subject and object in language have a unified core in the capacity for a certain level of mental representation. The capacity to represent oneself in play is a measure of the level of conceptual development in which the self can be taken as an object and other objects can be used for symbolic representation of the self (Piaget, 1952). Kathie's play incapacities at 3 years were exactly mirrored in speech, in her pronoun reversals and in her difficulties in achieving *I* as a stable concept and a stable grammatical form. Yet, this child at the age of 3 years had a rich vocabulary, if we make allowances for the restricted experience of a blind child, and her syntax did not jar the ear until we examined the sentences in which pronoun usage governed order and coherence. She was not retarded or in danger of autistic development.

Let us now observe Kathie between the ages of 4 and 5, as Evelyn B. Atreya and E.A. continued to follow her progress.

OBSERVATIONS AT 4 AND 5 YEARS OF AGE

Between the ages of 4 and 5, Kathie began to represent herself in doll play and, in a parallel development, we also began to see new complexities in syntax, a stabilization of pronoun usage and, finally, the emergence of *I* as a concept and a grammatical form.

At age $4\frac{1}{2}$ years, we got observations in doll play that parallelled, in all significant ways, the doll play of sighted children between the ages 2 and 3. Kathie was a solicitous mother to Drowsy and Pierre, her two dolls. She fed Drowsy from a toy nursing bottle (filling it herself and capping it with the nipple). She murmured endearments. To Drowsy: *Want to give me a kiss?—Bye bye, Drowsy.—Did you bump your head?* (Rubs it to make it feel better.) *She's crying. She wants her bottle.* She also spanked her dolls in anger and scolded them for misdemeanors. She toilet trained both dolls by placing them on her old potty chair.

Around the same time, Kathie acquired an imaginary companion she called "Zeen." Kathie carried on conversations with Zeen in two voices. When addressed by a friendly adult, Zeen was willing to extend the conversation. At lunch, when the observers were having coffee, E.A. asked what Zeen would like. Kathie, in an animated voice, said, *Here he comes. He's driving up the driveway driving a car. He has got to go home to make a cup of tea.*

It was Zeen who spilled the macaroni all over the kitchen floor; Kathie told her mother righteously when she herself was caught in the act.

After tracking Zeen for several months in our study, E.A. one day asked the direct question: "Where is *Zeen's* house?" Kathie said, *You gotta walk outside,* and then, *Wanna go for a walk?* E.A. accepted the invitation and Kathie took her for a walk to Zeen's house. Kathie told her that she would show her Zeen's sand box and Zeen's house, which had a door that you could open and close. It was a long walk to Zeen's house. And it was a cold day. E.A. complained of the sniffles and her need for a kleenex. Kathie said, *Here's a kleenex,* and produced an imaginary tissue, which she used to wipe E.A.'s nose. They walked for a long time and had many interesting encounters on the way. Finally, it dawned on E.A. that since Zeen was an imaginary person with an imaginary house, they were probably never going to get there. And they never did.

Around the same period, we received the first report of a dream. Kathie awoke one night very much upset and told her mother: *I stuck my foot in it and it turned on.* In the morning, Kathie reported her dream again but changed the detail to, *She bumped her foot.* Mother could give us no clues regarding this dream. While this may not have been Kathie's first dream, it was the first dream reported to her mother.

Verbatim speech records from visits at this time show an increase in the number of sentences that include a grammatically correct use of *I,* but there are still instances in which pronoun reversals appear.

At 4 years, 8 months, Mother reported that Kathie began to ask, *Today is what day?* And then, in a very rapid progress, it was reported to us that she began to learn the days of the week and the time concepts of "tomorrow" and "yesterday." As we were sorting data for this period, we made a discovery. The first record of use of the past tense appeared at the same time. Kathie had taken a walk to the outer limits of her home property. She reported when she came back, *I found Robinsons' house!*

One month later at 4 years, 9 months, we have the first report in our records of Kathie's ability to reconstruct from memory an event of the previous day. Kathie was playing with her mother's cigarette lighter. The next day Kathie's mother could not find the lighter and asked where it was. Kathie thought for a moment and said, *It's on the floor by the rocking chair.* (It was.)

As late as Kathie's fifth birthday there were still occasional lapses in her use of *I.* On the day of her birthday there was a routine visit to the doctor's office. Mother reported that Kathie told the doctor that it was her birthday. He asked her how old she was. Kathie: *She's four. No,* **I'm** *five years old.*

Here are a few samples of Kathie's conversations at the age of 5 years as reported by her mother:

(Kathie bumped into a little girl in the doctor's office.)
KATHIE: *Who is this?*
LITTLE GIRL: *Karen.*
KATHIE: *Where does your daddy work?*
LITTLE GIRL: *At Marshall's.*
KATHIE: *Does he work on a farm?* (Kathie's father did).

(Kathie overheard a mother spanking her baby during a visit to Kathie's home.)

KATHIE: *Don't spank the baby.* (The mother, embarrassed, said she wasn't hurting the baby.)

KATHIE: *Oh, did you do it gently and softly?*

(Kathie, at 5 years, 1 month of age, overheard the bus driver of her school bus say *Darn!*)

KATHIE: *Are you swearing?*

BUS DRIVER (embarrassed): *No.*

KATHIE (persisting): *Do you swear?*

At 5 years, 3 months, we have the following observations, which tie together concepts in language and in play. E.B.A. and a colleague were doing a videotape at Kathie's house to document play and language. At one point Kathie was feeding Drowsy, the doll, with the toy nursing bottle. She stopped for a moment and addressed the photographer: *Joy, what are you doing?* Joy said that she was taking pictures. Kathie said, *Oh, are you going to take my picture while I feed the baby?*

At another point, Kathie said that Drowsy was taking a nap. She whispered, *Don't wake him up!* Kathie began to make snoring noises as if pretending that Drowsy was asleep. *That's Drowsy*, she explained.

Later, everyone reviewed the tape in the kitchen. As Kathie heard the voices on the tape, she asked: *Evelyn, who is talking?* E.B.A. told her that it was Kathie talking to her mother. Kathie seemed to listen intently to the voices on the tape and to respond to them. She began to identify her own words, and when she heard herself snoring for Drowsy, she laughed out loud.

In these fragments from 5 years, 3 months of age, we see versatility in syntax, good pronoun usage, stable forms of *me* and *I*, and an objective concept of self that permits her to identify her own voice on tape and to laugh at her own clowning.

Comparisons of a Blind Child with a Sighted Child

In summary, Kathie's capacity for self-representation in play and the acquisition of the concept *I* finally did emerge in a coherent cognitive structure. Yet both were late acquisitions by sighted child expectations, which probably can be placed in the range from $2\frac{1}{2}$ to 3 years of age.

The relationship between self-representation and personal pronoun usage has not been rigorously examined in the sighted child literature. Zazzo (1948), whose longitudinal study of one child is unique in the literature of developmental aspects of pronoun usage, produced promising hypotheses, which he hoped would lead to controlled experimental research. His work has not yet been extended. While our own work was designed without knowledge of Zazzo's study and his hypotheses, there is close correspondence between his findings and ours on self-representation and the pronoun *I*.

In his study, "Image du corps et conscience de soi," Zazzo follows the gram-

matical transformations of self-reference pronouns in relation to the child's behavior toward his mirror image. The child was his son, Jean-Fabien, and the mirror
observations were recorded between the ages of 3 months and 2 years, 9 months.
(Photographs and home movies were also employed for picture identification, but
our summary will confine itself to mirror image.)

At 2 years, 3 months, Jean-Fabien made his first (and untutored) identification
of the baby in the mirror. After a moment's hesitation, he said, *Dadin*, the name
he used for himself. (From Jean-Fabien's behavior during this period, it appears to
us that the response *Dadin* is an identification of his image, but the *Dadin* in the
mirror is uncertainly himself—perhaps in the nature of "another Dadin.")

At 2 years, 4 months to 2 years, 5 months, Jean-Fabien used a syncretic form of
je (*ch'sais pas*). At 2 years 5 months, Zazzo reports, he had the pronouns *elle, i* (*je*
syncretic), *ça*. At $2\frac{1}{2}$ years, he began to use *moi* and *tu*.

At 2 years, 8 months, Jean-Fabien responded to his mirror image for the first time
with the phrase, *C'est moi*. At a later point in the essay, Zazzo adds that the phrase
C'est moi was accompanied by a gesture in which Jean-Fabian pointed to his own
chest. In all later variations in responding to his mirror image, the child used the
phrase, *Moi, Jean-Fabien*.

At 2 years, 8 months, the pronoun *je* was disengaged from syncretic forms, and
the author cites examples of discourse in which *je* was used inventively and in free
combination. During the same period, Zazzo reports in his later text, the momentary confusion before the mirror that preceded each self-identification had disappeared.

Zazzo's findings corroborate our own in essential aspects. The grammatical transformations of self-reference pronouns follow a progression that is linked with stages
in the evolution of the self-image; the non-syncretic *I* closes the sequence and
signifies the child's capacity to represent himself as an object in a universe of
objects. For the sighted child, and more so for the blind child, the achievement of
the concept *I* is a cognitive feat. The consistent, correct, and versatile employment
of the pronoun *I* tells us that the child has attained a level of conceptual development in which he not only endows himself with *I*, but recognizes that every *you* for
the child is an *I* for the other, and that he is a *you* to all other *I*s. This is a leap out
of his own skin, so to speak, and one that is normally facilitated and organized by
vision. Even when there are no mirrors and no pictures to consult, self-image
evolves through increasingly complex forms of mental representation in which the
body self is given objective form, a "double" as Zazzo suggests, an image of the self.

For the blind child, the constitution of a self-image and its representation through
I can appear in a protracted development. We have used self-representation in play
as the only means available to us to examine parallel representation of the self in
pronoun usage. If we can grant some equivalence to Kathie's self-representation in
play and imagination with Jean-Fabien's response to his mirror representation, we
can compare the characteristics of self-representation and pronoun usage in the
two children.

Following is a short summary:

Kathie, at 2 years, 2 months and Jean-Fabien at 2 years, 4 months, both employ a syncretic *I* and, more commonly, their own first names for self-reference. Jean-Fabien can name himself in the mirror. Kathie has no form of self-representation in her play.

At 2 years, 8 months, Jean-Fabien has *moi* and *tu* in his vocabulary. In the mirror, he identifies himself with the words, *C'est moi.* Kathie's *me* and *you* appear in echo responses, which inevitably lead to reversals. She cannot represent herself in play. At 2 years, 10 months, Jean-Fabien's *je* has completed the course of disengagement from syncretic usage, is used freely and inventively in discourse. The momentary confusion that had preceded mirror identification of himself has now disappeared, which indicates that he now feels at one with his mirror image. It is assimilated to *I.* Kathie's *I* is still employed in syncretic forms. *Me* and *you* are still embedded in set phrases as echo responses and appear as reversals. She cannot yet represent herself in play.

At 3 years, 6 months, Kathie employs *me* for the first time in our records.

At 4 years, 6 months, Kathie becomes a solicitous mother to her dolls and invents an imaginary companion.

At 4 years, 10 months, Kathie's *I* is now demonstrably a stable form, which is used inventively in discourse, but there are still occasional lapses.

From this concise summary, we can see that the two children whose *I* first emerged in syncretic form at 2 years, 2 months and 2 years, 4 months followed divergent paths in the acquisition of the nonsyncretic *I.* The sighted child travelled a route that brought him to a stable concept of *I* at 2 years, 10 months. The blind child's route brought her to the same point at the age of 4 years, 10 months. Jean Fabien's travels took him 6 months. Kathie's took her 2 years and 8 months.

The parallel developments in self-representation and pronoun usage from these two independent studies speak strongly in favor of Zazzo's view, which is also our own: the acquisition of personal pronouns goes beyond practice with grammatical tools. It goes beyond the influence of the language environment, which we can demonstrate through the incapacities of Kathie in self-reference pronouns while living in a home with six highly verbal family members. The hypothesis in these two independent studies links self-reference pronouns to self-image.

The blind child's delay in the acquisition of *I* as a concept and a stable form appears to be related to the extraordinary problems in constructing a self-image in the absence of vision. The blind child must find a path to self-representation without the single sensory organ that is uniquely adapted for synthesis of all perceptions and the data of self.

In infancy, most of the data of self are integrated into a body schema by submitting experience to visual tests. We need only reflect on the hands as a model. Through countless experiments before 6 months of age, the infant makes the discovery that "the hand" that crosses his visual field, "the hand" that he brings to his mouth, "the hand" that grasps an object is part of himself, an instrument that he controls. The games he plays with his hands before his eyes are experiments in self-discovery. It is vision that gives unity to the disparate forms and aspects of hands and brings about an elementary sense of "me-ness" for hands. Body image is constructed by means of the discovery of parts and a progressive organization of these parts into coherent pictures. In constructing a body image, vision offers a unique advantage that no other sensory mode can duplicate; the picture replicates exactly, and the picture by its nature can unite in one percept or a memory flash all the attributes and parts into a whole. Once the picture is there, it does not need to be reconstituted from its parts.

The blind child has no sensory mode available to him that will replicate his own body or body parts. He is obliged to constitute a body image from the components of nonvisual experience available to him, not one of which will give him through objective reference the sum of the parts. His tactile, auditory, vocal, kinaesthetic, and locomotor experience will give him a sense of the substantiality and autonomy of his own body, but these sensory modes bind him to egocentric body and self-experience and cannot lead him easily to the concept of self in which the self can be taken as an object, which is the indispensable condition for the nonsyncretic *I*. Self-image, which Zazzo suggests is a double, a replicate, a kind of mirror image of one's own person, is literally a picture of oneself. *I* is the externalization of that picture into a community of pictures each of which is an *I*.

For the blind child there is no single sense that can take over the function of vision in replicating body image. When Kathie, at 5 years, 3 months, identifies her own words and her voice on tape,[5] she has demonstrated a form of self-recognition that still offers imperfect comparisons with Jean-Fabien's identification of himself in the mirror at 2 years, 8 months. The voice on tape is an aspect of self, one of the components of self-image that can now be identified in objective form. But the voice does not replicate body image; the mirror image replicates exactly and instantly.

For the blind child, the level of inference required for the construction of the non-syncretic *I* goes beyond that of the sighted child. The blind child must infer from his own consciousness of himself as an entity a commonality with the consciousness of others who are *I*s; he must construct a world of human objects each of whom is an *I* to himself by granting forms of substantiality and "I-ness" to these human objects whom he has identified as having attributes similar to himself. He must do this without the one sensory mode that would describe, through the visual picture, the commonalities and the generalizations that lead to the concept *I*. Yet, when he does achieve *I* as a stable form and when he represents himself in play by means of a doll or an imaginary companion, he has indisputably externalized a form of self, reconstituted the self as an object. Our scientific imagination is strained to reconstruct the process.

The blind child's route to *I* and self-representation is a perilous one. Many blind children do not make it. In the blind child population a very large number of children at school age or later do not have *I* or any other self-reference pronouns

---

[5] Even as Jean-Fabien had had the mirror available to him for many months before he identified himself, Kathie had had experience with tape recorders in her home for some time before this occurrence. This need not have been her first identification of herself on tape, but it was our first observation.

in their vocabularies. From the study of Kathie and other healthy and adequate blind children, we can understand without difficulty why the pronoun *I* and forms of self-representation in play are delayed in comparison with sighted children. The more difficult problem is to understand how the blind child achieves this prodigious feat.

References

Fraiberg, S. Parallel and divergent patterns in blind and sighted infants. *Psychoanalytic Study of the Child,* 1968, *23*, 264—300.

Fraiberg, S. Intervention in infancy. *American Academy of Child Psychiatry, Journal, 10* (3), 381—405.(a)

Fraiberg, S. Smiling and stranger reaction in blind infants. In J. Hellmuth (Ed.), *Exceptional infant.* New York: Brunner/Mazel, 1971. Pp. 110—127.(b)

Fraiberg, S., The development of human attachments in infants blind from birth. *Merrill-Palmer Quarterly,* October, 1975. (In press).

Fraiberg, S., Siegel B., & Gibson, R. The role of sound in the search behavior of a blind infant. *Psychoanalytic Study of the Child,* 1966, *21,* 327—337.

Fraiberg, S., Smith, M., & Adelson, E. An educational program for blind infants. *Journal of Special Education,* 1969, *3* (2), 121—139.

Gesell, A., & Amatruda, C. *Developmental diagnosis.* Boston: Hoeber, 1947.

Piaget, J . *The Origins of intelligence in children.* New York: International Universities Press, 1952.

Ulrich, S. *Elizabeth.* (Introduction by S. Fraiberg, Commentary by E. Adelson.) Ann Arber: Univ. of Michigan Press, 1972.

Zazzo, R. Image du corps et conscience de soi. *Enfance,* 1948, *1,* 29—43.

III. Language in the Clinic

This section, as did the previous one, contains chapters that deal with practical problems. Nevertheless, the material is also of great importance to any psychobiological theory of language. Ingram's article is an extremely comprehensive overview of the entire spectrum of clinical speech disorders in pediatric practice. Fourcin's description of and comment on the case of Richard Boydell (who has provided an introduction of his own) deserves the reader's special attention. Here is one more piece of evidence that man can acquire a natural language in rather passive ways. Since the editor's first description of a child with congenital anarthria who gave every evidence of understanding even the most complicated sentences, several other cases have been described of subjects who were unable to speak (for various reasons) but whose language comprehension could be shown to be within normal limits. Mr. Boydell is of particular interest because he has also learned to express himself in writing. These cases clearly show the importance of testing comprehension independently from speech when examing patients handicapped from birth. Ryan stresses the highly predictable development of language in the mentally subnormal, a point that is of direct relevance to the planning of speech training of any particular individual in this category. There is obviously no point in trying to make a child say things in ways for which he is not ready because of a lack of prerequisite language stages. The chapter by Lefèvre is highly original and draws on clinical material that is simply not available in North America and Europe (at least not to the extent found in the author's home base). While malnutrition does not single out language as a target of failure, it is theoretically possible that the concomitant growth of abnormalities of the brain might be more troublesome for the proper development of language than for other types of skills. The situation, however, is more intricate, as the author points out. The final chapter, by Quirós and Schrager, is perhaps the most controversial of this volume. Although the editors do not share these authors' assumptions and biological presuppositions, the article deserves to be read carefully, since its point of view is by no means at odds with widely held opinions.

13. Speech Disorders in Childhood

T. T. S. Ingram

The study of speech disorders in childhood depends upon a knowledge of normal speech development. Major advances in the study of the development of linguistic skills in young children have been made in recent years. Unfortunately these still do not provide sufficient data on which to classify speech disorders according to phonological and linguistic criteria.

A clinical classification of speech disorders in childhood is presented and the variety of speech disorders defined within it are described in more detail. The dangers of making too close comparisons between acquired disorders of spoken language in the adult and disorders of spoken language affecting the developing child are emphasized.

Introduction

Any general review of speech disorders in childhood made within the compass of a chapter must necessarily be somewhat superficial; it cannot take full account of the many detailed scientific, linguistic studies of speech development in childhood that have taken place in recent years. Moreover, this chapter must be largely concerned with their medical aspects; although no account of disorders of spoken language would be complete unless some consideration were given to the increased knowledge of normal speech development, acquired in the past three decades (Bellugi, 1971; Bellugi & Brown, 1964; Berko, 1958; Bever, 1971b; Bullowa, 1967; T. T. S. Ingram, Anthony, Bogle, & McIsaac, 1971; Klima, 1964; Klima & Bellugi, 1966; Lenneberg, 1966; McCarthy, 1954; McNeill, 1966b, 1970; Schlesinger, 1971;

Weir, 1962). These authors and many others have elaborated and confirmed in experimental conditions many of the concepts about the development of spoken language put forward many years ago by Vygotsky (1934), Luria (1961, 1966), and Piaget (1932). They have resulted in new dimensions of developmental studies in psycholinguistics, which to a large extent have superceded the anecdotal accounts of speech development of children made by earlier workers, including the Sterns (Stern & Stern, 1928), Grégoire (1937), Guillaume (1925), Bühler (1930), Darwin (1877), and Lewis (1951), which have been well summarized by McCarthy (1954). For more recent work, see McNeill (1970).

A trend that is particularly welcome to the pediatrician interested in speech disorders is the increasing interest shown in sociolinguistics. The effects of environmental factors, including social class, education, and linguistic environment, on the development of spoken language have been intensively studied in England by Bernstein (1961, 1965, 1971b) and Robinson (1971), and in the United States by Hymes (1968, 1971), Labov (1966, 1970; Labov, Cohen, & Robins, 1965), and Cazden (1968, 1970). Numerous previous studies have demonstrated that children deprived in their early years of adequate linguistic stimulation tend to be slower to acquire spoken language than are those exposed to a rich linguistic environment. Institutionalized children, for example, show later and slower speech development than do children of similar intelligence coming from normal homes. The effects of deprivation seem to be intensified if the child suffers from retarded development because of inborn factors that result in general mental deficiency (Clarke & Clarke, 1960; Renfrew, 1964; Stevens, 1971), but the work of Bernstein, Hymes, Labov, and Cazden cited above has demonstrated with much more subtlety how different environments and different linguistic codes may profoundly affect the later spoken language of the child. Bernstein, for example, draws a distinction between the restricted code—the limited interpersonal language available to the child coming from a linguistically impoverished background, usually of low social class—and the elaborated code—the much more complex language capable of expressing abstract ideas available to the child coming from a linguistically sophisticated background (Bernstein, 1971a). Rather similar studies have been made in the United States by Ervin-Tripp (1971) and Cazden (1970).

The Neuropathology of Developmental Speech Disorders

Contemporaneously with the studies on the effects of speech development of environment, investigations have continued to be made on the underlying neuroanatomical and neurophysiological basis of spoken language in the child.

As yet, it is impossible to correlate neuroanatomical and neurophysiological maturation accurately with the development of behavior. The fundamental dichotomy between the thinking of neuroanatomists and neurophysiologists, on the one hand, and psychologists and linguists, on the other, persists (Hécaen, 1971). Moreover, attempts to explain abnormalities of speech development in terms of the brain lesions found in adult patients who have suffered loss of speech as a result of focal injury to the hemispheres have been conspicuously unsuccessful. The aplasia of the angular gyrus postulated by Brain to account for "developmental aphasia" in childhood has never been demonstrated. Even in the adult with a particular type of dysphasia, focal injuries may be found in a wide diversity of different situations, as shown in Figs. 13—1 and 2 (Conrad, 1964, Brain, 1965). A similar diversity of lesions was found by Russell and Espir (1961) in their studies of patients suffering from the effects of gunshot wounds sustained during the Second World War. The diversity of the situations of localized lesions that may cause speech disturbances is much easier to explain if the Pavlovian concept of analyzers and interanalyzer connections is accepted; interruption of a large number of different interanalyzer connections could result in loss of speech function. These ideas, in fact, mark a return to the original concepts of Charcot (1881), Kussmaul (1885), and Lichtheim (1884), who conceived of dysphasic disorders as being the result of interruption of particular nervous pathways between important "centers" in the hemispheres. It was perhaps inevitable that, extrapolating from these ideas, clinicians should have suggested that failure of the myelination of interanalyzer tracts might be responsible for evidence of disease of the central nervous system, in particular, syndromes of "minimal cerebral dysfunction." It has been shown, however, that many unmyelinated nerve tracts in the brain and spinal cords of infants function very similarly to those that are myelinated in adults (Ellingson, 1964). Nevertheless, the idea that the development of the hugely complex interconnecting tracts linking primary, secondary, and tertiary analyzers one with the other is somehow related to the development of higher nervous function in the child is an attractive one. It would be even more attractive if it were possible to correlate the maturational changes in the brain with milestones of motor, linguistic, adaptive, and social behavior, or, still more interestingly, the stages in conceptual thinking described by Piaget (1970; see also Flavell, 1970).

It is no coincidence that a number of authors have pointed out that many of the intellectual deficits and behavioral aberrations of brain-damaged children appear to be the result of a failure of intersensory integration—a concept that would be compatible with there being a failure of the development of interanalyzer connections. The theory is particularly interesting for it suggests that different tracts develop at different rates during late pregnancy and early childhood and that they are susceptible to damage to varying degrees. Thus the wide variety of clinical syndromes known to exist, might be produced by traumatic, hypoxic or toxic insults to the brain occurring at different maturational stages (Birch, 1964; Birch & Belmont, 1965; Birch & Lefford, 1963; Dobbing, 1968).

It is impossible to explain how children learn to use spoken language in neuro-physiological and neuroanatomical terms. It is still necessary to describe behavior in behavioralistic terms and brain function in terms of neuroanatomy and neuro-physiology. It is therefore possibly legitimate for some linguists and psychologists to go to the extent of assuming that young children have some innate, inborn facility that allows them to comprehend grammatical universals. Chomsky, for

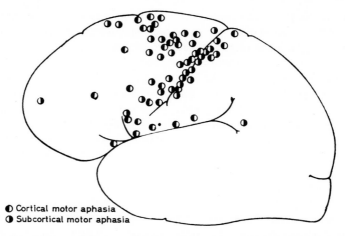

Figure 13–1. General view of all cases of motor aphasia in a series of fractures of the skull (from Conrad, 1954). The circles indicate the middle points of the trephine defect.

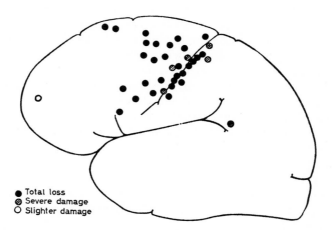

Figure 13–2. Cases of subcortical motor aphasia (according to the terminology Wernicke) in a series of fractures of the skull (from Conrad, 1954). The circles indicate the middle points of the trephine defects, and the symbols show the degree of speech disturbance immediately after the lesion. Note in both figures the distribution of the lesions in the superior frontal region in the neighbourhood of Penfield and Roberts's "supplementary motor area."

example, postulated the existence of a "language acquisition device" (LAD), which was universal and innate (Chomsky, 1965, 1968). Similar ideas were at one time expressed by McNeill (1966a), although he appears later to have changed his mind about the innateness of the child's ability to handle grammatical structures (McNeill, 1970). Lenneberg has suggested that it is theoretically possible that, to some extent, the ability to acquire spoken language may have biological foundations (Lenneberg, 1964, 1967). The idea of there being a LAD has been criticized severely by a number of workers, including Huxley (1969a, 1969b), Mehler and Bever (1968), and E. Ingram (1971). Ingram pointed out that the assumption of an innate linguistic drive could not be supported by current psychological and physiological work and that it did not form a useful part of any theoretical model designed to describe the development of spoken language.

It is clear that the developing spoken language of young children must be treated phenomenologically and described in appropriate linguistic and phonetic terms, and that in the present state of our knowledge it cannot be related directly to neuroanatomical or neurophysiological maturation. Once this is accepted, it is important to accept also that remarkably little is known about the underlying neuropathology of speech disorders. It is, in fact, only in the last three decades that serious systematic studies of these disorders, using linguistic criteria, have been made. This is hardly surprising when it is considered that the science of phonetics as we understand it today is barely 100 years old (Abercrombie, 1957; Firth, 1934), and the principles on which the International Phonetic Alphabet is based were formulated only in 1912 (Bloomfield, 1933; Firth, 1934). Studies of spoken language in terms of generative grammar were initiated only after the Second World War, largely stimulated by the exciting speculations of Chomsky (1957). Chomsky's attack on the somewhat traditional ideas of language and language development advanced earlier by Skinner (1957) marked the end of one era of research in linguistics and the beginning of another (Chomsky, 1959). The full implications of this revolution in linguistics for the study of speech development and speech disorders is yet to be seen (Lyons, 1970).

This chapter will be concerned with the prevalence of speech disorders in childhood, their significance, and their interpretation in terms of normal speech development. The common disorders will be described, and methods of assessment, with an emphasis on their medical aspects, will be considered.

The Assessment of Speech Development

Much recent work in linguistics (Bellugi, 1964, 1965, 1971; Bellugi and Brown, 1964; Klima, 1964; McNeill, 1970) has provided new insights into the ways in which speech development progresses in young children. Together with the increase in our understanding of the semantic aspects of language resulting from the work of Piaget and his disciples and the Russian authors, it is likely to be of major importance in helping to interpret deviation from the normal pattern of language development in children who suffer from speech disorders and in children who suffer from loss of language as a result of acquired brain injury or disease.

However, it is still impossible to assess completely, qualitatively or quantitatively, the maturation of spoken language in young children by using the experimental work that has been referred to, and, for the most part, rather arbitrary criteria have been employed in most research studies. Many of these derive from McCarthy (1930), for example those used by Templin (1957). In recent studies in the Department of Child Life and Health in Edinburgh (1974) (Table 13–1), criteria such as the mean length of 50 consecutive utterances produced by the child, the length of the longest utterance, the number of subordinate clauses, etc., certainly produce valid comparisons as children grow older (the mean sentence length, for example, becoming progressively greater), but as criteria they can hardly be said to give a great deal of insight into his ability to make grammatical formulations.

An increasing number of tests of language ability, as assessed by how children describe pictured situations or play with toy objects, has become available in recent years. For the comprehension of language, the Reynell Test is useful over the age range of 6 months to 6 years, and the Peabody Test (revised by Brimer & Dunn, 1963) is useful for children from 21 months to 18 years of age. The Reynell Test is helpful in testing expressive language, as are the Renfrew Language Attainment Scales. Anderson's Communicative Evaluation Assessment is a more general test of the child's ability to comprehend what is said to him and to communicate

TABLE 13-1   MEAN SCORES BY AGE FOR THE MAJOR LANGUAGE MEASURES BASED ON 50 SPONTANEOUS UTTERANCES PRODUCED IN FREE PLAY WITH TOYS.[a]

		$2\frac{1}{2}$ yr.	3 yr.	$3\frac{1}{2}$ yr.
		n = 55	n = 65	n = 76
	Percentage Intelligibility of Utterances	86.09	91.29	95.08
Length of Utterance	Average Number of Words per Utterance	3.76	4.88	5.74
	Number of Words in Longest Utterance	8.05	11.48	14.58
Sentence structure	Completence	28.09	37.92	43.36
	Complexity	24.98	41.82	56.32
	Clauses	23.89	36.95	46.01
	Subordinate Clauses	0.42	2.17	4.58
Grammar	Subordinating Conjunctions	0.27	1.18	2.59
	Prepositions	7.69	11.57	14.99
	Inflections	17.55	27.23	35.08
	Auxiliaries	7.00	12.48	16.38
	Tenses other than Simple Present	5.40	11.48	15.71
	Combined Grammar Score	37.80	64.18	84.70
	Recognition Vocabulary	28.40	40.54	49.21

[a]Data based on McCarthy (1930).

using spoken language. There are many psychological tests with a larger component of cognitive evaluation. These include the Snyders-Oomen Test, the Illinois Linguistic Tests, the Weschler Intelligence Test, which has a performance and a verbal scale, and its junior number suitable for children from the ages of 3 to 5, (the WPPSI), the Goodenough Draw-A-Man Test, which, as shown by Mason (1967), depends largely upon the child's ability to name parts of the body if they are to be represented in drawing.

These tests and also some tests of general intelligence such as the Merrill Palmer and the Stanford Binet, which contain a large number of verbal items, are of the greatest value in providing quantitative and qualitative assessments of a child's language ability and relating them to the maturity of his other sensorimotor skills.

There are a number of tests of phonological development. One devised by Renfrew has been standardized in England (Renfrew, 1964). There are a large number of American tests that have not been standardized in England. The Edinburgh Articulation Test has been standardized on a representative population of Edinburgh children; it consists of a naming game in which the child is asked to name pictures of well-known objects. A study is made of all the consonants and consonant clusters commonly used in English in different positions. Vowels are not studied, for they vary greatly in different social classes and in different regions, and so would be difficult to evaluate on a purely maturational basis. Many of the words give a number of consonantal items (Figs. 13−3, 4, 5), so that it is possible in a period of about 10−15 min to obtain 68 items from most children between the ages of 3 and 6. The raw scores obtained on this test can be converted into "articulatory ages" or "articulatory quotients" using a table devised as a result of the standardization of the test on the representative population sample of Edinburgh children.

There is also a qualitative analysis of the speech sounds, their usual maturational patterns having been studied in the 500 children who formed the population sample uopn whom the test was standardized. This gives some idea of the nature of the child's phonological maturation. If he is proceeding according to a normal maturational pattern, the sounds he realizes should occur more or less in a vertical distribution. On the other hand, if he suffers from dysarthria attributable to neurological or structural abnormalities of the articulatory organs, the pattern of speech sounds produced is likely to be scattered more horizontally (Fig. 13−6). This test has been found to be of great value in clinical circumstances. It has the drawback, however, that it tests the child's word sound production in single words only and not in connected speech—a much more difficult matter to attempt (T. T. S. Ingram et al., 1971).

The Edinburgh Articulation Test was an offshoot of a larger research project designed to examine healthy children of average or superior intelligence who were slow to develop spoken language, and to compare their educational achievements later with a group of comparable children with normal speech as regards social class, age, and intelligence. The hypothesis that a high proportion of children with slow speech development would have difficulties in learning to read and spell was confirmed; the fact that these difficulties were relatively specific was shown

Average 4·0-year-old performance

Name _____ WILLIAM _____ Sex __ M. _____ Test given by _____ AA.

Address _____ EDINBURGH _____ Place of Test _____ EDINBURGH

Date of Birth _____ 30/12/62 _____ Date of Test _____ 24/11/66

Birth Rank _____ 3rd. _____ Social Class _____ III

monkey	℞ ŋk	ŋ'k ✓	sleeping	sl	sℓℓ X	finger	f	f ✓
tent	t	t ✓		p	p ✓		ŋg	ŋŋg ✓
	nt	n? ✓	wings	ŋz	ŋz ✓	thumb	θ	f X
fish	ʃ	ʃt ✓	garage	g	g ✓	watch	w	w ✓
train	tr	trr X		r	r ✓		tʃ	?ʃ ✓
umbrella	m	M X		dʒ	dʒ ✓	string	✱ str	stər ✓
	b	bʌ	aeroplane	pl	pℓ ✓		ŋ	ŋŋ X
	r	ʒ	spoon	sp	sʌp ✓	three	θr	fər X
	l	ʒ		n	n ✓	teeth	θ	f X
milk	m	m ✓	toothbrush	θbr	isbʌr X	pencil	p	p ✓
	lk	ℓkʰ ✓		ʃ	ʃ X		ns	n?s ✓
stamps	℞ st	st ✓	red	r	r ✓		l	ℓ ✓
	mps	m?s ✓		d	d ✓	yellow	℞ j	ℓ X
queen	℞ kw	kw ✓	bottle	tl	tʌL ✓		l	ℓ ✓
clouds	℞ kl	kℓ ✓	birthday	rθd	rfd X	sugar	℞ ʃ	ʃ X
	dz	dʒ X	horse(ie)	h	ʒ ✓		g	g ✓
Christmas	kr	kər X	feather	ð	ʒ ✓	Indian	n	n ✓
	sm	sm X	elephant	l	ℓ ✓		d	d
	s	ʃ X		f	f		j	j
bridge	br	br ✓		n	n		n	n
	dʒ	dʒʒ X		t	t	matches	tʃ	?ʃ ✓
flower	fl	fℓ ✓	soldier	s	ʃ X		z	z ✓
chimney	tʃ	tʃ ✓		ldʒ	ldʒ ✓	scissors	z	z X
	mn	mʌr X		r	r ✓	desk	d	d ✓
smoke	sm	smm X	glove	gl	kℓℓ X		sk	ssk ✓
	k	?kʰ ✓		v	v ✓			

✱ accepted local adult form.

Total Right = 46

Standard Score = 103.

Figure 13—3. *Edinburgh Articulation Test.* Results obtained in the quantitative sheet from a "normal" child 4-year old.

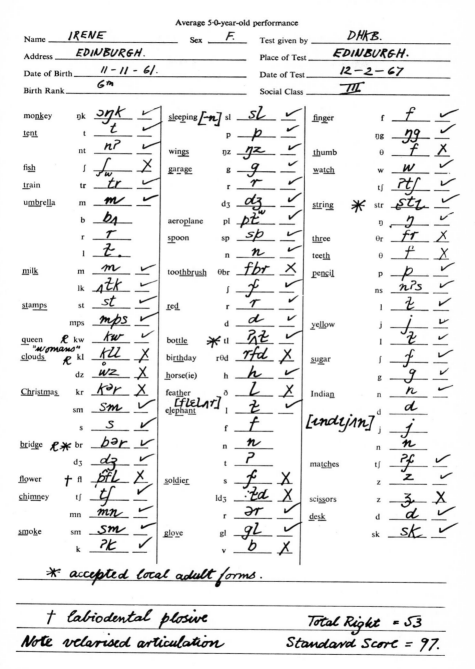

Figure 13—4. *Edinburgh Articulation Test.* Results obtained on the quantitative sheet from a "normal" child 5-years old.

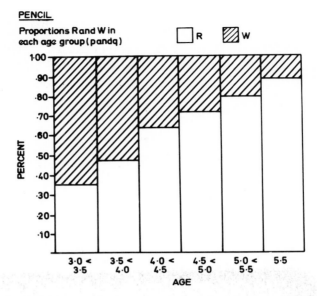

Figure 13—5. Histogram showing the proportion of a representative group of children by age who correctly pronounced the final l in *pencil.*

by the fact that whereas in 40% of these children (and in only about 4% of the controls) performance in reading and spelling was a year or more retarded, the children in the control group did not score quite so highly in tests of arithmetical ability at the age of seven years (T. T. S. Ingram *et al.*, 1973).

The Prevalence of Speech Disorders

Speech disorders are common in childhood in England. Miss Muriel Morley, in a pioneer survey in Newcastle, found that 14% of 5-year-old children had serious articulatory difficulties; these were so severe in 4% that the children were un-intelligible to their teachers (Morley, 1957). In Nottingham more than 7% of children between the ages of 5 years, 3 months and 6 years, 2 months had what was termed "baby speech"; two years later the proportion of these children, then between the ages of 7 and 8 with baby speech had fallen to less than 1% (Grady & Daniels, 1964). In a huge national study of 11,000 children of age 7, 14% were found to have retarded speech development (Pringle, Butler, & Davie, 1966). In the childhood population of the Isle of Wight it was found that of a small but representative sample of children between 9- and 11-years old, 6.8% had defects of articulation (Rutter, Tizard, & Whitmore, 1970); 6.2% showed "poor complexity of language;" and in the total population of children in the same age group .8 per 1000 were considered to have severe developmental language dis-

EDINBURGH ARTICULATION TEST—QUALITATIVE ASSESSMENT SHEET

	Phonetic reali-sation	Adult form	Minor variations	Almost mature	Immature			Very immature		Atypical substitutions	
st<u>ring</u>	-ŋ	ŋᵊ ŋg						n ɲ		g	
<u>s</u>oldier	s-	θs	ṣ ʂ ş		ʃ ç θ		ɬ	c t		h	
Christma<u>s</u>	-s	ns	ṣ ʂ ş		θ f ç		ɬ	– t h ʔ			
sci<u>ss</u>ors	-z-	dz gz	ẓ ʐ ʑ	s	ṣ ð ʂ j ş ʒ		ɬ ʒ̇	ɟ d		t h ʔ	
matche<u>s</u>	-z	dz ðz	ẓ ʐ ʑ	s	ṣ ð ʂ j ş ʒ			– ɟ h d ʔ		t	
<u>sm</u>oke	sm-	tsm smm θsm səm sm(m)	ṣm(m) ʂm(m) şm(m)		θm mm fm mm çm		ɬm	m̥ m		s p f b	
<u>sp</u>oon	sp-	tsp səp θsp	ṣp ʂp şp		θp fp çp		ɬp	p p̂f		ʍ f	
<u>st</u>amps	st-	tst pst	ṣt ʂt şt		θt çt		ɬt	t		sk s sl	
<u>sl</u>eeping	sl-	tsl sll səl	ṣl(l) ʂl(l) şl(l)		θl sr ʃl ɬl sw tl sɥ			s ṣ θw l ʂ tl ş		f p t ʍ	
Chri<u>stm</u>as	-sm-	səm	ṣm ʂm şm		θm hm ɬm fm m̥m çm			f m ʔm		ht kð	
pe<u>nc</u>il	-ns-		nṣ nʂ nş		nθ ~s nɬ nç			nt nh		θ h	
<u>st</u>amp<u>s</u>	-mps	mfs mpts	mpṣ mpʂ mpş		mpθ ~ps mpɬ mp mpç			ms ps		nts ~p	

Figure 13–6. One of five pages.

orders. (It is important to note, however, that these included some children who were mentally retarded.) A somewhat similar figure for the prevalence of severe developmental language disorders in children of school age was found in Edinburgh as a result of a survey by questionnaire directed to teachers, social workers, school medical officers, and speech therapists. The prevalence, excluding mentally retarded children, was .75 per 1000 (T.T.S. Ingram, 1963c).

In the United States an early investigation of 4,862 children in Madison, Wisconsin, was reported to show that 5.69% had speech defects severe enough to be detected by an outside observer (Blanton, 1916). A rather later investigation in the same city was reported to the 1931. White House Conference. This gave a prevalence of 7% of children with significant speech disorders. An investigation carried out by means of questionnaires in 48 other urban areas, reported at the same Conference, gave a mean prevalence of 6.9% of children of school age with significant speech defects, but it was noted that there were great variations in the prevalence reported from different towns and cities. Mills and Streit (1942) found that 33.4% of 1196 children in the first three grades of school in Holyoke, Massachusetts, had speech defects. Most of these were considered to be mild, but in 12.6% of the children they were considered to be "serious."

In Iowa it was found that of 30,000 individually tested school children, 5.7% had defective speech, 0.7% stuttered, and 3.6% had "voice problems" (the latter being a high assessment compared to most other surveys) (Johnson, 1942). In Ohio, Hawk reported that 9.5 per cent of elementary school children had significant speech defects (Hawk, 1945). Irwin reported that 7.7% of elementary school children in Cleveland, Ohio, suffered from speech disorders (R. B. Irwin, 1948). He found that a higher proportion of children in kindergarten suffered from articulatory and language disorders than did those in elementary schools—hardly a surprising discovery when one considers that many of the speech disorders he reported were probably associated with retarded development, which might be expected to improve with maturation; he did, however, also include in his estimate children who suffered from stuttering abnormalities of voice, and severe language difficulties.

In Newcastle, England, a careful study was made on the incidence and the prevalence of stuttering in children of school age by Andrews and Harris (1964). They reported that the incidence of stuttering was between 3 and 4% among school children and that any one time approximately 1% of the school population showed speech dysrhythmia—manifest as slurring, or prolongation of syllables, stuttering, blocking, or speech arrest at the beginning of utterances.

The Importance of Speech Defects

It is clear from these studies reported from many different areas that a relatively high percentage of children suffer from speech defects. A high proportion of pre-school children and young elementary school children, studied by Sheridan, 1972, suffered from speech disorders which could be regarded as developmental, in the sense that they might be expected to disappear as the children grow up. Nevertheless, a significant proportion continue to show abnormalities of voice, rhythm, articulation, or language during their school years and are likely to require therapy.

Speech defects are not only important in themselves; children who suffer from speech defects are frequently frustrated by their inability to communicate intelligibly to their families and other children. Often they are subjected to the merry teasing of their school fellows and are made very unhappy. Moreover, a high proportion of children with retarded speech development have later difficulties in learning to read and spell, even though their speech disorder may seem to have been resolved by the time they go to school (T. T. S. Ingram *et al.*, 1973). In the Isle of Wight survey, it was found that 14% of children who showed specific difficulties in learning to read and spell had abnormalities of articulation at the time they were studied, and that 15.1% had "poor complexity of language compared to 6.8% and 6.2% in control series" (Rutter *et al.*, 1970). T. T. S. Ingram and Reid (1956) found that there was a history of slow speech development in almost half of the 78 children of school age whom they studied in a department of child psychiatry; these children were of at least average intelligence, but suffered from specific difficulties in learning to read and spell. It was interesting to observe in this latter study that in a high proportion of the patients the cause of referral was not specifically educational difficulties but, rather, emotional stress; this was considered by the authors to be secondary to the educational difficulties. This emphasizes the need for the early ascertainment, assessment, and treatment of children who show abnormalities of speech. Moreover, these children should not be lost touch with after speech therapy has ceased; contact should be maintained with them either directly or through the educational psychologists throughout their early years at school.

Despite the importance of speech disorders in childhood and the frequency with which they occur, they have received scant attention from pediatricians until recent years. It is still impossible to delineate them accurately in terms acceptable to linguists or phoneticians, though increasing numbers of pioneering studies of children with complex speech disorders are being made—for example the detailed description of the unintelligible speech of a 10-year-old boy reported by Beresford (1972). It is, in fact, only relatively recently that a comprehensive account of the changes that occur in consonants and consonant clusters in the preschool years in normal children has been produced (T. T. S. Ingram et al., 1971).

The Classification of Disorders of Speech in Childhood

There is no single satisfactory classification of disorders of spoken language in childhood. Classification by etiology or cause is unsatisfactory because the causes of disorders are frequently multiple or, especially in the case of children, unknown. For example, simple defects of articulation in a child may be due to his being mildly intellectually subnormal, to his being environmentally deprived, to his being hard of hearing, or to his being genetically predisposed to be slow to develop spoken language, including articulation. Frequently it is found that a number of the above factors are present in any individual child. The causes of disorders of spoken language in the adult may be equally complicated.

Classification by the type of disorder of language ability is also complicated. It has been shown, for example, that children who stammer commonly have a degree of retardation in the development of spoken language. In children, defective articulation (the production of speech sounds) is frequently the presenting abnormality, but closer examination will almost always show that development of spoken language, as indicated by tests of vocabulary, grammatical complexity, and the length of utterances, is also immature (Sheridan, 1971). Similarly an adult who suffers from gross impairment of the ability to produce spoken language as a result of a cerebrovascular accident (stroke) usually shows abnormalities of articulation, as well as difficulties in word-finding, constructing grammatically correct sentences, and, often, understanding what is said to him.

In these circumstances, a classification based on the major function of language ability that is disturbed and on associated clinical characteristics has been found useful, if not theoretically completely satisfactory.

T. T. S. Ingram (1959a) suggested a classification for disorders of language ability in children which may also be used to cover disorders of language ability in adults. This is not an ideal classification for either children or adults because so many disorders are complex and their origin is multifactorial, but it does allow for a broad classification of disorders of language ability, which may be modified to some extent according to need.

The classification is as follows:

1. Disorders of voicing (abnormalities of voice production, commonly due to disease of the larynx or affecting the larynx—usually "dysphonia").

2. Dysrhythmia (stammer, hesitation, blocking, repetition of syllables, due to a failure of the synchronization of respiratory and articulatory movements during speech).

3. Dysarthria (disorders of articulation due to abnormalities of structure or of function of the articulatory organs or related structures).

a. Due to structural abnormalities (for example, cleft palate, absence or underdevelopment of the tongue, abnormalities of related structures, such as dental malocclusion or palatopharyngeal disproportion, or an inadequate nasal airway due to gross enlargement of the adenoids or congenital defects of the nose).

b. Defects of innervation of the lips, tongue, and palate, or related organs (there may be paresis, unco-ordination, or involuntary movements of the lips, tongue, and palate or related structures).

4. Secondary speech disorders (in childhood these consist typically of retardation of speech development with no demonstrable abnormality of the structure or function of the articulatory organs) due to

a. Mental defect.

b. Hearing impairment.

c. Severe psychiatric disorders, e.g., infantile autism, psychosis, and elective mutism.

d. Severe social deprivation (much commoner in the child than the adult).

5. The specific developmental speech disorder syndrome (confined to children).

a. Articulation only. (Children affected with this disorder show "developmental" difficulties in articulation. They are unable to pronounce correctly the later acquired sounds that they should have in their repertoire. Only on very detailed testing will retardation of spoken language be demonstrated. Generally they are described as "having words but unable to pronounce them".)

b. Developmental disorders of articulation with retardation of spoken language. (Children in this category not only demonstrate defects of the articulation of speech sounds but are also slow to use spoken language. On test they show low scores in vocabulary, grammar, and, commonly, auditory memory.)

c. Articulatory abnormalities, difficulties in using spoken language, and difficulties in comprehending what is said. (Children in this category are much more severely affected, show more articulatory abnormalities than do children in (a) and (b) and can be shown to have difficulties in comprehending what is said to them as well as in using spoken language.)

d. Very severe retardation of articulatory development, associated with gross retardation of the development of spoken language and the comprehension of language. (Many of these children fail to recognize speech sounds until the third or fourth year or even later and have been referred to as suffering from "central deafness".)

6. Patients suffering primarily from language disorders (predominantly adults).

a. Patients with developmental retardation of spoken language with disproportionately mild difficulties in articulation (seen rarely in childhood).

b. Patients with severe difficulties in word finding, constructing sentences, and describing abstract concepts in words (dysphasia—most often found in adult patients).

c. Patients with difficulties in perceiving what is said to them as well as in constructing phrases and sentences indicative of their thinking, particularly their abstract thoughts (receptive dysphasia—most commonly seen in adult patients).

7. Mixed disorders of spoken language (this category is reserved for patients in whom it is virtually impossible to make a definitive primary diagnosis of the type of speech that is predominantly disturbed—for example, adults who suffer from impairment of comprehension and difficulties in using spoken language, associated with speech dysrhythmia and severe dysarthria, following a stroke).

It will be seen that the first category is concerned with abnormalities of voice production, the second with disorders produced by a lack of synchronization of breathing with the movements of the articulatory organs. In Categories 3, 4, and 5, disorders of articulation are the presenting feature. In Category 3, "dysarthria," the articulatory abnormalities are directly attributable to faults in the structure or innervation of the lips, tongue and palate or related organs. In the majority of patients in Category 4, though not all those in Category 4c, there is retarded development of articulation, which is usually the striking presenting feature, though it is associated with general retardation of the development of all other aspects of language ability.

Similarly in Category 5, "specific developmental speech disorder syndrome," especially 5a,b, the presenting feature is retardation of articulatory development; on detailed testing, however, using the many tests of spoken language that are available, it is found that children in these categories will have been slow to acquire the ability to use complex grammatical structures, will produce sentences shorter than average for their age, and will show limited vocabularies and immature patterns of language. In patients in Category 5b it is not uncommon to find that there are defects in passive vocabulary on test; these children score poorly on tests of comprehension even though no clinical evidence of difficulties in comprehension may have been found in the course of routine examination. In Categories 5c,d the development of articulation and spoken language is still more retarded than in Categories a and b, and, in addition, there is impairment of comprehension of spoken language, which has usually been obvious to parents and is apparent on clinical examination as well as on specialized testing.

In Category 6, the predominant finding is one of retarded language development, or the loss of language ability, though there may be associated abnormalities of articulation.

It is not the aim in what follows to give a comprehensive description of all types of speech disorders, but rather to indicate the diversity of the speech disorders commonly encountered in clinical practice.

Description of the Different Disorders of Spoken Language in Childhood

DYSPHONIA (HOARSENESS OR IMPAIRMENT OF VOICE)

This is the presenting feature in from 3 to 4% of children referred to specialist speech clinics in hospitals. Most frequently dysphonia results from recurrent or chronic laryngitis occurring in the early years, or it may be the result of chronic changes due to misuse of the voice, as in excessive shouting. Dysphonia may also occur in children suffering from papillomata of the larynx (multiple, usually benign tumours). Very rarely dysphonia may date from birth; it is then usually associated with paralysis of the vocal cords, the cause of which is obscure.

In children suffering from dysphonia an assessment by an otolaryngologist is essential, and laryngoscopy is required to aid the identification of the disease of the larynx causing the voice disorder. Speech therapists, however, can often contribute greatly to the diagnosis of voice disorders merely by listening to the child's voice quality. Sound spectrography can be very helpful in the diagnosis of disorders of the voice and has probably not been sufficiently employed in the past (Birrell, 1954; Greene, 1964).

Hysterical dysphonia is rare before puberty. Dysphonia may also be a complication of central neurological disease, for example, dyskinetic cerebral palsy, in which unwanted involuntary movements of the larynx as well as of the muscles of the trunk, limbs, tongue, palate, and respiratory muscles often occur. In this type of cerebral palsy voice quality may be further altered by the fact that the child speaks uncoordinately on inspiration as well as expiration.

Dysphonia occurs in up to 4% of patients in some speech clinics devoted to children suffering from speech disorders. Since a high proportion of these patients are "shouters" with a history of early upper respiratory tract infections frequently dating from infancy, it is hardly surprising that many come from Social Classes IV and V ("semiskilled and unskilled workers"—Registrar General's Classification of Social Class by Occupation). Mothers in high tenements frequently say, for example, "I don't need to look out of the window to see if he is there—I can always hear him."

Treatment of disorders of the voice due to shouting and chronic inflammation is difficult. If there is any evidence of persistent infection, long-term antibiotic treatment is probably indicated, but this may be only partly effective in relieving the condition, especially when nodules of the vocal cords have developed. Ideally the vocal cords should be rested, and the child should be persuaded to communicate by whisper rather than by using his voice, but this is a very difficult thing for young children to achieve.

SPEECH DYSRHYTHMIAS (DISORDERS OF THE RHYTHM OF SPEECH)

These disorders are caused by a failure of coordination between the activity of the respiratory and the articulatory musculature. The common manifestations are hesitation, stammer (or stutter), blocking, and unwanted prolongations of syllables.

Normal speech production requires that respiratory activity be subordinate to the needs of articulated speech. Speech pulses, stress patterns, and the need to take breath are coordinated from quite an early age in the healthy child, as has been described (Bullow, 1967).

Any involuntary interference with the normal control of the respiratory mechanism during speech is likely to interfere with the normal patterns of breathing that occur during the production of spoken language, and to result in a failure on the part of the individual to control the timing of his speech pulses or to modify his stress patterns.

This may be manifest in the unwanted prolongation of word sounds (prolongations), which may occur in any part of a phrase or sentence, in the arrest of speech, which occurs most often at the beginning of phrases or sentences (hesitations), or in the repetition of syllables, which occurs most often at the beginning of sentences or phrases, repetitions that constitute "stammer" or "stutter." In most patients it is found that prolongations, hesitations, and repetitions occur together and that they are loosely grouped together under the word "stammer" or "stutter," which freely is used as an inclusive term.

It is impossible in a chapter even of this length to consider fully all the vast literature on the causes of speech dysrhythmia. Books have been written about them, interpreting the condition in terms of psychoanalytic theory (Barbara, 1965), and in terms of aberrant development due to faulty parental handling (Johnson, 1959a, 1959b). Other authors have stressed the high incidence of a family history of speech dysrhythmia in affected patients (Jameson, 1955; Johnson, 1955). Johnson points out that nonfluencies, that is, interruptions in the normal flow of spoken language, occur remarkably commonly in normal adults and even more frequently in children 2- to 5-years, a period when language maturation is proceeding very rapidly. He has suggested that undue attention paid to nonfluencies at this crucial time may make the child unduly aware of them and, by producing emotional tension, exacerbate the tendency to speech dysrhythmia. Parents who know of a family history of stammering may be particularly liable to pay attention to their young children's nonfluencies, and it is exactly their offspring who are likely to be genetically predisposed to stammer (Johnson, 1959a; Moncur, 1951, 1955). Johnson calls this process "the negative evaluation of the child's nonfluencies by the parents' identification of these as stuttering." Johnson's work has been subjected to considerable criticism, but it has been the basis for many theories concerned with the origin of speech dysrhythmia and has provided rationales for a number of systems of therapy.

A full review of current theories of the cause of stammering, and one of the most detailed studies of a large series of patients, was that made by Andrews and Harris (1964). They considered "stutter" as possibly being inherited as a Mendelian dominant characteristic in a proportion of patients. The expression of the dominant characteristic varied from patient to patient according to environmental circumstances and the way the child was handled, but they emphasize that the causes of stammering are probably multifactorial and that a great deal more work requires to be done before the importance of the genetic component in stammering can be evaluated.

THE SYMPTOMS AND SIGNS OF SPEECH DYSRHYTHMIA

As indicated above, nonfluencies, including prolongations, hesitations, blockings, and repetitions, occur frequently as a normal phenomenon in young children at a stage of rapid speech development. These nonfluencies are generaly regarded as manifestations of "cluttering," which is regarded as a normal stage to be distinguished from stammering. In fact it is very difficult by clinical observation to distinguish clutter from stammer, and it is necessary to be cautious in taking for granted that the conditions are necessarily different. It may be reasonable, for example, to regard clutter as nonpathological speech dysrhythmia and stammer as pathological speech dysrhythmia—the major difference being that in pathological speech dysrhythmia there is interference in communication using spoken language and the child is aware of his speech difficulties, whereas in the stage of clutter his ability to communicate using spoken language is usually not significantly impaired and he does not regard his speech difficulties as being in any way abnormal. In practice it is often impossible to tell anxious parents whether their child at the age of 2 or 3 will stammer later, but it is reasonable to point out to them that the child is a great deal more likely to show persistent speech dysrhythmia if they continually draw his attention to his prolongations, repetitions, hesitations, and blockings. Nevertheless, in spite of the best handling, a number of children who show severe clutter certainly proceed to show chronic speech dysrhythmia.

Dysrhythmia may occur at any time, but the most frequent periods are at the age of 2 or 3 when its onset occurs with cluttering, at the age of 5 when the child first goes to school, at the age of 7–8, and much less commonly in adolescence or in adult life, though children who have shown dysrhythmia may show recurrences at any time during the process of maturation. Children who show dysrhythmic features early are more likely to become "chronic stammerers" than are those who develop symptoms at a later age, but there is a great variation in the clinical course they follow. What is remarkable is that the majority of patients who show speech dysrhythmia do so during childhood and that their symptoms do not generally last for more than a few months, though there may be later relapses. The persistent chronic stammerer occurs in a ratio of about one to three compared to what might be called "transient stammerers." Thus, though as many as 3 or 4% of children stammer at some time in their lives, at any one time not more than 1% of the childhood population is likely to be showing speech dysrhythmia. There is considerable evidence that stress may precipitate speech dysrhythmia in those who have shown it at an earlier age; acquired disease of the central nervous system or severe emotional stress, such as occurs under battle conditions, may precipitate a recurrence of symptoms that may have been in abeyance for many years. The first onset of speech dysrhythmia after the age of 11 is relatively uncommon; 50% of patients show dysrhythmia that might be regarded as excessive or "pathological" before the age of 5. Andrews and Harris (1964) described three patterns in the development of stammering:

1. *Transient developmental stammering*—"a transient period of difficulty in the smooth articulation of speech between the ages of two and four years," at the time when children are developing speech. This appears to be the same as cluttering as defined earlier and "development stuttering" as described by Métraux (1950) and T. T. S. Ingram (1959a).

2. *"Remitting stutterers"*—those children who show speech dysrhythmia for a period of between 6 months and 6 years and then show remission. In these patients symptoms first appear between the ages of 3 and 11, the mean age being $7\frac{1}{2}$. It was

found by Andrews and Harris that males in this group tend to stammer for longer than females.

3. *"Persistent stutterers"*—this group comprises about 1% of the population. Commonly speech dysrhythmia appears between the ages of 2 and 8, persisting until the age of at least 15 and quite frequently into adult life. Patients in this group provide the large body of "chronic speech dysrhythmics" of "chronic stutterers" who require most clinical help. Males outnumber females by two to one, and it is in this group that real distress in adult life may result.

The clinical course followed by patients in this third group is not constant, but the pattern described by Bloodstein (1950) certainly occurs in the majority. He defines four phases in the development of persistent speech dysrhythmia. During the first phase there is a repetition of speech sounds and sometimes of two or more syllables at the beginning of phrases; prolongations of speech sounds and hesitations may occur but are less frequently found. Dysrhythmic symptoms are more frequent when the child is excited, especially when he wants to say a great deal quickly and seems to have "pressure of talk." To begin with, dysrhythmia is intermittent; gradually, however, the periods during which it is present lengthen and the periods of remission shorten. The onset of this phase occurs most commonly in the preschool stage.

By the time the second phase has been reached, the periods of remission have practically disappeared, though there may be considerable variation in the severity of symptoms from time to time. As in the first phase, repetitions, especially at the beginnings of sentences and phrases, are the most marked feature, but prolongations and hesitations and "blocking"—in which speech becomes arrested in mid-phrase—also occur with increasing frequency. The child seems to try harder and harder to keep his speech going and as he does so manifests associated involuntary movements of the limbs and trunk with grimacing and sometimes quite bizarre postures. He becomes increasingly aware of his difficulties in using spoken language as a medium of communication and may substitute other words for words he finds particularly difficult to produce.

The second phase merges gradually into the third phase, the characteristic feature of which is that the repetitions, blockings, and prolongations become more frequent and severe, and repetition of individual syllables may be associated with repetition of whole words or even occasionally phrases. The child becomes progressively anxious in the talking situation and shows a greater liability to "become stuck" when excited. He begins to be concerned about any situation in which he has to use spoken language.

In phase four the fully developed picture of dysrhythmia has appeared. Substitution of difficult words is made increasingly frequently, a tendency to reply whenever possible by gesture or by using monosyllables is obvious, and situations in which speech is likely to be used are avoided. For example, a child who stammers when he reads (and not all children do) may ask to go to the lavatory as his turn comes up to read aloud in class. Such children may be under very great emotional stress purely because of their symptoms, and it is probable that this has misled many clinicians to interpret anxiety as being the provoking factor of the speech disorder. The fourth stage has been particularly well described by Travis (1959).

It is suggested that a strong family history of persistent speech dysrhythmia, the presence of overanxious parents, or the existence of obviously adverse psychosocial backgrounds favor the persistence of speech dysrhythmia. But even when speech symptoms do remit in the preschool period, there is still a possibility that they will recur at a later age, most commonly between the ages of 6 and 10, often apparently as a result of anxiety provoked by difficult school situations (Andrews & Harris, 1964).

There are even more treatments for stammer than there are theories of causation. Treatments have varied from hypnosis to psychoanalysis and from electro-shock to relaxation. The difficulties of evaluating the work of therapists who believe fervently in their own methods of treatment are obvious in a condition in which emotional factors are so important (Glauber, 1958; Mason, 1960; Moore, 1946; Van Riper, 1954, 1959). Experiments using "delayed feedback," in which the patient's speech is fed back to him after a delay of a fraction of a second, have been of great interest, for in a high proportion of patients they result in the restoration of a normal speech rhythm (paradoxically, many people with relatively few non-fluencies show many more prolongations, hesitations, repetitions, and blockings when presented with delayed feedback than they do without).

It is always difficult to describe how best to manage a preschool child showing marked dysrhythmic symptoms. By the time they bring their offspring to the clinic, the parents are usually acutely anxious and often the child himself is beginning to realize "there is something wrong with my talking"—yet he is really too young to cooperate fully in direct therapy. In most cases the best that can be done to help the child is to advise the parents and anybody else who cares for the child to ignore his speech symptoms to the maximum extent, try to understand what he says, and take no special measures to correct his dysrhythmia. This is often very difficult advice for parents and teachers to accept, but there is no doubt that recurrent nagging or fussing will exacerbate any dysrhythmic tendency that may exist in a young child, an older child, or even an adult. It is usually fairly easy, for example, to produce stammer in an adult with a history of stammering in childhood, even though he may have been in remission for twenty or thirty years, by appropriate provoking behavior.

There should be a full and frank discussion about the possible and probable causes of the child's speech difficulties and the parents reactions to them; the parents should be told about the likely prognosis as accurately as possible. In many cases a frank discussion at this stage seems to be reassuring and results in some relaxation in the general family anxieties about the child's speech with resultant improvement in his dysrhythmia. At the same interview it should be explained to parents that even if the stammer persists, (and it should be emphasized that it might), effective individual treatment will be possible at a later age when the child's ability to co-operate in therapy has improved.

A major advance in the treatment of stammering has undoubtedly been the introduction of training in so-called "syllable-timed speech." This consists of teaching patients to speak syllable by syllable, stressing them equally and evenly so that pulses tend to occur rhythmically. It is difficult for many children to learn to use syllable-timed speech, and they are very aware of the fact that it is "different" from normal speech. Many, after a period of two or three weeks of intensive training, relapse; but in a significant proportion syllable-timed speech is used successfully and gradually becomes less obviously "odd," as it merges with more normal speech patterns. When using syllable-timed speech very few patients show marked dysrhythmia, and even if they do not use it in everyday life many feel that it is a form of producing spoken language that they can fall back upon in situations of stress in which they are likely to stammer. Experience has shown that syllable-timed speech is usually best taught to the child in a group situation over a 2- or 3-week period, during which intense daily instruction is given. It is essential thereafter that there should be an adequate follow-up with reinforcement of the original instruction. Moreover, unless parents and other members of the family are prepared to co-operate in reminding the child to use syllable-timed speech and are prepared to accept it as preferable to his dysrhythmic speech, it is almost certain that he will cease to use the technique quite soon. Though training patients in syllable-timed speech and maintaining their use of it is time-consuming and demanding for the therapist, the patient, and the patient's relatives, it appears to hold great promise for a proportion of older children who suffer from disabling, chronic speech dysrhythmia (Andrews & Harris, 1964).

DYSARTHRIA (DISORDER OF ARTICULATION DUE TO ABNORMALITIES OF THE LIPS, TONGUE, PALATE, OR RELATED ORGANS, OR THEIR NEUROLOGICAL CONTROL)

In this category are included abnormalities of speech sound production attributable to abnormalities of the function or the structure of the lips, tongue, palate, or related structures such as the teeth and jaws. There may be a failure of the normal function of these organs because of neurological disease, which may be present at any level from the hemispheres to the cranial nerves or even the neuromuscular junctions, as in myasthenia gravis, or the muscles themselves, for example, in facio-scapulo-humeral dystrophy. These neurological disorders, which cause abnormalities of the voluntary movements of the lips, tongue, and palate during speech, form the first subgroup of dysarthric disorders.

The second comprises disorders that are the result of structural abnormalities. The differentiation between disorders due to structural abnormalities and those due to neurological disease is not always as simple as might appear. There is considerable evidence, for example, that malocclusions of the jaws may be the result of abnormalities of muscle tension, which in turn are due to neurological disease. A good example, perhaps, is the effect that simple tongue thrusting, which may be inherited as a Mendelian dominant trait, can have in pushing the upper anterior incisors forward (Hopkin, 1972; Hopkin & McEwan, 1955). Nevertheless, the distinction between dysarthria due predominantly to neurological dysfunction and dysarthria due to structural or anatomical abnormalities is one that is worth making in clinical practice. Within the second subgroup, comprising anatomical abnormalities, it is possible to differentiate dysarthria due to abnormalities of the articulatory organs themselves, for example cleft palate or lingual hypoplasia (Fig. 13—7). (Interestingly enough, isolated clefts of the lip are rarely associated with marked dysarthria unless there are considerable associated malformations of the dental arches.) In contrast to this group of patients, in whom the organs themselves are anatomically abnormal, the one patient whose dysarthria is due to abnormalities of related structures, for example malocclusion of the jaws or palatal disproportion—the name given to the situation when the palate is normal in size but the nasopharyngeal aperture is unduly large and there is an excess of nasal escape, as in unrepaired cleft palate. This condition may be contrasted with hyporhinophonia due to an excessively small nasopharyngeal aperture which may be found as a result of adenoidal enlargement or, very occasionally, due to actual skeletal deformities as in Crouzon's Disease. In these conditions the normal speech sounds cannot be produced even though the actual function and structure of the lips, tongue, and palate themselves, the articulatory organs, are normal.

Many dysarthric disorders have very characteristic defective sound systems and a well-trained speech therapist can often make an accurate diagnosis as to the nature of the underlying neurological abnormality as a result of listening to the child's speech.

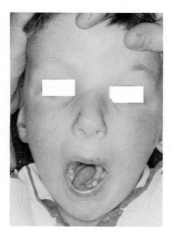

Figure 13—7.   Lingual hypoplasia after surgical release of the tongue from the floor of the mouth. The child's speech was intelligible prior to operation.

SPEECH DEFECTS IN CEREBRAL PALSY

The slow, labored pattern of the speech of the child suffering from cerebral palsy with paretic involvement of the bulbar musculature is characteristic. He speaks more slowly than normal children and has a greater difficulty in changing the position of his lips, tongue, and palate to produce new sounds, so that sound groupings requiring major changes in the position of the lips, tongue, and palate are particularly difficult for him to achieve. On the qualitative score sheets of the Edinburgh Articulation Test there tends to be an apparently almost random scatter of "errors," but a close study shows that these profiles tend to be very similar from child to child suffering from spastic cerebral palsy.

The pediatrician studying such a child will often elicit an early history of feeding difficulties; not infrequently tube feeding may have been required for a prolonged period following birth. Often there is a tendency to regurgitation, slow feeding from the bottle, and apparent difficulties in swallowing. Feeding on semisolids may be easier or more difficult than feeding on liquids, but the majority of patients are rather slow to learn to chew solid materials. Drooling that persists for longer than in the normal infant is almost a constant feature and may persist into later childhood, though there is usually a tendency for drooling to diminish in amount in adolescence if not earlier. On neurological examination there is usually a poverty of facial movement, invariably bilateral though not necessarily symmetrical, and a greater or lesser degree of loss of voluntary movement patterns in the lips, tongue, and palate. Some children, for example, may not be able to protrude the tongue voluntarily at all. In others attempts to protrude the tongue result in an almost tremulous anterior movement, or a very brief and partial protrusion before the tongue is involuntarily withdrawn into the mouth. The palate moves poorly when the child is asked to utter consonant sounds such as *r*. Further evidence of poor palatal movement may be obtained by carrying out X-ray palatography using soft tissue radiography when the child is at rest and saying *n* and *e* or *a*, for in the latter positions the palate should be fully elevated. This technique, however, gives limited information about the palatal movements that occur in continuous speech. This is important, for it is as much the need for rapid changes of position as the ability to move the organ through a full range that impairs articulation.

In contrast to the paralysis or paresis of voluntary movement of the tongue and face, it is quite remarkable to observe the extent to which involuntary activities involving extensive movements of the lips, tongue and palate may be carried out. For example, in coughing and sneezing quite full movements of the palate occur in a high proportion though not in all affected patients, and facial movements may in fact be excessive when the child smiles or shows distress. Similarly it is always a little surprising to the clinician who has demonstrated to his complete satisfaction that the child cannot voluntarily move his tongue to any significant extent to see his tongue come forward involuntarily and lick his lips when he is in the process of feeding. It was the observation of this phenomenon of apparently full involuntary movements in patients showing paresis of voluntary movement that led Jackson (1873) to some of his most fundamental observations on the nature of impairment of movement as a result of disease of the brain.

Dysarthria occurs relatively rarely in children suffering from congenital or acquired unilateral hemiplegia, but it does occur occasionally for reasons that are very difficult to understand unless one assumes that there are associated lesions in the brain stem as well as damage or developmental abnormalities in one or both hemispheres (Fig. 13—8).

In contrast, severe dysarthria is almost invariable in patients showing clinical evidence of bilateral hemiplegia, usually with gross structural changes in both hemispheres due to developmental abnormalities of the brain occurring at an early age, to severe brain damage occurring at the time of birth, or—increasingly frequently in recent years—to severe head injury or damage to the brain associated with vascular lesions occurring in the early years of life, to encephalitis, or to meningitis, which would have killed affected patients before modern methods of treatment were available for them.

In diplegic cerebral palsy the degree of involvement of the bulbar musculature varies considerably. Even in some mildly affected patients in whom paresis of voluntary movement appears to be confined to the lower limbs, it is not unusual to find mild dysarthria; when the upper limbs are affected there is nearly always dysarthria, which may be severe if the diplegia is extensive and associated with the feeding difficulties and drooling described above (Table 13—2) (T. T. S. Ingram, 1966a; Ingram & Barn, 1961).

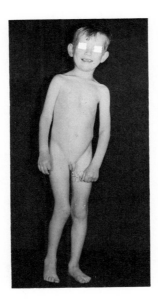

Figure 13—8. Child suffering from congenital right hemiplegia associated with moderately severe dysarthria due to paresis of the lips, tongue and palate.

TABLE 13–2 TYPES OF SPEECH DISORDER IN 122 DIPLEGIC PATIENTS BY EXTENT OF LIMB INVOLVEMENT

Extent of limb involvement	No abnormality of speech	No speech	Dysarthria only	Retardation only	Dysrhythmia only	Dysphasia only	Not exclusive categories				Total
							Dysarthria + other speech defects	Retardation + other speech defects	Dysrhythmia + other speech defects	Dysphasia + other speech defects	
Paraplegia	22	1	6	6	1	1	13	13	2	1	49
Triplegia	2	0	3	1	0	0	3	3	0	0	9
Tetraplegia	6	21	16	8	1	0	14	13	3	1	64
Total	30	22	25	15	2	1	30	29	5	2	122
Approx. %	24	18	20	12	2	1	24	23	4	2	100

In ataxic cerebral palsy without associated diplegia the weakness and unco-ordination of voluntary movements so obvious in the limbs, especially in severely affected patients, is also present in voluntary movements of the lips, tongue and palate. This may affect feeding in infancy, but rarely causes difficulties anything like as severe as those found in severe diplegic cerebral palsy. Dysarthria may not be evident for quite a long time in ataxic patients, for in a significant pro-portion there is a considerable delay in their developing spoken language, even when their comprehension appears intact and they are of reasonable intel-ligence. When speech does appear it shows the same characteristic scanning quality as is found in the speech of patients suffering from acquired ataxia, though this may not be really noticeable until the child is using sentences of four or five words. There is a tendency for patients to have considerable difficulties in the accurate articulation of consonant clusters, particularly in the middles of words; another curious characteristic is that vowel formants are rather inconsistent, vary-ing even in the same word at different times in different sentences, or even the same sentence. Speech tends to be a little slow.

On neurological examination the pediatrician will find the classical features of weakness, incoordination, intention tremor, hypotonia, and unsteadiness in the limbs and trunk. Careful observation will reveal similar abnormalities in the face, palate, and tongue, and intention tremor on protrusion of the tongue is not very difficult to observe with practice. If the child can deviate the tongue laterally toward the corners of the mouth the intention tremor becomes even more apparent.

In ataxic diplegia the nature of the speech disorder will depend upon a number of different factors. The nature of the dysarthria varies according to the relative severity of the ataxic and the diplegic components in affected patients. When the ataxia is predominant and the diplegia mild, the speech disorder is very similar to that found in ataxic patients. On the other hand, when the spastic diplegia is more important than the ataxia, the speech is more like that found in diplegic cerebral palsy. In the majority of patients, however, the disorder is manifest by a mixture of the scanning, slow speech characteristic of the ataxic and the slow, labored speech of the spastic with the characteristic difficulties in producing consonants and consonant clusters accurately that have been described. In addi-tion, since a high proportion of these patients are mentally retarded, there is likely to be delayed and slow speech development.

Ataxic diplegia is the characteristic type of cerebral palsy associated with hydrocephalus; this means that in a high proportion of cases there is the curious, but characteristic, language disorder that has been described as "cocktail party chatter." Many children affected by hydrocephalus have a very high verbal output, which at first hearing is rather impressive. On closer examination, however, it will be found that the child's spoken language consists largely of repetitions of what he has heard adults saying and is in itself repetitious and very often irrelevant to any subject another child or an adult is attempting to discuss with him. It is perhaps a reflection upon the vanity of adults that they are so frequently delighted by the speech of hydrocephalic children and regard them as "clever"—merely because these children produce repetitively large portions of what the adults have said to them (T. T. S. Ingram, 1963a; Ingram & Naughton, 1962).

In dyskinetic cerebral palsy the same sudden, involuntary changes of tone and involuntary movements that disrupt attempted voluntary movements in the limbs affect the lips, tongue, and palate. Dysarthria affects a higher proportion of patients suffering from dyskinesia than from any other type of cerebral palsy except bilateral hemiplegia. Moreover, the dysarthric disorder tends to be very severe and particularly frustrating to patients in this category of cerebral palsy, because more of them are of average, near average, or superior intelligence than are those in the other categories. Thus their desire to communicate is greater and their ability to do so using spoken language, and frequently even using writing, is often more severely impaired. In children suffering from dyskinesia of any significant degree a history of feeding difficulties in infancy is almost constant. Initially these occur in the immediate postnatal period during the time that the immediate effects of perinatal injury or kernicterus are apparent, but they frequently persist for months or even into adult life. The picture of the badly affected, intelligent patient suffering from choreoathetoid cerebral palsy, drooling from the mouth, requiring considerable help in feeding, showing quite violent movements on any voluntary effort, and struggling desperately to utter a few single intelligible words in response to anybody talking to them is a most distressing one. I believe that in the past speech therapists have sometimes been too active in trying to help children suffering from dyskinetic cerebral palsy to produce spoken language and have succeeded in increasing their sense of frustration rather than in improving their powers of communication. (Figs. 13—9, 10, 11).

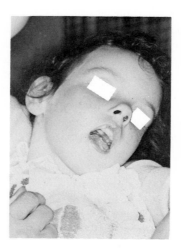

Figure 13—9. Child suffering from severe dyskinetic cerebral palsy of age 2, showing reflex mouth-opening and involuntary movements of tongue and palate.

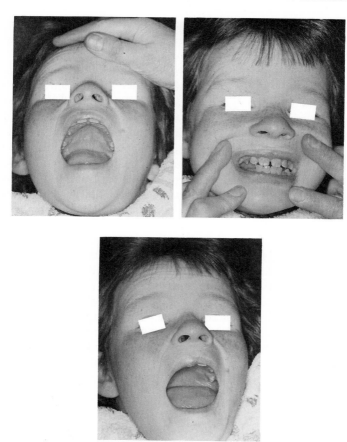

Figure 13—10. Girl suffering from severe dyskinetic cerebral palsy showing involuntary movement of face, tongue and palate. Tongue thrust is evident.

It is impossible to give a full account of the vast variety of sound distortions, irregularities, omissions, and abnormalities of intonational patterns and rhythm that occur in dyskinetic cerebral palsy. They are characterized by their variability from moment to moment as the patterns of involuntary movement of the lips, tongue, and palate, and the associated involuntary movements of the larynx and respiratory musculature, which have been referred to, occur. Explosive speech is not a bad description of the difficulties that many children have in initiating their first syllable and their inability to control the word sound uttered. This may or may not be followed by a sequence of other syllables, depending upon the degree of associated dysrhythmia and involuntary glottal closure and the violence of associated body movements. On the qualitative chart of the Edinburgh Articulation Test, the characteristic pattern in dyskinesia, in patients who are not so severely affected that the test is impossible for them, is an almost random distribution of sounds with an almost complete absence of consonant clusters and the later-acquired consonant sounds.

It should be emphasized that dysarthria is not the most important cause of the abnormalities of spoken language in cerebral palsy. Retardation of speech development, due in the majority of cases to associated mental defect, sometimes with associated hearing impairment especially in severe tetraplegic diplegia and in dyskinesia, and often a degree of linguistic deprivation in the environment in infancy and early childhood are more frequent and important causes of speech disorders. In addition, a proportion of patients, particularly those suffering from acquired right hemiplegia, suffer from true dysphasia, and this may also appear as a new phenomenon in children suffering from congenital right hemiplegia following a severe focal epileptic attack, particularly if there has previously been extensive cortical sensory loss. Presumably further brain damage has occurred. There are probably other associated problems in patients suffering from cerebral palsy, such as abnormalities of self-monitoring and auditory feedback, about which very little is known as yet and which are extremely difficult to study.

The complexity of the speech disorders in cerebral palsy requires the full diagnostic resources of a team of speech therapist, pediatric neurologist, and child psychologist, and often the help of a phonetician whth a fully equipped laboratory at his disposal and of an audiologist is invaluable. In a high proportion of cases, however, the close study of a patient by a pediatric neurologist and a speech therapist working together can sort out, to a large extent, the relative importance of retardation of speech development secondary to mental retardation or hearing

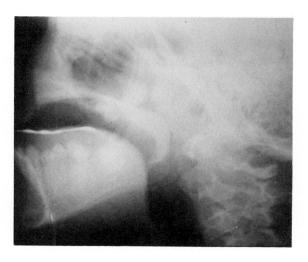

Figure 13–11. Child suffering from dyskinetic cerebral palsy, showing tongue (coated with barium) thrusting as he attempts to produce *l, e,* and *Q* (*th*) sounds.

impairment, dysarthria and dysphasia. Moreover, the correlation of the information that the speech therapist can provide by a detailed analysis of the child's speech with observations or the nature of the movement disorder found in the lips, tongue, and palate in dysarthric patients can add greatly to an understanding of the nature of the child's difficulties in producing spoken language. Such a combined study is really essential if the planning of therapy is to be helpful. Moreover, when therapy is planned it is important to relate it to the total needs of the child for other therapy, education, and enlarging environmental experience.

OTHER NEUROLOGICAL DISORDERS

In the same way as disorders of voluntary movement, which occur in cerebral palsy, tend to produce rather characteristic patterns of articulatory abnormalities and clinical symptoms and signs, so do other neurological disorders (Figs. 13—12, 13, 14). In the Moebius syndrome (nuclear agenesis—Fig. 13—15) their severity varies according to the extent of the involvement of the cranial nerve nuclei and the extent and severity of the lower motor neurone paresis in the lips, tongue, and palate. For example, a very different picture will be apparent when the face and palate are paretic but the tongue is spared than when the face moves normally, the palate is mildly affected, and the tongue is virtually paralysed. When the palate is affected, nasal escape is always present; there is very commonly a history of the nasal escape of milk and later semisolids during feeding in infancy; and there are difficulties in swallowing, frequently with a history of choking, regurgitation or inhalation of food stuffs, and drooling (Fig. 13—16). Drooling is even more severe when the tongue is also involved, and a tendency for salivation to be uncontrollable is, of course, more marked if the child cannot purse his lips to diminish its flow from

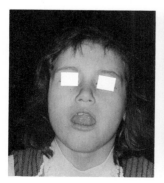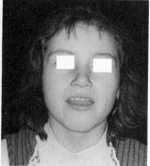

Figure 13—12. Child 8-years old, who suffered from encephalitis affecting the brain stem at the age of 11 months, with abnormal movements of the tongue.

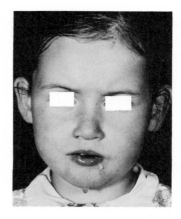

Figure 13—13. Typical drooling in a child who suffered from encephalitis affecting the brain stem at the age of 11 months causing abnormality of tongue movement.

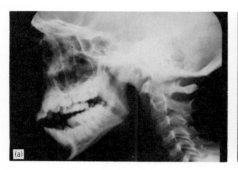

Figure 13—14. The palatal paresis in the child in Fig. 13—13 was confirmed by palatography. There is no difference in the position of the palate when the child utters *n* (a) and *e* (b) sounds.

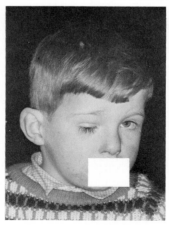

Figure 13—15. Nuclear Agenesis. When the child deviated his eyes to one side the contralateral eye lid closed.

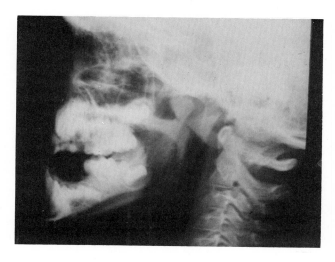

Figure 13—16. X-ray palatogram showing a short hypoplastic palate which cannot close the naso-pharyngeal aperture.

the mouth. A detailed neurological study of the movements of the lips, tongue, and palate is nuclear agenesis is essential if the speech therapist is to have a rational basis on which to plan therapy. But because the defects of movement in this condition are relatively consistent, the defects of articulation that are found are also rather constant and vary much less than they do, for example, in spastic cerebral palsy. When there is palatal paresis, there will be persistent nasal escape. When the lips are paralyzed, there will tend to be an absence of plosives. When the tongue is very weak, labial and dental sounds are conspicuous by their absence. Severely affected children have a very limited repertoire of consonants and consonant clusters and in many cases can be helped to only a limited extent by speech therapy. The effects of palatal paresis, however, may be greatly minimized bu diminishing the size of the nasopharyngeal aperture by pharyngoplasty, an operation that should probably not be carried out until the child is over the age of 7 or 8.

In myasthenia gravis of the onset type the findings are rather characteristic, both from the point of view of the child's speech patterns and from the point of view of his neurological findings. Characteristically speech is least abnormal at the beginning of sentences and when the child is fresh and not tired. As the day advances and he becomes more fatigued, his speech deteriorates; whereas quite long sentences may have been correctly articulated at breakfast time, by lunch time the ends of long sentences are becoming "slurred and slow," as they are described by many parents. What they notice, in fact, is that the child is having difficulty in producing consonants and consonant clusters, particularly those that require the greatest amount of voluntary movement from the lips, tongue, and palate. In addition there is often a diminution in the airstream towards the end of sentences, which means that the voice tends to "fade out." Thus the child ceases to make plosives, labiodental sounds, and then fricatives, and his voice becomes quieter towards the end of sentences. By evening his speech may be still more abnormal. Such a history is quite characteristic and is surprisingly often elicited. A rather similar history is found in many patients suffering from weakness of the lips, tongue and palate as a result of facio-scapulo-humeral dystrophy or congenital dystrophia myotonica, but it is more striking in myasthenia gravis than in these conditions. Moreover, clinically the conditions are relatively easily distinguished on the basis of the history and the neurological findings and by use of the "Tensilon" (edrophonium) or "prostigmine" (neostigmine) Tests, which when indubitably positive, clearly establish the diagnosis of myasthenia.

STRUCTURAL ABNORMALITIES

Similar considerations as regard diagnosis are true for structural abnormalities causing dysarthria. A careful phsyical examination, an assessement of the function on test of the articulatory organs and the health of other related structures, is essential.

The speech therapist will certainly be able to diagnose the nature of defects of velarization by assessing the abnormalities of the child's vocal resonance, the degree of nasal escape or nasal obstruction occurring during speech, and will be able to give an accurate account of the nature of the particular abnormalities of tongue movements that account for the pattern of abnormal word sounds pro-duced. But this must always be confirmed by a direct observation of the organs themselves and by seeing what happens when a child is moving them on request. Such observations may have to be made using radiological techniques. Very full accounts have been presented of sophisticated methods of clinical examination of the actions of the lips, tongue, and palate in situations other than speech by Bosma (1957; Bosma & Lind, 1960; Logan & Bosma, 1967). These may be supplemented by detailed observations made by an orthodontist with great advantage especially in patients suffering from cleft lip and palate, hypomandibulosis, and other types of malocclusion of the jaws, particularly when the relationship between the jaws is changing in the course of maturation (Dixon, 1966; Hopkin & McEwan, 1955). Often, however, as in cleft palate, agenesis or hypoplasia of the tongue, or gross enlargement of the tonsils and adenoids, the medical diagnosis is easy.

A good example of the way in which cooperation between a speech therapist, surgeon, orthodontist, and pediatric neurologist interested in speech disorders may help in the diagnosis of a patient is a case in which a child showed nasal escape following what appeared to have been an adequate repair of the palate and had associated abnormalities of tongue movement. The pediatric neurologist sus-pected that there was some impairment of palatal movement secondary to pharyngitis, which proved to be the case; the pediatric surgeon pointed out that there was a small fistula, which it was possible to demonstrate, showing enlarge-ment and allowed escape of air when the intra-oral pressure was increased; and the orthodontist pointed out that he suspected the increasing malocclusion that he noted must be due to tongue thrust. The pediatrician suggested that this might be secondary to the fact that the child had frequent sore throats and was avoiding using the body of the tongue, especially far back in the mouth. Treatment of the pharyngitis produced considerable improvement in palatal movement, a small dental plate served to cover the fistula's opening, and tongue thrust diminished considerably once the child's pharyngitis had improved (Figs. 13—17, 18).

Nasal escape may occur as a result of cleft palate, hypoplasia of the palate, impairment of movement of the palate as found in submucous cleft of the palate even

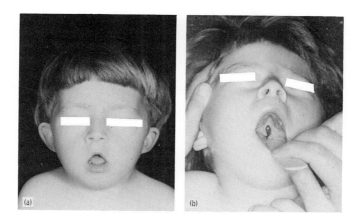

Figure 13—17. Child suffering from cleft palate ad fistula of hard palate. "Compensatory" tongue movements contributed to his speech disorders after repair (b).

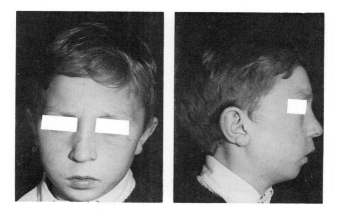

Figure 13—18. Maxillary hyperplasia with hypomandibulosis associated with apparent tongue thrust and hypernasality.

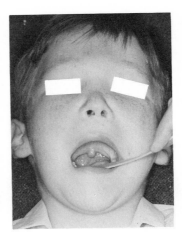

Figure 13—19. Congenital short hypoplastic palate with overgrowth of adenoids inferiorly.

though the organ may appear to be intact at first sight. Scarring of the palate following infection or injury is another less common cause of defective palatal movement (Fig. 13—19).

The palatal disproportion syndrome is a much commoner condition than is generally realized and is often compensated for by enlargement of the adenoids, against which the palate may close. Thus nasal escape may only occur following adenoidectomy. Parents are rarely grateful if their child, who has been operated upon because he has sounded "all stuffed up," leaves the hospital without his adenoids and with a clear nasal airway, but talking as if he had a cleft palate (Fig. 13—20). Thus care should be taken to assess the size of the nasopharynx

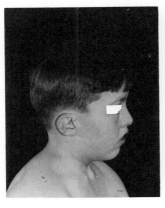 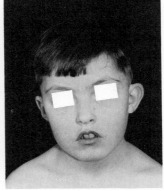

Figure 13—20. Typical "adenoidal facies," associated with mouth breathing and hyperhinophonia. It is often wise to carry out X-ray palatography before deciding to perform adenoidectomy.

and the relative size of the adenoids before operation is carried out. Often it is possible to carry out a partial adenoidectomy, leaving the lower part of the adenoids against which the palate can close but removing the upper part of the adenoids, which are likely to obstruct the Eustachian tubes when inflamed (Birrell, 1960). When nasal escape persists following operation for cleft palate or after adenoidectomy, a considerable reduction in nasal escape may be achieved by pharyngoplasty or by other operations (Batchelor, 1966). Accounts of the nature of the speech disorders encountered in children suffering from clefts of lip and palate have been presented by Morley (1962) and by T. T. S. Ingram (1966b). A much more extensive coverage, including a consideration of more recent work, is contained in Grabb, Rosensten, and Bzoch (1971).

The importance of dental malocclusion as a cause of speech defects has been much disputed. There is no doubt that the structure of the face and the occlusion of the jaws are greatly influenced by the orofacial musculature and that the activity of the tongue plays a crucial part in producing forward protrusion of the anterior incisors in many patients in whom this occurs. On the other hand, a tendency to the inheritance of occlusal characteristics is very obvious in many families (under-bite or overbite in common language, skeletal malformations 1, 2, and 3 in technical parlance), often being obvious in the parents of a child brought to a speech clinic with a speech defect apparently associated with malocclusion of the jaws (Burkitt & Lightoller, 1927; Hopkin, 1972; Hopkin & McEwan, 1955; Lightoller, 1926). It seems probable that both genetic inheritance of abnormal occlusion of the jaws and secondary malocclusion due to the atypical formation of orofacial musculature or the abnormal action of the tongue may produce malocclusion. This may explain why malocclusion of the jaws is seen relatively commonly when there is gross weakness of the orofacial musculature, as in some patients suffering from nuclear agenesis or dystrophia myotonica congenita or cerebral palsy. It would also explain why in other patients there appears to be no abnormality of the orofacial musculature whatsoever, though there is quite marked underbite or overbite, hypomandibulosis or overdevelopment of the maxilla with an enlarged nasopharyngeal aperture and nasal escape during speech (Figs. 13—21, 22).

There are other abnormalities of structures related to the lips, tongue, and palate that may cause speech disorders. A few of these, which have been seen in recent years in the Speech Clinic of the Royal Hospital for Sick Children, Edinburgh, may be mentioned. They include chronic and recurrent parotitis, choanal atresia, with almost complete obstruction of the nasal airway, a dermoid cyst of the nasopharynx, sarcoma of a tonsil, the presence of foreign bodies in both nostrils, the presence of a palatal tooth, and unrecognized perforation of the soft palate as a result of trauma. Nevertheless, the commonest associated abnormalities are anatomical, affecting velarization or occlusion of the jaws, and are the effects of acquired diseases. The commonest of these are pharyngitis, adenoiditis, and tonsillitis. These conditions are particularly liable to affect speech when inflammation is associated with enlargement of the tonsils and adenoids.

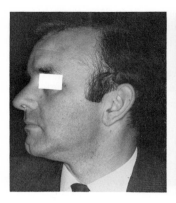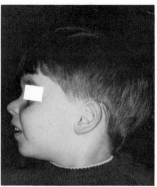

Figure 13–21. Typical facial appearances in fathers and sons showing long, wide maxillae, with palatal dysproportion and hypernasality.

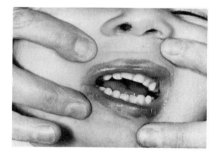

Figure 13–22. Malocclusion. "Open bite" with tongue thrust. Child was a thumb sucker.

Clearly, diagnosis of the disorders depends upon a careful clinical examination, supplemented when necessary by further radiological studies. Soft tissue rays are of particular value in helping to estimate the size of adenoids and the extent of the restriction of palatal movement secondary to adenoidal enlargement and inflammation of the nasopharynx. Repeated cephalometry using carefully standardized techniques helps to determine the patterns of growth of the jaws and related structures and has been used extensively, especially in patients who suffer from cleft palate with or without cleft lip.

The effects of abnormalities of organs and structures associated with the lips, tongue, and palate vary greatly according to their situation and extent. It is unwise, for example, to assume because there is malocclusion of the jaws that a speech defect is necessarily due to it. It may be true that because there is a large space between the upper and lower incisors when the mouth is shut, there is room for the tongue to protrude between them during speech, but it is equally possible that the malocclusion has been caused by the same abnormalities of movement of the tongue and orofacial musculature that are responsible for the defective articulation (Hopkin, 1962). Similarly, even in a gross anatomical abnormality such as cleft lip and palate it is unwise to assume that all the articulatory abnormalities are the direct result of the lesion. Numerous studies have demonstrated that the whole pattern of tongue and orofacial movements that occur during speech are altered when this condition is present. This has been demonstrated by many authors, most of the earlier important studies being referred to by T.T.S. Ingram (1966b).

Secondary Speech Disorders

The heading "Secondary Speech Disorders" is used to comprise a rather diverse group of conditions, which present themselves as abnormalities of spoken language without there being evidence of any abnormality of the structure or function of the lips, tongue, or palate. For the most part these disorders are manifest as retardation of speech development, though particular disorders responsible for the speech defect may produce particular articulatory manifestations or typical linguistic abnormalities. It will be seen from the classification in Table 13—3 that five major causes of secondary speech disorder are recognized, but it should be emphasized that these may occur in combination and that the list is by no means exclusive.

TABLE 13—3   CRUDE CLASSIFICATION OF SECONDARY SPEECH DISORDERS

1. Associated with mental defect.
2. Associated with hearing defect.
3. Associated with true dysphasia.
4. Associated with psychiatric disorders.
5. Associated with environmental deprivation or other adverse factors in environment.
6. Combinations of the above. (The commonest)

Secondary Special Readers

MENTAL RETARDATION

Undoubtedly the commonest cause of retardation of speech development secondary to disease is that found in association with mental retardation, whether the retardation is the result of a genetically determined condition such as mongolism or phenylketonuria, is due to teratogenic factors occurring in early pregnancy, or is the result of perinatal brain damage. Parents are often very unwilling to recognize the extent of the backwardness of their mentally retarded children and are liable to concentrate on their speech defects rather than upon their general retardation of behavior development. Thus it is hardly surprising to find that a rather large number of children who suffer from mental retardation are referred to speech clinics. Of children with severely retarded speech development, 55% were found to be mentally retarded in a consecutive series referred to the Speech Clinic of the Royal Hospital for Sick Children, Edinburgh (T.T.S. Ingram, 1964b). Another factor that favors their being referred to a speech clinic is, however, that a significant proportion of mildly or moderately severely mentally retarded patients have virtually normal milestones of early motor development (Illingworth, 1967). Unfortunately some doctors seem to believe that normal motor milestones indicate that the child is likely to be of average or nearly average intelligence. A large number of studies have been made of the phonology of the speech of mentally retarded children since the pioneering work of O. C. Irwin (1942; Irwin & Spiker, 1949). In any large group of patients, the severity of the delay in speech maturation tends to be inversely proportional to the intelligence quotient, as shown in Table 13–4. Very few idiots use spoken language as a means of communication, even when they are adult. The verbal communication of imbeciles is very limited (Karlin & Strazzula, 1952; Matthews, 1959). Sirkin and Lyons (1941) studied 2522 institutionalized mentally retarded patients. They found that 17% had no speech and 50% had marked speech defects; patients with intelligence quotients of over 69 were found to have defective speech in 31% of cases (Sirkin & Lyons, 1941). Lenneberg (1964) found that there was a closer relationship between the development of motor skills and language development than there was between language development and intelligence quotients using standard tests, a finding that has been replicated in normal children more recently by Neligan and Prudham (1969a, and 1969b). In patients of below average intelligence, tests of vocabulary, sentence length, and articulation tend to correlate quite well. A number of authors have pointed out that the phonological patterns, grammatical structures, and other characteristics of the speech of mentally retarded older children and adults are strikingly similar to those found in very young children of average intelligence, and the pattern of phonological development does not deviate from that found in normal younger children (Bangs, 1942) (see Table 13–4.)

TABLE 13–4   AGE OF SPEECH ACQUISITION[a]

Activity	IQ 15–20	IQ 26–30	IQ 51–70
Babbling	25 months	20.4 months	20.8 months
Word use	54.3 months	43.2 months	34.5 months
Sentence use	153 months	93 months	89.4 months

[a] *Karlin and Strazzulla 1952.*

There used to be a tendency to consider that gross retardation of the development of spoken language was inevitable in mental defectives and that it was irremediable. There has been a change in attitude in recent years. The extent to which moderately severely backward children may be helped by speech therapy has been demonstrated by many workers and especially by Renfrew in the United Kingdom (Renfrew, 1964). The effect of training children in the understanding of words implying spatial and temporal relationships is of obvious importance, not only because of the fact that it facilitates their communication using spoken language but also because it seems likely in the light of recent Russian and French work that an increased vocabulary and repeated demonstrations of what is implied by words and phrases such as *under, on top of, forward, backward, later,* and *soon* and the use of tenses may encourage conceptual development. Evidence for this is inevitably rather slender so far.

The fact that many patients suffering from cerebral palsy suffer from mental retardation has been mentioned. It should also be remembered that a significant proportion of patients who are mentally retarded suffer from other abnormalities, including hearing loss, structural abnormalities of the lips, tongue, and palate, including cleft palate; merely because a patient is found to be mentally retarded there is no reason why the same careful, joint assessment by a pediatrician and a speech therapist should not be carried out as is done for children suffering from other types of speech disorder.

SECONDARY SPEECH DISORDERS DUE TO HEARING LOSS

Increasing numbers of very young children are referred to speech clinics either because during routine screening examinations by health visitors or local authority doctors babies seem to be inattentive to sounds or show abnormal babbling patterns or because their parents are afraid there may be hearing impairment because of family history. The increase in numbers of such patients referred emphasizes that facilities for the testing of hearing of very young children should be available in speech clinics; this, in turn, makes it necessary that either the pediatrician or the speech therapist should be trained in the techniques of testing the hearing of young children or that audiologists should be available to undertake this. Recent development of sophisticated apparatus designed to test hearing in children and other patients who cannot cooperate fully has marked a considerable advance in the diagnosis of hearing loss at an early stage. In particular more extensive use of EEG and crossed acoustic audiometry promises to be helpful in small babies (Henderson, 1975).

With many patients the pediatrician is able to elicit a history suggesting that potential causes of hearing loss may have been present. There may be a family history of hearing loss, and this should always be sought with some care. Very occasionally there are signs of conditions associated with hearing loss. The author well remembers the repeated visits of an attractively made-up mother with her daughter, who had atypical speech development and a suspicion of hearing loss; it was the fifth or sixth visit before the mother appeared with her hair "un-dyed," revealing a central white patch in the mid-forehead, which indicated not only why she had her hair colored, but also suggested very strongly the presence of Waardenburg's syndrome, in which this characteristic feature is associated with hereditary deafness (Fig. 13—23). In other patients there may be a history of premature delivery, neonatal apnoea, or, more significantly still, hyperbilirubinaemia. Chronic and recurrent otitis media is remarkably common in infancy and is still far too often treated by ineffective eardrops. It is impressive to note how frequently one obtains a history of "he seemed to have sore ears when he was a baby," or even "when he was little his ears were always discharging," or "he was never free of colds and he was always stuffed up, and when he was stuffed up he never seemed to hear" in children who present damaged middle ears and serious hearing loss at the age of 3 or 4, usually with gross retardation of speech development. This is particularly liable to occur in patients in the lower social classes who are probably at a disadvantage in any case so far as speech development is concerned because of the relative lack of stimulation for language development in their environments.

Though the pediatrician will always ask the mother when he takes the history about her exposure to rubella, it is surprising how frequently this is denied, it later being discovered that she was in contact with the disease in early pregnancy. Examination of the child suffering from deafness due to rubella will almost invariably reveal rubella retinopathy, and in many patients where there is deafness due to the effects of perinatal injury, abnormal neurological signs indicating the presence of brain damage will be evident (Stark, 1966). Frequently the effects of early otitis media are all too apparent on otoscopy, and there may also be associated anatomical abnormalities that predispose to middle ear infection, such as cleft palate (T. T. S. Ingram, 1966a; Miller, Court, Walton, & Knox, 1960; Nylen, 1961).

Less common causes of hearing loss are virus infections and so-called "allergic" or "autoimmune" reactions in childhood. Deafness may occur in the course of meningitis, and in older series of patients was reported to occur in between 10 and 20% of patients with a history of this condition. Hearing loss is still not uncommon as a complication of measles and may be due in this condition to associated otitis media or to nerve deafness when there is associated involvement of the central nervous system. Deafness associated with mumps may also occur. Increasing

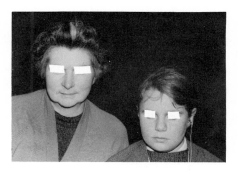

Figure 13—23. Waardenburg syndrome (white forelock and hereditary nerve deafness). Mother and daughter (5-years old).

numbers of patients suffer from unilateral hearing loss as a result of cranial trauma (Maran, 1966).

As indicated above, the routine testing of the hearing of infants has resulted in an improvement in the recognition of hearing loss at an early age. Quite simple tests may be employed in screening for impaired hearing (Sheridan, 1948, 1964). Most testers have found that it is much easier to test the hearing of children up to the age of about three months than it is later, for thereafter they show a decreasing tendency to respond to repetitive stimuli consistently.

In spite of the fact that ascertainment has improved, a surprisingly large number of children come to speech clinics at the age of 2–4 with fairly obvious impairment of hearing. Almost 10% of a recent series of children with very slow speech development of ages between 3 and 6, referred to the Royal Hospital for Sick Children, Edinburgh, were found to have serious hearing loss, which should have been diagnosed much earlier.

The speech therapist will often recognize high-tone hearing loss because of the omission of consonants and consonant clusters in which high frequencies are particularly important, such as *f, th, pt, sh,* and *s,* but many patients who suffer predominantly from high-tone deafness also have impairment of hearing for lower frequencies, and when hearing loss is severe speech defects tend to be much less characteristic.

In many textbooks it is stated that conductive deafness results in hearing loss that is relatively similar in its severity throughout the frequencies from 125 to 8000 Hz. This is not always so, however, and in a small proportion of patients who suffer from middle ear disease, high-tone deafness very similar in type to that found in so-called "nerve deafness" may be found (Ingram, 1966b; Nylen, 1961; Spriestersbach, 1955).

Speech therapists and audiologists are more aware than clinicians of the characteristic searching behavior, the apparently increased visual awareness, especially in the periphery of their visual fields and the tendency to turn their heads from side to side almost continuously to inspect their environments, which are characteristic features of children suffering from hearing loss. When this is severe, children tend to rely on the gestures of people communicating with them and on lip reading. When they do attempt to produce spoken language, it is often obvious that the sounds they produce are those that involve gross movements of the lips, such as *o, m, w,* and *u* sounds.

Even when experts attempt to assess the hearing of young children using the most sophisticated apparatus, they may be unable to reach a definitive diagnosis; in these circumstances it is important to begin appropriate training without waiting for a precise assessment, so that speech development may be encouraged when the child is still very young. In some patients the provision of appropriate hearing aids will enable the child to make good progress, but in older children training may be very much more difficult, with or without hearing aids. In the early stages of training, the child must be treated largely indirectly by parent counseling; this is a field in which, to date, British speech therapists have not been allowed to assist to the extent they could. Many teachers of the deaf still feel that the care of such patients is their particular preserve.

The same environmental and inborn characteristics that modify the development of adaptive and social behavior of children also affect their linguistic development. Similarly, environmental stress is liable not only to cause behavioral abnormalities but also disorders of speech, as has been described in patients particularly predisposed to speech dysrhythmia.

PSYCHIATRIC DISORDERS AND SPEECH DEFECTS

In any speech clinic it is found that a relatively high proportion of the children referred suffer predominantly from maladjustment and psychiatric symptoms; their speech symptomatology is of relatively minor importance. Perhaps the commonest example of this is the small child who has been grossly overprotected from his earliest days, who has been prevented from developing any personal independence or interpersonal relationships with children of his own age, and who has had a very limited environmental experience; his doting parents, sometimes accompanied by their own parents, complain that his speech is "babyish," a few months before he is due to go to school. Many such children show normal language ability on tests and average or superior scores on tests of passive vocabulary. But they tend to use immature forms of speech and immature patterns of articulation. They may prefer to themselves by name or as *me* rather than *I*, and speak of *doggies* and *horsies* even at the age of $4\frac{1}{2}$ years or more. On the other hand, they usually respond very rapidly to speech therapy which is commonly given in a group situation and benefit from nursery or nursery school placement.

Another group of children who come to speech clinics is also clearly recognizable: this consists of those who suffer from the effects of severe environmental and often parental deprivation. There are many causes for this. The mother may have seen very little of her child because of physical or psychiatric illness requiring hospitalization, because she is single or separated from her husband, or in financial straits that have made it necessary for her to go out to work. The parents may have a very large family; in these circumstances it is not uncommon for one of the children to be "squeezed out" and to fail to have as close a relationship with his parents and his siblings as do the other members of the family, so that he grows up in a rather solitary, and often emotionally neglected, state. Emotional maladjustment is very liable to occur in such circumstances and is frequently accompanied by considerable retardation of the development of spoken language, which may be demonstrated in the low scores obtained on tests of active and passive vocabulary, tests of the ability to express himself using spoken language, and on tests of articulation.

Similarly, children who are significantly emotionally immature are likely to have retarded speech development, even though they may be of average or even superior intelligence. In some cases emotional immaturity is accompanied by retardation of physical development. In these circumstances it often seems somewhat unreasonable that they should be treated by educational authorities according to their chronological age rather than according to the stage of skeletal and emotional development they have achieved. There are striking differences in the stages of physical, emotional, and intellectual development in any group of children of similar age entering school for the first time (aged 5 in the United Kingdom); some of the children look and behave as if they were little more than 3-years old, whereas others seem like normal 7- or 8-year olds. Perhaps more account should be taken of the great natural variation in the rate of physical, emotional, and behavioral development that occurs in healthy children who a few years later will be found to be of average intelligence. These immature children are expected to conform to behavioral patterns according to their chronological age, and when they fail to do so are liable to be regarded as "backward." Since it is so important in their early school years that their speech should not appear "babyish," their parents often bring them to speech clinics in the vain hope that the speech therapist can make their speech sound normal in the course of a month or two immediately before school entry. When possible, it is often advisable to retain such children in nurseries or in nursery schools until they are $5\frac{1}{2}$ or 6 years of age, rather than expose them to the stress of formal schooling before they are ready for it.

It is always important in a speech clinic for the speech therapist and pediatrician to ask themselves what are the underlying reasons parents may have for bringing their child to the clinic. Not infrequently the answer is that the parents are fearful that the child may be mentally retarded and find it difficult to admit this to themselves, or they are aware of his immature behavior, his temper tantrums, his solitariness, or the fact that perhaps he masturbates excessively or is excessively clinging to his mother. In other cases still more serious anxieties have precipitated the child's referral.

ELECTIVE MUTISM

Elective mutism is probably not a single syndrome. The term is applied to children who speak in a certain limited number of circumstances, for example in the home and perhaps in a small group of playmates, but not in other circumstances. Children who show "elective mutism" very often speak quite freely in their home environment but never speak outside it and may remain utterly mute for months or years in other circumstances, including their schools.

Elective mutism most often appears in the early school years. It is said in the literature on the subject that more boys than girls suffer from this condition, though this is not the author's experience. There may or may not be a history of slow speech development.

In the majority of such patients there are other symptoms of emotional disturbance, usually those associated with withdrawal—a failure to play with other children, a reluctance to enter into organized activities in school, a failure to play their part in any group activity. There tends to be an overdependence upon parents and other members of the family (Haskill, 1964; Trammer, 1934).

Most elective mutes are suffering from neurotic disturbances of which their mutism is but a part. There are usually very basic maladjustments between the mute child and his parents, the other members of his family, and neighbors, teachers and others who come into contact with the child. Frequently in large families it is found that the elective mute is very much "the odd man out," but it is not uncommon to find that one or the other parent of a child suffering from elective mutism has also been solitary in childhood. In one particular patient the father was found to have shown retarded speech development and been regarded as "backward" at school; he had made no real friends until he entered the army at the age of nineteen. He recalled with considerable distress his feelings of fear when he was forced by circumstances to come into close contact with his fellow human beings. His daughter spoke freely and easily at home, but had been unable to make any friends outside her home environment. When she went to school she remained mute for three years, until she was referred to the speech clinic of the Royal Hospital for Sick Children, Edinburgh, and the Department of Psychological Medicine. Intensive therapy by these departments was arranged, and after a few weeks of in-patient treatment the child spoke for the first time—actually telling her speech therapist to "go away," much to the therapist's delight.

In a minority of patients who suffer from elective mutism, however, it is found that the condition is a manifestation of a severe psychotic personality disorder, usually of schizophrenic type. Such children have a poor prognosis. They are usually found to be quite severely maladjusted at the time of their referral to a speech clinic, and their maladjustment seems to increase in severity as they grow older, rather than diminish as in the case of children suffering from "neurotic" elective mutism.

It is important that elective mutism should be recognized for what it is, when children suffering from it appear at a speech clinic. Usually it is found that in the home environment the various obtainable measures of spoken language and comprehension of speech are within average limits. Fundamentally, the disorder should be regarded as a manifestation of psychiatric disease, rather than primarily as a disorder of spoken language. Therefore the child psychiatrist can be expected to do much more for the majority of patients who suffer from elective mutism than can the speech therapist, though the speech therapist may be able to help in encouraging the child to express himself (or more often herself) once the major problems of adjustment have been lessened.

SPEECH DISORDERS ASSOCIATED WITH CHILD PSYCHOSIS

The first full description of the syndrome of infantile autism was that given by Kanner (1943). He presented a description of strange, withdrawn, solitary children with obsessive tendencies, difficulties in forming personal relationships even within their families, and markedly retarded speech development, as well as other rather characteristic behavioral patterns. Following his first description, he has modified his views as to which symptoms and signs constitute the syndrome of "autism" (Kanner, 1965). After Kanner's initial description of children suffering from "autism," many other studies have been made of the characteristic symptomatology shown by patients similar to those he described.

Creak *et al.* (1961) suggested that there were nine principal points by which the syndrome of infantile autism could be recognized (Table 13—5). These criteria are unsatisfactory, however, for if one analyzes the behavior of children suffering from cerebral palsy or mental retardation or "minimal cerebral dysfunction," it will be found that a high proportion show more than four of the manifestations of "autism" as thus defined. There is a very great overlap in the abnormal behavioral characteristics of patients who might be regarded as suffering primarily from a severe personality disorders that may be conveniently called "autism" or "Kanner's syndrome," and children showing other evidence on neurological examination of cerebral dysfunction. It may be a convenient description of their behavioral manifestations to say that they suffer from "autistic features," but it is probably more realistic to consider the possibility that "autism" in childhood may in some patients be the result of brain damage, while in others it is a manifestation of a severe inherited personality disturbance unaccompanied by any clinical signs of motor or sensory dysfunction (T. T. S. Ingram, 1969).

When a childhood psychosis has been present since infancy, speech development is usually very slow and a proportion of affected patients never learn to use spoken language as a means of communication. On the other hand, when the psychosis first appears in early childhood, as it may, there is often a marked reduction in the amount of spoken language produced by the child and a slowing of further language acquisition. When some spoken language is acquired, it may not be used as a means of communication; there is a marked tendency among autistic children who talk to themselves or to some unreal person whom they visualize. In contact with other speaking children or adults, autistic children echo what has been said to them or produce meaningless remarks derived from the linguistic content of the person who is speaking to them. When the autistic child is alone, it is frequently fround that he appears to have "latched on" to a particular small segment of the spoken language he has recently been exposed to and either repeats it or plays with its linguistic content in a very self-contained manner for long periods, hours after he has heard what was said (Cunningham, 1966; Rutter, 1966; Wolff & Chess, 1964).

There are a number of very detailed studies of the speech of autistic children. One of the best is that of Cunningham (1966). He describes the speech of one autistic child as follows:

> *There was much less speech giving information or communicating meaning to others than in normal children with the same mean sentence length; there was more immediate repetition of his own remarks or the experimenter's, though delayed repetition was rare. Affirmation was indicated by the repetition of the question. Personal pronouns tended to be reversed so that he might use "me"*

instead of "you." Sentences were more often grammatically incomplete than with younger children who used sentences of corresponding length. There appeared to be some difficulty in understanding speech. He scarcely ever asked questions. There was a general shortage of all kinds of pronouns.

TABLE 13–5   NINE POINTS FOR RECOGNITION OF INFANTILE AUTISM SYNDROME[a]

1. Gross and sustained *impairment of emotional relationships* with people. This includes the more usual aloofness and the empty clinging (so-called symbiosis) and also abnormal behavior towards other people as persons, such as using them, or parts of them, impersonally. Difficulty in mixing and playing with other children is often outstanding and long-lasting.

2. *Apparent unawareness of his own personal identity* to a degree inappropriate to his age. This may be seen in abnormal behavior towards himself such as posturing or exploration and scrutiny of parts of his body. Repeated self-directed aggression, sometimes resulting in actual damage, may be another aspect of his lack of integration (see also Point 5), as also the confusion of personal pronouns (see Point 7).

3. *Pathological preoccupation with particular objects* or certain characteristics of them, without regard to their accepted functions.

4. *Sustained resistance to change in the environment* and a striving to maintain or restore sameness. In some instances behavior appears to aim at producing a state of perceptual monotony.

5. *Abnormal perceptual experience* (in the absence of discernible organic abnormality), implied by excessive, diminished, or unpredictable response to sensory stimuli, for example, visual and auditory avoidance (see Points 2 and 4), or insensitivity to pain and temperature.

6. Acute, excessive and seemingly illogical *anxiety*. This is a frequent phenomenon and tends to be precipitated by change, whether in material environment or in routine, as well as by temporary interruption of a symbiotic attachment to persons or things (compare Points 3 and 4, and also 1 and 2). (Apparently commonplace phenomena or objects seem to become invested with terrifying qualities. On the other hand, an appropriate sense of fear in the face of real danger may be lacking).

7. *Speech* may have been lost, or never acquired, or may have failed to develop beyond a level appropriate to an earlier stage. There may be confusion of personal pronouns (see Point 2), echolalia or other mannerisms of use and diction. Though words or phrases may be uttered, they may convey no sense of ordinary communication.

8. *Distortion in motility patterns*, e.g., (a) excess as in hyperkinesis; (b) immobility as in catatonia; (c) bizarre postures, or ritualistic mannerisms, such as rocking and spinning (themselves or objects).

9. *A background of serious retardation* in which islets of normal, near normal or exceptional intellectual function or skill may appear.

[a] *After Creak* et al. *1961.*

Thus a reduced length of sentences, a greater number of grammatically incomplete sentences, and a general reduction in the amount of spoken language, which might all be ascribed to retardation of speech development, are present. However, the reduced use of pronouns, the persistent difficulty in using them correctly, and the great tendency of these children to repeat their own and other people's remarks are rather characteristic of infantile autism.

In its classical form, as described by Kanner (1971), infantile autism is not difficult to diagnose, but when the condition is atypical or if a child suffering from brain damage manifests "autistic features," it may be very difficult to determine the extent to which his personality disorder is responsible for his difficulties in spoken language. Moreover, the extent of any underlying brain damage and its importance are difficult to assess. When infantile autism is not present with all its classical features, there is often great difficulty in the differential diagnosis between auditory imperception, peripheral hearing loss, mental retardation, and "central deafness." Since many of these conditions may coexist with one another in children who are suffering from the effects of brain damage, the diagnosis is made even more difficult. It is virtually impossible, for example, in the case of a birth-damaged, mentally retarded child with temporal-lobe epilepsy and high-tone hearing loss, who shows "autistic features," to determine the relative importance of the various etiological factors. In such circumstances it is very much more important to assess the patient's needs in the sphere of management than to make a precise academic diagnosis however clever this may be (Wing, 1966).

The treatment of children who suffer from "Kanner's syndrome" or from conditions in which many autistic features are manifest should be in the hands of an experienced child psychiatrist. Direct speech therapy may have some place in management, but the speech therapist's major role is usually to organize environmental circumstances so that they stimulate an increase in the child's use of spoken language (Connel, 1966).

ACQUIRED DYSPHASIA IN CHILDHOOD

As indicated above, it is important to distinguish between retardation of the development of spoken language that occurs in childhood and loss of language functions that may result in adults following brain disease. If the dominant hemisphere of a child is severely damaged at the time of birth or before he has begun to use spoken language, dysphasia (the term used by neurologists concerned with adult patients when they refer to the impairment of the comprehension of spoken language or the reduced ability of their patients to speak intelligibly) cannot occur, for the young child has not yet acquired any significant ability to use spoken language that he could lose (T. T. S. Ingram, 1959b). Damage to either hemisphere at the time of birth or in early childhood may be associated with retarded speech development, but it is most unfortunate that the term developmental dysphasia has been applied to this condition (Basser, 1962).

Dysphasia in young children may occur, but its manifestations are rather different from those found in adult patients whose language development has been complete. In the latter, the only possible effect on their ability to use spoken language is a reduced ability to comprehend and/or to produce intelligible spoken language. In the young child who has developed some spoken language, but whose linguistic development is incomplete, brain damage, especially if it occurs in the dominant hemisphere, has different effects. The major result of brain injury, if it affects speech, is to produce a delayed and slower development of spoken language, though there may be some loss or impairment of the child's receptive and expressive linguistic abilities. The effects of brain damage depend greatly upon the age of the child and the stage of linguistic development he has reached. In a child 10-years old or more, the clinical picture is likely to be very similar to that found in adults when damage to the brain causes dysphasic syndromes. If the damage occurs at the age of 6 months, it is likely that the child's speech will not show any significant abnormality; most children who suffer from congenital hemiplegia who are of average intelligence have relatively normal speech development. But if the child is in the process of acquiring speech, at the age of perhaps 3 or 4, there will be a combination of loss of acquired speech faculties and a retardation of subsequent speech development (Guttman, 1942). This is most often manifest not so much as an abnormality of spoken language but as a reduction in the amount of spoken language produced by the child. Children who suffer from interruption of their language development at this age tend subsequently to be remarkably silent, to respond in conversation by single words or very simple phrases, and to use an excess of gesture. Their behavioral characteristics are perhaps more striking than any particular peculiarity of the spoken language they produce. They rarely show evidence of impairment of the ability to comprehend what is said to them.

When they go to school, however, the full effects of the disturbance of language development and loss of the language they have acquired become apparent. They have the greatest difficulties in learning to read and spell, and it is these educational problems that usually result in affected patients being referred to specialized clinics. Alajouanine and Lhermitte (1965) studied a large series of children who suffered from brain damage that affected their use of spoken language; "Every child showed peculiar behavior of psychomotor inhibition resulting in a reduction of oral and written language and in a reduction of gesture activities. Spontaneous speech was nearly nil. To get these children to speak it was necessary to multiply incentives and encouragements to repeat questions and orders." They noted that logorrhoea, not an infrequent manifestation of language disorders in adult patients suffering from brain disease, was very infrequent in childhood, and they found it difficult to identify the recognized syndromes of dysphasia described in adult patients. Younger children tend to show a more marked reduction in the amount of spoken language they produce than do older children and, though many more brain-damaged children than adults whose speech is affected by brain injury appear to make a good recovery, a high proportion show what Alajouanine and Lhermitte term "some phonetic disintegration." Moreover, it seems possible that there is a marked impairment in the child's later development of abstract concepts as expressed in language and complex concepts requiring "inner language" for their formalization. Thus even when children appear to have recovered their ability to speak normally, it must be remembered that there may be underlying fundamental defects of conceptualization and that educational difficulties may result.

Speech therapy may help a great many children with impairment of spoken language as a result of acquired disease or trauma to the brain by encouraging them to speak, however deviant their spoken language may be, and to have confidence in themselves. In this sense the activities of the speech therapist with children are not very different from those with adult patients. The therapist can, however, help very considerably in a more direct manner to correct the "phonetic disintegration" described by Alajouanine and Lhermitte when this is present, by helping the child to increase the intensity of his self-monitoring.

The pediatrician has a considerable part to play in ensuring that undue stresses are not placed upon the child suffering from acquired dysphasia. His rôle is particularly important because teachers and others who come into contact with the child are likely to assume that because the child's spoken language is relatively fluent he should be able to learn and to behave like other children. In fact, in many cases it will be found that children who manifest symptoms and signs of acquired childhood dysphasia have major difficulties in the school situation and are also liable to show somewhat liable behavioral patterns when placed under stress. They may display excessive reactions of rage or depression and, like similarly affected adults, to laugh, cry, or lose their tempers more easily than unaffected people. The pediatrician must make sure that the child's teachers are aware of the fact that the child may have very real difficulties in learning to read and spell and sometimes in doing arithmetic and that he is not lazy, stubborn, or "bloody-minded."

To ensure that parents, teachers, and others who come into contact with the child understand the nature of his difficulties is one of the most important tasks of the pediatrician, for it may mean the difference between a child who is relatively well adjusted, even though he may be a little behind in his educational achievements, and a child who is clearly handicapped—who has been regarded as lazy, difficult, or negativistic and who as a result of the treatment he has received has become grossly maladjusted. Often this maladjustment is shown by abnormalities of behavior, such as stealing, attacking other children, truancy, temper tantrums, and being exhibitionistic in school. If children suffering from the indirect effects of brain damage are fully studied from the medical, psychological, and social points of view, it is usually possible to interest those coming into contact with them, especially teachers, to the extent that they are prepared to take an immense amount of trouble to help them. On the other hand, if their difficulties are not understood, they are liable to suffer a series of very traumatic experiences, which may continue to affect them into adult life.

Environmental Conditions and Speech Disorders

Though some consideration has already been given to the effects of environment on speech development, it would be inappropriate to omit "environmental conditions" from a section concerned with "secondary speech disorders." The environment in which a child grows up is so important to his speech development that it is virtually an integral part of it; even the articulatory characteristics of his parents will be carried by the child through life. Bernard Shaw's Professor Higgins may have been a somewhat mythical figure, but skilled phoneticians who have never met the parents may often identify the places where they were brought up from the speech of their offspring. This is an indication of how important the speech of parents is to the child's development of spoken language. Children developing speech imitate. In healthy families this imitation is encouraged and part of the encouragement is the "expansion," of utterances so clearly described by Klima and Bellugi (1966) and other contemporary authors. This tendency to expand the child's statements and to correct their grammaticality in the process is not universal. It is, in fact, particularly characteristic of parents in Social Classes I, II, and III and rather uncharacteristic of parents in Social Classes IV and V (Bernstein, 1960). These expansions and corrections are of great importance in stimulating the child's language.

Clearly, if a child is exposed merely to what Bernstein terms "the restricted code," he is not likely to develop an elaborate spoken language of his own describing ideas that are of no interest to his family. One of the most unhappy children I have ever had to treat was the son of an unintelligent milk delivery man; the boy's IQ was assessed as about 150, and he was mocked by his parents for his interest in the works of Descartes, Hume, and other moral philosophers. On the other hand, if a child is significantly mentally retarded, the stress placed upon him by parents of the upper social classes with educational ambitions may be quite intolerable, result in his becoming increasingly anxious and developing abnormalities of speech or language as part of his more general maladjustment.

Increasing numbers of immigrants are referred to clinics dealing with children suffering from speech disorders. In the majority of these patients, the language used at home is other than English. A particularly extreme example occurred when a child was referred for "lack of speech" who came from an isolated farm cottage where his refugee Latvian parents and grandparents cared for him. Until the age of 5 he had met practically no English-speaking children. Fortunately, there was on the staff of the hospital at the time he was referred a psychologist with some knowledge of Latvian, who was able to assure the Senior School Medical Officer concerned that "though the child's English is certainly very retarded in development, his Latvian is well up to age." Whether this report was of much practical help is unknown; the child was never seen again!

Most young preschool children exposed to two languages learn them both. They learn them both more easily if the situations in which each of the languages is used are kept consistent. Thus a child talking to his father who is English-born will talk in English, and to his mother who is French-born he will talk French. When the whole family is together, the language generally used will be adopted by the child as well as by his parents. When situations become confused, for example, when the parents talk together in one language one day and another the next, or when parents alternate in the language in which they talk to the child, he is very liable to become confused and produce parts of one language in the middle of a complex sentence containing the vocabulary of the other. Situations in which each spoken language is used should be kept apart. Most children exposed to three or more languages seem slow to develop language skills in all of them in their early years.

The effects of environmental deprivation on speech development have been referred to, but it should be emphasized that children who suffer from speech disorders are particularly liable to suffer from environmental deprivation. For example, children who are mentally retarded, who suffer from severe cerebral palsy, or who are immobile because they suffer from spina bifida, are particularly liable not to be talked to because they cannot move about with their parents, or are not in a position, because of their general environmental deprivation, to talk interestingly or to answer back (Cazden, 1970).

The mixture of intrinsic and extrinsic factors that contribute to a gross delay in the development of spoken language is probably best seen in children who are admitted to institutions for the mentally retarded, run on old-fashioned lines (fortunately these are becoming fewer). Patients in these institutions have extraordinarily limited contact with people using spoken language in any meaningful way. There is a lack of stimulus for them to develop linguistically. Yet it has been shown repeatedly that mentally defective patients given adequate and appropriate stimulus, especially when they are young, can be trained by dedicated therapists or teachers to a remarkable extent and that their poverty of language can be remedied even at a relatively late age (Fraser, 1972). Speech therapists are showing greatly increased interest in mentally retarded patients in insitutions because they find some respond dramatically and their spoken language develops remarkably.

Specific Retardation of Speech Development

Between 30 and 40% of the children who are referred to hospital speech clinics are of average intelligence, are healthy, come from unexceptionable home backgrounds, and yet are slow to develop spoken language. In a high proportion of patients there is a history of other relatives being slow to learn to speak and having difficulties in learning to read and spell. Ambidexterity or left-handedness is found more frequently in these families than is expected in most (Bever, 1971a). In Scotland it is possible to identify a number of families who are particularly likely to produce children with retarded speech development, educational difficulties, and sinistrality or ambidexterity. These include the Kerrs, the MacDonalds, the Mac-

Gregors, the Macleans, the Campbells, the Scotts, and their related clans. An extended discussion of this curious finding has been presented elsewhere (T. T. S. Ingram, 1964b). In other cases it seems probable that patients have suffered brain damage at the time of birth or later, which has resulted in retardation of their speech development without other obvious neurological abnormalities being present. Nevertheless it is probable that the vast majority of intelligent, healthy children who show evidence of retarded speech development do so because of genetic factors. There is scope for genetic research in this category of speech disorder.

Many more boys than girls show the syndrome. The ratio varies in different series of patients from between 2 to 1 and 5 to 1 in favor of the male.

Whatever the reason for their retarded speech development, patients show rather consistent abnormalities of speech. When these are mild, they predominantly affect articulation; though the child's vocabulary, comprehension, and use of grammatical forms may be up to age, what he says is more difficult to understand than it should be because of multiple errors of articulation. The sounds affected vary from child to child according to the severity of his retardation, but the pattern is a remarkably consistent one. It conforms to the pattern of word sound acquisition described as a result of the analysis of the speech of 500 children that led to the creation of the Edinburgh Articulation Test (T. T. S. Ingram *et al.*, 1971). The consonant sounds and consonant clusters that are acquired late are always missing, and, according to the severity of the disorder, sounds acquired earlier and earlier are also either omitted or substituted, very often inconsistently and according to the place in the word where they occur.

If specific retardation of speech development is more severe, then the child will show a larger number of omissions and substitutions of consonants, and on the Edinburgh Articulation Test his quantitative score will in general be lower than in children considered to be mildly affected. Moreover, quite apart from his difficulties in saying words, it will be found that he was late to develop spoken language and that the development of his language and phonology has been slower than in normal children. In this group of moderately severely affected patients, comprehension of spoken language appears to be normal, though on sophisticated testing it is very often found to be a little defective. What is important is that, in this somewhat arbitrarily determined subgroup, children are much more immature, so far as phonological development is concerned, and show definite retardation on tests of language output such as the Reynell Test or the Renfrew Test. They are also retarded in their spoken language when it is compared with that of normal children by the criteria devised by McCarthy (1954), Reynell (1969), Templin, (1957). The mean number of words in their utterances is smaller than it should be, they use fewer subordinate clauses, their use of prepositions is immature, and so forth. This merely emphasizes that their speech is immature rather than deviant; though its subsequent development may be very much slower than it would be in a normal child who had begun to speak at an average age, it will, in fact, probably develop to an adult level in time (Table 13–6).

TABLE 13-6 CLASSIFICATION OF THE DEVELOPMENTAL SPEECH DISORDERS SYNDROME

Severity	Description	Other terms
Mild	Retardation of acquisition word sounds. Language normal.	Dyslalia.
Moderate	More severe retardation word sound acquisition and retarded spoken language development. Comprehension normal.	Developmental expressive dysphasia.
Severe	Still more severe retardation word sound acquisition and spoken language development. Impaired comprehension of speech.	Developmental receptive dysphasia. Word deafness. Auditory imperception.
Very severe	Gross failure of speech development. Impaired comprehension of language and significance of other sounds. Often apparent deafness.	Auditory imperception. Central deafness.

In more severely affected children it is not only spoken language that is affected but also the comprehension of what is said (Ingram, 1964a). This category contains patients considered to suffer from "severe degree of the specific developmental speech disorders syndrome." Parents usually give good evidence, however circumstantial, that the child's hearing for sounds other than those of speech has always been acute, but they have very often been puzzled and worried by the fact that though the child can apparently hear and behaves in an intelligent manner in other ways, he does not seem to be able to comprehend the content of what they are saying. They also, of course, observe that the child says nothing himself.

Such patients occur less frequently than those mildly or moderately affected, but they are probably more frequent in the community than has been recognized, and it is likely that a significant proportion have been wrongly diagnosed in the past as mentally retarded, autistic, or suffering from hearing impairment, or have been treated as if they suffered from a serious psychiatric disorder. Parents usually describe how the child will do what they ask him to do if they gesture and how the child himself gestures as a means of communication. Some of these children, even when their hearing has been demonstrated to be normal on test, appears to derive more from lip-reading than they do from hearing the sounds of spoken language.

Inevitably in these circumstances the development of spoken language is very slow, and the ages at which the child says his first recognizable words, makes phrases, and makes sentences (if he ever does) are very much later than those of children in the previous two categories reaching equivalent milestones. Moreover, the more severely children are affected by retarded speech development the longer speech development takes, as noted above. Thus children in this category are severely handicapped from the point of view of spoken language and education.

The majority will have rather limited speech by the time they enter school and a high proportion (Mason, 1970) inevitably have difficulties in learning to read and spell (Table 13—7).

A small proportion of patients in this category are more severely affected than the rest; they frequently appear to be deaf during their first year or more of life and are slow to react to sounds in general. It is often possible to demonstrate that the hearing of such children is within normal limits but their powers of word sound discrimination are impaired. Frequently they tend to rely on gesture and sometimes on lip-reading rather than on verbal input when communicating with other people. Children suffering from the developmental speech disorders syndrome of this degree have extremely slow speech development; it is very uncommon to find an adult with a history of a very severe degree of this syndrome with any degree of verbal fluency or capability of expressing himself using spoken lan-

Table 13—7   Classification of Symptomatology III: Specific Developmental Dyslexa and Dysgraphic

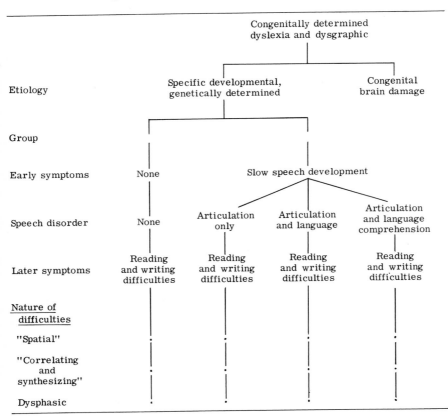

guage. Because of the secondary or associated difficulties in learning to spell, many such patients remain virtually illiterate (Fig. 13—24).

A very small number of children, perhaps one in 50,000 of the childhood population, are still more severely affected. In infancy and early childhood they have difficulty both in localizing and in recognizing the nature of sounds in their environment. They behave in many respects as if they were deaf, though characteristically parents are able to give circumstantial accounts of rare episodes in which the child has certainly reacted to quite quiet sounds. Such patients have been said to suffer from "severe auditory imperception" or "central deafness." In most respects they do behave like children with severe peripheral hearing impairments, but prolonged observation almost always results in the finding that on one or more occasions the child has responded to noises in the environment. I well remember spending approximately an hour with a child who was subsequently demonstrated

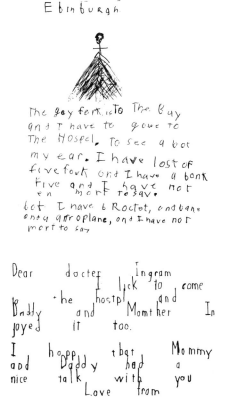

Figure 13—24. Specimens of the spontaneous written work of two hearing, 10-year old children who had been late to speak.

to suffer "central deafness" and being on the point of telling her parents that I thought she was deaf. The click made by my ballpoint pen, however, as I put it in my pocket was certainly perceived by the child, who looked down having localized it correctly, to see what made the noise—the first indication of hearing, let alone localization of a sound stimulus noted in the clinic. Many children who suffer from "central deafness" are diagnosed and treated as if they suffered from peripheral deafness, for they may be 2 or 3 years of age before they begin to respond to sounds and of school age before they begin to discriminate between speech sounds and start to comprehend what is said to them even to a limited extent. Children in this category are quite frequently referred to schools for the deaf, and it is only in recent years that teachers of the deaf have recognized them and treated them by different methods. It is very doubtful if hearing aids or other forms of auditory amplification are of any assistance; experience suggests that in many cases they may be harmful (Ewing, 1930; Gordon, 1964; T. T. S. Ingram, 1964b; Worster-Drought & Allan, 1928–1929).

A family history of slow speech development, of difficulties in learning to read and spell, and of sinistrality or ambidexterity is obtained in a high proportion of patients who suffer from the specific developmental disorders syndrome. Weakness of lateralization of handedness and footedness is characteristic. On the "Phi Test," which gives an indication of visual field dominance, it is a frequent finding in children who suffer from the syndrome, as it is in children with specific learning difficulties, that they are slow to lateralize to one or the other side the apparent movement of a control light that flickers alternately with two lateral lights (McFie, 1952).

In a small proportion of patients there is no other member of the family known to be affected, but there are indications in the personal history of the patient and on neurological examination that brain damage may have occurred at or about the time of birth or in infancy. The fact that such patients show abnormal neurological signs, such as an increase of involuntary associatied movements, or an isolated extensor plantar response, or mild asymmetries of the muscle tone and tendon jerks (often termed "soft signs" in the United States), has led to their being included in the group of children considered to show minimal cerebral dysfunction. It is easy, however, to raise objections to this term being used in any diagnostic sense, for the brain dysfunction is clearly anything but minimal, and the minor abnormalities of voluntary movement and of muscle tone are of no great significance in themselves (T. T. S. Ingram, 1963b; Paine, 1963; 1966).

In other patients there is both a history of other members of the family suffering from retarded speech development or educational difficulties and a history suggestive of birth injury, with minor abnormal neurological signs. It seems possible in such cases that congenital brain damage or injury sustained in infancy as a result of disease or trauma may have precipitated the symtoms of retarded speech development in a child genetically predisposed.

It is important also that the effect of environmental factors on children who suffer from the syndrome of specific retardation of speech development should not be underestimated. Affected children are much more vulnerable to adverse environmental influences than are children with normal speech development. The fact that they cannot converse using spoken language frequently means that parents and brothers and sisters tend not to talk to them because of the lack of "feedback." Thus there is deprivation of normal exposure to spoken language. When they go to school, children who are severely affected are in still greater difficulties, and there is a tendency for them to withdraw from the society of other children of their own age, especially if they are teased about their articulatory difficulties, and to become solitary and uncommunicative. Secondary difficulties in learning to read and spell, frequently attributed by teachers to laziness or cussedness or backwardness, mean that they are looked upon as and feel "different" from their classmates. Secondary anxieties, emotional stress, and associated behavior abnormalities contribute to the very complex clinical picture that is often found by the time affected children reach hospital clinics.

Assessment of patients who suffer from the specific developmental speech disorders syndrome of any severity provides major problems in clinical, psychological and speech aspects. The clinician has to be careful to make sure that the retardation of speech development is not secondary to mental retardation, hearing loss, psychiatric disorder, or adverse environmental factors. The psychologist is presented with a child whose ability to perform on many tests of intelligence that involve a significant verbal component is necessarily limited; if the syndrome is severe, the child may have difficulty in comprehending the instructions even for nonverbal items. The speech therapist frequently finds that the child has so little speech that a detailed assessment of the nature of the language disorders is very difficult to determine. Frequently it is only after a prolonged period of study and repeated discussions of their findings by the pediatrician, speech therapist, and psychologist that an adequate assessment can be made and reasonable plans for future management devised. Such management depends upon the severity of the child's symptoms and the degree of impairment of his comprehension of spoken language. For those who are mildly affected and whose predominant problems are in the production of word sounds, it is often possible merely to hold a "watching brief." Specific speech therapy may never be required. In more severely affected children, it is highly important that a speech-stimulating environment, such as is found in a well-run nursery or nursery school, should be provided. Children with severe difficulties in comprehension may benefit from a regime that really amounts to auditory training, and for the most severely affected children education rather similar to that provided for deaf children, but without auditory amplification, is often indicated.

To date, adequate training and education facilities for children severely affected by the specific retardation of speech development syndrome have not been made available to the extent required in the United Kingdom, and apart from Moore House, and the John Horniman Schools, all in England, there are few schools or training establishments devoted specifically to children suffering from severe language disorders.

"Mixed" Speech Disorders

It is not proposed to discuss "mixed" speech disorders in any detail, for the problems of assessment were discussed when dysarthria associated with cerebral palsy was described. The frequency with which speech disorders due to other causes may be exacerbated by environmental influences is often overlooked, however, and even when the cause of a speech disorder appears obvious, the possibility of additional contributory, exacerbating causes should always be considered. Children who suffer from cleft palate, for example, frequently have associated hearing impairment due to coexisting middle-ear disease which adds a component of impaired comprehension of spoken language to their difficulties in speech production. This in turn is likely to lessen the amount of spoken language to which they are exposed because people find them not only difficult to understand but also difficult to 'get through to." Thus the child, in addition to his physical handicaps, lacks the stimulus of being exposed to a normal talking environment. Similar problems are found in children who suffer from severe speech disorders secondary to mental retardation, hearing loss, or cerebral palsy.

The Diagnosis and Management of Children Suffering from Speech Disorders

In the past it has been all too common for speech therapists to work in isolation and for them to be expected to diagnose as well as to treat all children referred to them. Adequate backing from pediatricians, neurologists, audiologists, psychiatrists, psychologists, social workers and medical specialists has often been lacking.

Speech therapists are entitled to expect that children referred to them shall have had a detailed medical assessment, involving history-taking, clinical examination, and necessary investigations, and, when indicated, psychological and other specialist studies should have been completed. The speech therapists, for their part, should assess their patients, using standardized tests of articulation, spoken language, and comprehension. The need and type of treatment to be given should be discussed with the medical staff, the psychologists, and the teachers concerned, and the aims of treatment should be clearly stated. The days of diagnosis by hunch and treatment by intuition are past.

In ideal circumstances, the speech therapist should work closely with a pediatrician, pediatric neurologist or neurologist, and psychologist in a general speech clinic, and with an otolaryngologist or audiologist in clinics in which hearing impairment is the major problem. Similarly, the therapist is a member of a team so far as the management of patients suffering from cleft lip or palate are concerned—the team often consisting of a plastic surgeon, orthodontist, pediatrician, psychologist, and speech therapist.

Unfortunately, outside hospitals many children suffering from speech defects are treated by speech therapists working with very limited contact with doctors and psychologists, few of whom, at least in the United Kingdom, have any great expertise in the diagnosis of children suffering from speech disorders or knowledge of how best to help the speech therapist and provide necessary information. The situation, however, is gradually improving as it is realized by school medical officers that they have a part to play in the assessment of children suffering from speech disorders, and as speech therapists insist increasingly upon having an adequate medical history taken and examination available before treatment is undertaken.

It is to be hoped that in the future speech disorders in childhood will be recognized as requiring a team approach similar to that employed for children suffering from behavior disorders in child guidance clinics. Certainly the increased awareness of the importance of disorders of speech in childhood shown by doctors, teachers and psychologists in recent years holds great promise for the future.

Acknowledgments

I should like to thank the speech therapists with whom I have worked during the past 20 years, and especially the present Senior Speech Therapist of the Royal Hospital for Sick Children, Edinburgh, Miss Ann Henderson. They have done their best to teach me. The late Miss Catherine Brydone took care of the photographs used as illustrations for this chapter. Miss Ursula Burnet typed the manuscript cheerfully and checked the references. Professor J. O. Forfar has, as always, been encouraging in the chapter's preparation.

References

Abercrombie, D. *Elements of general phonetics*. Edinburgh: Edinburgh Univ. Press, 1967.

Alajouanine, T., & Lhermitte, F. Acquired aphasia in children. *Brain*, 1965, *88*, 633–662.

Andrews, G., & Harris, M. The Syndrome of Stuttering. In *Clinics in Development Medicine*. No. 17. London: Spastics Society & Heinemann, 1964.

Bangs, J. L. A clinical analysis of the articulatory defects of the feeble minded. *Journal of Speech Disorders*, 1942, 7, 343.

Barbara, D. A. *New directions in stuttering: Theory and practice*. Springfield, Ill.: Thomas, 1965.

Basser, L. S. Hemiplegia of early onset and the faculty of speech with special reference to the effects of hemispherectomy. *Brain*, 1962, *85*, 427–460.

Batchelor, A. D. R. Role of surgery in the treatment of clefts of lip and palate. In C. M. Drillien, T. T. S. Ingram, & E. M. Wilkinson (Eds.), *Causes and natural history of cleft lip and palate*. Edinburgh: Livingstone, 1966.

Bellugi, U. The emergence of inflections and negation systems in the speech of two children. Paper presented at the meeting of the New England Psychological Association, 1964.

Bellugi, U. The development of interrogative structures in children's speech. Rep. No. 8, Center for Human Growth and Development, University of Michigan, 1965.

Bellugi, U. Simplification in children's language. In R. Huxley & E. Ingram (Eds.), *Language acquisition: Models and methods*. New York: Academic Press, 1971. Pp. 95–119.

Bellugi, U. & Brown, R. The acquisition of language. *Monographs of the Society for Research in Child Development*, 1964, *29*, 1–192.

Beresford, R. Deviant Language Acquisition: the phonological aspect in the child with delayed speech. In M. Rutter & J. A. M. Martin (Eds.), *Clinics in developmental medicine*. No. 43. London: Spastics Society & Heinemann, 1972. Pp. 161–167.

Berke, J. The child's learning of English morphology. *Word*, 1958, *14*, 150–177.

Bernstein, B. Language and social class. *British Journal of Sociology*, 1960, *11*, 271.

Bernstein, B. Social structure, language and learning. *Educational Research*, 1961, *3*, 163. 163–176.

Bernstein, B. A socio-linguistic approach to social learning. In J. Gould (Ed.), *Penguin survey of the social sciences*. Baltimore: Penguin, 1965.

Bernstein, B. Language and roles. In R. Huxley & E. Ingram (Eds.), *Language acquisition: Models and methods*. New York: Academic Press, 1971. Pp. 67–71. (a)

Bernstein, B. A socio-linguistic approach to socialisation; with some reference to educability. In D. Hymes & J. Gumperz (Eds.), *Directions in socio-linguistics*. New York: Holt, 1971. (b)

Bever, T. G. The nature of cerebral dominance in speech behaviour in the child and adult. In R. Huxley & E. Ingram (Eds.), *Language acquisition: Models and methods*. New York: Academic Press, 1971. Pp. 231–261 (a)

Bever, T. G. Remarks made in discussion after various papers. In R. Huxley & E. Ingram (Eds.), *Language acquisition: Models and methods*. New York: Academic Press, 1971. (b)

Birch, H. G. The problem of brain damage in children. In H. G. Birch (Ed.), *Brain damage in children: The biological and social aspects*. Baltimore: Williams & Wilkins, 1964.

Birch, H. G., & Belmont, L. Auditory-visual integration in brain-damaged and normal children. *Developmental Medicine and Child Neurology*, 1965, *7*, 135–144.

Birch, H. G., & Lefford, A. Intersensory development in children. *Monographs of the Society for Research in Child Development*, 1963, *38*, 1.

Birrell, J. F. Hoarseness in childhood. *Speech*, 1954, *18*, 40–47.

Birrell, J. F. *The ear, nose and throat diseases of children*. London: Cassell, 1960.

Blanton, S. A survey of speech defects. *Journal of Educational Psychology*, 1916, *7*, 581.

Bloodstein, O. Conditions under which stuttering is reduced or absent: a review of the literature. *Journal of Speech Disorders*, 1950, *14*, 295; *15*, 29.

Bloomfield, L. *Language*. London: Allen & Unwin, 1933.

Bosma, J. F. Deglutition: pharyngeal stage. *Physiological Review*, 1957, *37*, 275.

Bosma, J. F., & Lind, J. Roentgenologic observations of motions of the upper airway with establishment of respiration in the newborn infant. *Acta Paediatrica*, 1960, *49* (Suppl. 123), 18.

Brain, R. *Speech disorders: Aphasia, apraxia and agnosia*. (2nd ed.) London: Butterworth, 1965.

Brimer, M. A., & Dunn, L. M. *Manual for the English Picture Vocabulary Test*. London: National Foundation for Educational Research in England and Wales, 1963.

Bühler, C. *The first year of life*. New York: John Day, 1930.

Bullowa, M. The onset of speech. Paper presented at the meeting of the Society for Research in Child Development, March, 1967.

Burkitt, A. N., & Lightoller, G. S. The facial musculature of the Australian aboriginal. *Journal of Anatomy*, 1927, *61*, 14.

Cazden, C. B. Three socio-linguistic views of the language and speech of lower class children—with special attention to the work of Basil Bernstein. *Developmental Medicine and Child Neurology*, 1968, *10*, 600–611.

Cazden, C. B. The neglected situation in child language research and education. In F. Williams (Ed.), *Language and poverty—Perspectives on a theme*. Chicago: Markham, 1970. Pp. 81–101.

Charcot, J. M. *Diseases of the nervous system*. 1881. (Engl. transl. by G. Sigerson) New York: Hafner, 1962.

Chomsky, N. *Syntactic structures*. The Hague: Mouton, 1957.

Chomsky, N. Review of B. F. Skinner, *Verbal behavior. Language*, 1959, *35*, 26.

Chomsky, N. *Aspects of the theory of syntax*. Cambridge, Mass.: MIT Press, 1965.

Chomsky, N. *Language and mind*. Chicago: Harcourt, 1968.

Clarke, A. D. B., & Clarke, A. M. Some recent advances in the study of early deprivation. *Journal of Child Psychology and Psychiatry*, 1960, *1*, 26.

Connell, P. H. Medical treatment in early childhood autism. In J. K. Wing (Ed.), *Early childhood autism.* London: Maxwell, 1966.

Conrad, K. New problems of aphasia. *Brain,* 1954, 77, 491.

Creak, M., *et al.* Schizophrenia syndrome in childhood—Progress report of a working party. *Developmental Medicine and Child Neurology,* 1961, 3, 501—503.

Cunningham, M. A. A five year study of the language of an autistic child. *Journal of Child Psychology,* 1966, 7, 143.

Darwin, C. The biography of an infant. *Mind,* 1877, 2, 285.

Dixon, D. A. Abnormalities of the teeth and supporting structures in children with clefts of lip palate. In C. M. Drillien, T. T. S. Ingram, & E. M. Wilkinson (Eds.), *The causes and natural history of cleft lip and palate.* Edinburgh: Livingstone, 1966. Pp. 178—205.

Dobbing, J. Vulnerable periods in developing brain. In A. N. Davison & J. Dobbing (Eds.), *Applied neurochemistry.* Oxford: Blackwell, 1968.

Ellingson, R. J. Cerebral electrical responses to auditory and visual stimuli in the infant—human and sub-human. In P. Kellaway & I. Petersen (Eds.), *Neurological and electroencephalographic correlative studies in infancy.* New York: Grune & Stratton, 1964.

Ervin-Tripp, S. Social backgrounds and verbal skills. In R. Huxley & E. Ingram (Eds.), *Language acquisition: Models and methods.* New York: Academic Press, 1971. Pp. 29—39.

Ewing, A. W. G. *Aphasia in childhood.* London: Oxford Univ. Press, 1930.

Firth, J. R. 1934. The word "phoneme." In J. R. Firth (Ed.), *Papers in linguistics.* London: Oxford Univ. Press, 1934. Pp. 1—2.

Flavell, J. H. Concept development. In P. E. Mussen (Ed.), *Carmichael's manual of child psychology.* (3rd ed.) New York: Wiley, 1970. Pp. 983—1059.

Fraser, W. Modifications of language situations in an institution for profoundly retarded children. *Developmental Medicine and Child Neurology,* 1972, 14, 148—155.

Glauber, I. P. The psychoanalysis of stuttering. In J. Eisenson (Ed.), *Stuttering: A symposium.* New York: Harper, 1958.

Gordon, N. The concept of central deafness. In C. Renfrew & K. Murphy (Eds.), *The child who does not talk.* Clinics in Developmental Medicine No. 13. London: Spastics Society & Heinemann, 1964. Pp. 62—64.

Grabb, W. C., Resensten, S. W., & Bzoch, K. R. *Cleft lip and palate.* Boston: Little, Brown, 1971.

Grady, P. A. E., & Daniels, J. C. *A survey of the incidence of speech defect in children.* Nottingham, Eng.: Univ. of Nottingham, Inst. of Education, 1964.

Greene, M. C. L. *The voice and its disorders.* London: Pitman, 1964.

Grégoire, A. *L'apprentissage du langage.* Vol. I. Paris: Droz, 1937.

Guillaume, P. *L'imitation chez l'enfant.* Paris: Alcan, 1925.

Guttman, E. Aphasia in children. *Brain,* 1942, 65, 205.

Haskill, S. Elective mutism. In C. Renfrew & K. Murphy (Eds.), *The child who does not talk.* Clinics in Developmental Medicine No. 13. London: Spastics Society & Heinemann, 1964. Pp. 150—154.

Hawk, E. A. A survey and critical analysis of speech needs in the elementary schools of Ohio city of 15,000 population. Summarized in L. E. Travis, *Handbook of speech pathology.* London: Peter Owen, 1959. Pp. 248.

Hécaen, H. Sentence production in normal children, adolescents, and in patients with diffuse and unilateral cerebral disease. In R. Huxley & E. Ingram (Eds.), *Language acquisition: Models and methods.* New York: Academic Press, 1971. Pp. 277—283.

Henderson, A. G. Electrophysiological tests of hearing. *Developmental Medicine and Child Neurology,* 1975, 17, 96—98.

Hopkin, G. B. Mesiocclusion—A clinical and roentgenographic study. Unpublished doctoral dissertation, University of Edinburgh, 1962.

Hopkin, G. B. Orthodontic aspects of the diagnosis and management of speech defects in children. *Proceedings of the Royal Society of Medicine, Laryngology,* 1972, 65, 409.

Hopkin, G. B., & McEwan, J. D. Speech defects and malocculusion—A palatographic investigation. *Dental Practitioner*, 1955, 6, 123.

Huxley, R. Language: Chimpanzees and children. In P. Wolff & R. MacKeith (Eds.), *Planning for better learning*. Clinics in Developmental Medicine No. 33. London: Spastics Society & Heinemann, 1969. Pp. 90—99. (a)

Huxley, R. Research in language development. In P. Wolff & R. MacKeith (Eds.), *Planning for better learning*. Clinics in Developmental Medicine No. 33. London: Spastics Society & Heinemann, 1969. Pp. 77—89. (b)

Hymes, D. Linguistic problems in defining the concept of the tribe. *Proceedings, Spring Meeting, American Anthropologist, 1967*. Pp. 23—78.

Hymes, D. Competence and performance in linguistic theory. In R. Huxley & E. Ingram (Eds.), *Language acquisition: Models and methods*. New York: Academic Press, 1971. Pp. 3—28.

Illingworth, R. S. *The development of the infant and young child—Normal and abnormal*. (3rd ed.) Edinburgh: Livingstone, 1967.

Ingram, E. The requirements of model users. In R. Huxley & E. Ingram (Eds.), *Language acquisition: Models and methods*. New York: Academic Press, 1971. Pp. 147—159.

Ingram, T. T. S. A description and classification of common speech disorders. *Archives of Disease in Childhood*, 1959, 34, 444—455. (a)

Ingram, T. T. S. Specific developmental disorders of speech in childhood. *Brain*, 1959, 82, 450—467. (b)

Ingram, T. T. S. Ataxia and ataxic diplegia in childhood. In G. Walsh (Ed.), *Cerebellum posture and cerebral palsy*. Clinics in Developmental Medicine No. 8. London: Spastics Society & Heinemann, 1963. Pp. 70—82. (a)

Ingram, T. T. S. Chronic brain syndromes in childhood other than cerebral palsy, epilepsy and mental defect. In M. Bax & R. MacKeith (Eds.), *Minimal cerebral dysfunction*. Clinics in Developmental Medicine No. 10. London: Spastics Society & Heinemann, 1963. Pp. 10—17. (b)

Ingram, T. T. S. The prevention of severe language disorders in childhood. Report presented to the Dysphasia Sub-committee of the Scottish Paediatric Society, Edinburgh, 1963. (c)

Ingram, T. T. S. Auditory imperception and related disorders. *Proceedings of the Royal Society of Health*, 1964, Sections 40—42. (a)

Ingram, T. T. S. Late and poor talkers. In C. Renfrew & K. Murphy (Eds.), *The child who does not talk*. Clinics in Developmental Medicine No. 13. London: Spastics Society & Heinemann, 1964. Pp. 77—83. (b)

Ingram, T. T. S. The neurology of cerebral palsy. *Archives of Disease in Childhood*, 1966, 41, 337—357. (a)

Ingram, T. T. S. In C. M. Drillien, T. T. S. Ingram, & E. M. Wilkinson (Eds.), *Causes and natural history of cleft lip and palate*. Edinburgh: Livingstone, 1966. (b)

Ingram, T. T. S. Developmental disorders of speech. In P. J. Vinken & G. W. Bruyn (Eds.), *Handbook of clinical neurology*. Vol. 4. Amsterdam: North-Holland Publ., 1969.

Ingram, T. T. S., Anthony, N., Bogle, D. A., & McIsaac, M. *The Edinburgh Articulation Test*. Edinburgh: Livingstone, 1971.

Ingram, T. T. S., & Barn, J. A description and classification of common speech disorders associated with cerebral palsy. *Cerebral Palsy Bulletin*, 1961, 3, 57.

Ingram, T. T. S., Mason, A. W., & McIsaac, M. Specific difficulties in learning to read and spell associated with a history of slow speech development, 1974.

Ingram, T. T. S., & Naughton, J. A. Paediatric and psychological aspects of cerebral palsy associated with hydrocephalus. *Developmental Medicine and Child Neurology*, 1962, 4, 287—292.

Ingram, T. T. S., & Reid, J. F. Developmental aphasia observed in a department of child psychiatry. *Archives of Disease in Childhood*, 1956, 31, 161—172.

Irwin, O. C. The developmental status of speech sounds in ten feeble-minded children. *Child Development*, 1942, 13, 29.

Irwin, O. C., & Spiker, C. C. The relationship between the IQ and indices of infant speech sound development. *Journal of Speech and Hearing Disorders*, 1949, 14, 335.

Irwin, R. B. Ohio looks ahead in speech and hearing therapy. *Journal of Speech and Hearing Disorders,* 1948, *13*, 55.

Jackson, J. H. On the anatomical and physiological localisation of movements in the brain. *Lancet,* 1873, *1*, 84, 162, 231.

Jameson, A. M. Stammering in children—some factors in the prognosis. *Speech,* 1955, *19*, 60—67.

Johnson, W. *The Iowa remedial education program: Summary report.* Iowa City: 1942.

Johnson, W. *Stuttering in children and adults.* Minneapolis: Univ. of Minnesota Press, 1955.

Johnson, W. *The onset of stuttering.* Minneapolis: Univ. of Minnesota Press, 1959. (a)

Johnson, W. Perceptual and evaluation factors in stuttering. In L. E. Travis (Ed.), *Handbook of speech pathology.* London: Peter Owen, 1959. Pp. 897—915. (b)

Kanner, L. Autistic disturbances of affective contact. *Nervous Child,* 1943, *2*, 217.

Kanner, L. Infantile autism and the schizophrenias. *Behavioral Science,* 1965, *10*, 412.

Kanner, L. *Child psychiatry.* Springfield, Ill.: Thomas, 1971.

Karlin, I. W., & Strazzulla, M. Speech and language problems of mentally deficient children. *Journal of Speech Disorders,* 1952, *17*, 286.

Klima, E. S. Negation in English. In J. A. Fodor & J. J. Katz (Eds.), *The structure of language.* Englewood Cliffs, N.J.: Prentice-Hall, 1964. Pp. 246—323.

Klima, E. S., & Bellugi, U. Syntactic regularities in the speech of children. In J. Lyons & R. Wales (Eds.), *Psycholinguistic papers.* Edinburgh: Univ. of Edinburgh Press, 1966. Pp. 183—213.

Kussmaul, A. In *Ziemssen's Handbuch der speziellen Pathologie und Therapie, Leipzig,* 1885, *12*.

Labov, W. *The social stratification of English in New York City.* Washington, D.C.: Center for Applied Linguistics, 1966.

Labov, W. The study of language in its social context. *Studium Generale,* 1970, *33*, 30—87.

Labov, W., Cohen, P., & Robins, C. A preliminary study of the structure of English used by Negro and Puerto Rican speakers in New York City. Columbia Univ. Co-operative Research Project No. 3091, New York, 1965.

Lenneberg, E. H. The capacity for language acquisition. In J. A. Fodor & J. J. Katz (Eds.), *The structure of language.* Englewood Cliffs, N.J.: Prentice-Hall, 1964.

Lenneberg, E. H. The natural history of language. In F. Smith & G. A. Miller (Eds.), *The genesis of language.* Cambridge, Mass.: MIT Press, 1966.

Lenneberg, E. H. *Biological foundations of language.* New York: Wiley, 1967.

Lewis, M. M. *Infants' speech.* London: Routledge & Kegan Paul, 1951.

Lichtheim, L. On aphasia. *Brain,* 1884, 7, 433.

Lightoller, G. S. The modiolus and muscles surrounding the rima oris, with some remarks about the panniculus adiposus. *Journal of Anatomy,* 1926, *60*, 1.

Logan, W. J., & Bosma, J. F. Oral and pharyngeal dysphagia in infancy. *Pediatric Clinics of North America,* 1967, *14*, 47—61.

Luria, A. R. *The role of speech in the regulation of normal and abnormal behaviour.* Oxford: Pergamon, 1961.

Luria, A. R. *Higher cortical functions in man.* (Engl. transl. by B. Haigh) London: Tavistock, 1966.

Lyons, J. *New horizons in linguistics.* London: Pelican, 1970.

McCarthy, D. *Language development of the pre-school child. Institute of Child Welfare Monographs,* 1930, No. 4.

McCarthy, D. Language development in children. In L. Carmichael (Ed.), *Manual of child psychology.* (2nd ed.) New York: Wiley, 1954.

McFie, J. Cerebral dominance in cases of reading disability. *Journal of Neurology, Neurosurgery and Psychiatry,* 1952, *15*, 194.

McNeill, D. The creation of language by children. In J. Lyons & R. Wales (Eds.), *Psycholinguistic papers.* Edinburgh: Edinburgh Univ. Press, 1966. Pp. 95—132. (a)

McNeill, D. Developmental psycholinguistics. In F. Smith & G. A. Miller (Eds.), *The genesis of language.* Cambridge, Mass.: MIT Press, 1966. Pp. 15—84. (b)

McNeill, D. The development of language. In P. A. Mussen (Ed.), *Carmichael's manual of child psychology,* (3rd ed.) New York: Wiley, 1970. Pp. 1061—1161.

Maran, A. G. D. The causes of deafness in childhood. *Journal of Laryngology,* 1966, *80,* 495.

Mason, A. A. *Hypnotism for dental and medical practitioners.* London: Secker & Warberg, 1960.

Mason, A. W. Specific (developmental) dyslexia. *Developmental Medicine and Child Neurology,* 1967, *9,* 183—190.

Matthews, J. Speech problems of the mentally retarded. In L. E. Travis (Ed.), *Handbook of speech pathology.* London: Peter Owen, 1959.

Mehler, J., & Bever, T. G. The study of competence in cognitive psychology. *International Journal of Psychology,* 1968, *3,* 273.

Métraux, R. Speech profiles of the pre-school child 18—54 months. *Journal of Speech Disorders,* 1950, *15,* 37.

Miller, F. J. W., Court, S. D. M., Walton, W. S., & Knox, E. G. *Growing up in Newcastle upon Tyne.* London & New York: Oxford Univ. Press, 1960.

Mills, A., & Streit, H. Report of a speech survey, Holyoke, Massachusetts. *Journal of Speech Disorders,* 1942, *7,* 161.

Moncur, J. P. Environmental factor differentiation: stuttering children from non-stuttering children. *Speech Monographs,* 1951, No. 18, 312.

Moncur, J. P. Symptoms of maladjustment differentiating stutterers from non-stutterers. *Child development,* 1955, *26,* 91.

Moore, W. E. Hypnosis in a system of therapy for stutterers. *Journal of Speech Disorders,* 1946, *11,* 117.

Morley, M. E. *The development and disorders of speech in childhood.* Edinburgh: Livingstone, 1957.

Morley, M. E. *Cleft palate and speech.* Edinburgh: Livingstone, 1962.

Neligan, G., & Prudham, D. Norms for four standard developmental milestones by sex, social class and place in family. *Developmental Medicine and Child Neurology,* 1969, *11,* 413—422. (a)

Neligan, G., & Prudham, D. Potential value of four early developmental milestones in screening children for increased risk of later retardation. *Developmental Medicine and Child Neurology,* 1969, *11,* 423—439. (b)

Nylen, B. O. Cleft palate and speech. *Acta Radiologica, Supplementum,* 1961, *203.*

Paine, R. S. Discussion of group reports. In M. Bax & R. MacKeith (Eds.), *Minimal cerebral dysfunction.* Clinics in Developmental Medicine No. 10. London: Spastics Society & Heinemann, 1963. Pp. 97—98.

Paine, R. S. Neurological grand rounds: minimal chronic brain syndromes. *Clinical Proceedings, Children's Hospital, Washington, D.C.,* 1966, *22,* 21.

Piaget, J. *The language and thought of the child.* (2nd ed., Engl. transl. by M. Gabainn) London: Routledge & Kegan Paul, 1932.

Piaget, J. Piaget's theory. In P. E. Mussen (Ed.), *Carmichael's manual of child psychology.* (3rd ed.) New York: Wiley, 1970.

Pringle, M. L. K., Butler, N. R., & Davie, R. *11,000 seven-year-olds—First report of the National Child Development Study (1958 cohort).* New York: Longmans, Green, 1966.

Renfrew, C. Assessment of the poor talker. In C. Renfrew & K. Murphy (Eds.), *The child who does not talk.* Clinics in Developmental Medicine No. 13. London: Spastics Society & Heinemann, 1964. Pp. 84—91.

Reynell, J. *Reynell Developmental Language Scale.* Windsor, England: National Foundation for Educational Research Publ. Co., 1969.

Robinson, W. P. Social factors in language development in primary school children. In R. Huxley & E. Ingram (Eds.), *Language acquisition: Models and methods.* New York: Academic Press, 1971. Pp. 49—66.

Russell, W. R., & Espir, M. L. E. *Traumatic aphasia.* London & New York: Oxford Univ. Press, 1961.

Rutter, M. Early childhood autism: behavioural and cognitive characteristics. In J. K. Wing (Ed.), *Early childhood autism.* London: Maxwell, 1966.

Rutter, M., Tizard, J., & Whitmore, K. *Education, health and behaviour.* London: Longmans, Green, 1970.

Schlesinger, I. M. Learning grammar: from pivot to realisation rule. In R. Huxley & E. Ingram (Eds.), *Language acquisition: Models and methods.* New York: Academic Press, Pp. 79—93.

Sheridan, M. D. *Child's hearing for speech.* London: Methuen, 1948.

Sheridan, M. D. Development of auditory attention and the use of language symbols. In C. Renfrew & K. Murphy (Eds.), *The child who does not talk.* Clinics in Developmental Medicine No. 13. London: Spastics Society & Heinemann, 1964. Pp. 1—10.

Sheridan, M. D. & Sinclair H. Sensorimotor action patterns as a condition for the acquisition of syntax. In R. Huxley & E. Ingram (Eds.), *Language acquisition: Models and methods.* New York: Academic Press, 1971. Pp. 121—135.

Sheridan, M. D. Reported evidence of hearing loss in children of 7 years. *Developmental Medicine and Child Neurology,* 1972, *14,* 296—303.

Sirkin, J., & Lyons, W. F. A study of speech defects in mental deficiency. *American Journal of Deficiency,* 1941, *46,* 74.

Skinner, B. F. *Verbal behavior.* New York: Appleton, 1957.

Spriestersbach, D. C. Assessing nasal quality in cleft palate speech of children. *Journal of Speech and Hearing Disorders,* 1955, *20,* 266—270.

Stark, G. D. Rubella retinopathy. *Archives of Disease in Childhood,* 1966, *41,* 420—423.

Stern, C., & Stern, W. *Die Kindersprache.* (4th Ed.) Leipzig: Barth, 1928.

Stevens, N. *The educational needs of severely subnormal children.* London: Arnold, 1971.

Templin, M. C. *Certain language skills in children, their development and inter-relationships. Institute of Child Welfare Monographs,* 1957, No. 26.

Trammer, H. Echter Mutismus bei Kindern. *Zeitschrift für Kinderpsychiatrie,* 1934, *1,* 30.

Travis, L. E. The unspeakable feelings of people with special reference to stuttering. In L. E. Travis (Ed.), *Handbook of speech pathology.* London: Peter Owen, 1959, Pp. 916—946.

Van Riper, C. *Speech correction.* Englewood Cliffs, N.J.: Prentice-Hall, 1954.

Van Riper, C. Symptomatic therapy for stuttering. In L. E. Travis (Ed.), *Handbook of speech pathology.* London: Peter Owen, 1959, Pp. 878—896.

Vygotsky, L. S. *Thought and language.* 1934. (Engl. Transl. by E. Hanfmann & G. Vakar) Cambridge, Mass.: MIT Press, 1962.

Weir, R. H. 1962. *Language in the crib.* The Hague: Mouton, 1962. *White House conference on child health and protection—Special education.* New York: Century, 1931.

Wing, J. K. Diagnosis, epidemiology and aetiology. In J. K. Wing (Ed.), *Early childhood autism.* Oxford: Pergamon, 1966. Pp. 3—49.

Walff, S., & Chess, S. A behavioural study of schizophrenic children. *Acta Psychiatrica Scandinavica,* 1964, *40,* 438.

Worster-Drought, C., & Allan, I. M. Congenital auditory imperception (congenital word deafness): with a report of a case. *Journal of Neurology and Psychopathology,* 1928—1929, *9,* 193.

14. Language Development in the Absence of Expressive Speech

A. J. Fourcin

with an introduction by
Richard Boydell

In 1962 a child was described (Lenneberg, 1962) who had a severe congenital anarthria (inability to make speech sounds) but who was found to have perfectly good comprehension of spoken language. Similar cases have been discovered since that time. The present article gives further evidence for the primacy of language comprehension over language expression and also adds an important new aspect to congenital anarthria: it is shown here that expressive capacities may develop subclinically, so that the anarthric person, having acquired comprehension passively, may be prevented from expression until a medium or vehicle is developed that enables him to engage actively in verbal interchange. In the Introduction to this chapter, the anarthric victim himself tells his own story. He was able to express himself in English for the first time in his life at about 30 years of age, at which time he was given a few days of instruction in the use of a foot-operated electric typewriter. Syntax and semantics were perfect at that time. In the second part of the chapter, the author discusses the theoretical implications of these clinical facts [*Editor*].

Introduction

Like every child, I was born without language. Unfortunately, I was also born with cerebral palsy which, in my case, means that, although my intelligence is unimpaired, I have a very severe speech defect and no use in my hands and arms. So, to start with, I acquired an understanding of language by listening to those around me. Later, thanks to my mother's tireless, patient work I began learning to read and so became familiar with written, as well as spoken, language. As my interests developed—particularly in the field of science—I read books and listened to educational programs on radio and, later, television which were at a level that was normal, or sometimes rather above, for my age. Also when people visited us, either other children or my parents' friends, I enjoyed listening to the conversation even though I could only play a passive role and could not take an active part in any discussion or argument. Even this may, however, have had its compensation, for I was often reminded of the rhyme:

> There was an old owl who lived in a tree
> And the more he heard the less said he
> And the less he said the more he heard
> Now wasn't he a wise old bird!

But, even so, it was sometimes very frustrating not to be able to express my own opinion except to my parents afterward; as they were, at that time, the only people who had the patience to try to understand my speech. This incidentally, made it extremely frustrating for my parents when other people could not, or would not, believe that my intelligence was normal; such as the Education Officer who saw me when I was about 6-years old and couldn't be bothered to listen to me reading from one of the school books my mother had bought specially to ensure that my education was at a normal level.

As a result of this sort of attitude I was denied any formal education. So my mother, and later my father, gave me lessons every day using proper school textbooks to make it as much like school education as possible. This continued until I was old enough to study on my own. As well as reading books and listening to radio and television to continue my general education, I read the news paper every day to keep in touch with current affairs.

Then, at the age of 30, I started using the POSSUM typewritter and, for the first time in my life, had the opportunity to express myself and make some use of the knowledge acquired over the years. The first benefit was the ability to correspond with friends and relatives. Then the Spastics Society installed Possum typewriters in some of their schools and centres, and invited me to help the students in the use of the equipment through correspondence. So not only was two-way communications possible for the first time, but I was also able to help others through personal effort. The use of the POSSUM typewriter enabled me, in 1967, to go to the Spastics Society's further education centre where, after passing an aptitude test, I started working for the Ford Motor Company as a Computer Programmer using the latest development in POSSUM equipment, the word-store typewriter, which is not only faster, but also much less tiring, than the earlier machines. Also indirectly, POSSUM helped me to expand the ability to communicate into the field of amateur radio; after passing the requisite examinations I obtained my transmitting licence with the callsign G3VOA. Morse code provides the alternative to the defective speech, with a foot operated *morse key based on my first POSSUM control, and the POSSUM typewriter is used to keep the detailed log of all contacts made as required by law. So having acquired language without the ability to speak or write, I can, at long last, make good use of it.*

RICHARD BOYDELL

Comment

Richard Boydell, who wrote the introduction to this note, is now 38-years old; he is a congenital quadriplegic spastic with severe athetosis and has a bilateral high-frequency hearing loss (40 dB at 1 kHz). He has been able to type by making use of a foot-controlled electric typewriter developed by R. Maling (manufactured by Maling Rehabilitation Systems Ltd., Beicer Road, Aylesbury, U.K.). Until he obtained the typewriter at the age of 30, he was, as he has written, entirely unable to communicate in depth. His speech was, and is, extremely difficult to understand and only sufficient as a vehicle for the most basic requirements of day-to-day living with his parents and people on terms of close acquaintance. In consequence, his first letter, produced after 9 days work with the new typewriter and addressed to Mr. Maling, came rather as a shock to his parents and friends, since it was not only elegantly phrased but also made a suggestion for the improvement of the machine that was subsequently incorporated by its designer. Since that time Dick Boydell's main achievement has been to become a professional computer programmer and to be accepted as a qualified member of the British Computer Society. This degree of success in communication is, of course, dependent on the typewriter—which is now available without charge for patients in the United Kingdom from the National Health Service—but the ability to use the machine derives from Dick Boydell's intrinsic intelligence and perceptual language ability.

Dick Boydell's ability to process language is entirely built on the training in childhood he received from his mother. He was an only child, and his mother was able to devote a great deal of time to the development of his speech comprehension. By holding the child with his head supported in her arm, she was able to assess his responses to her speech by his head and body movements. This proximity of mother to child, which was necessary to assess the child's response, was also important, in view of his hearing loss, in ensuring that the sounds were at sufficient intensity to be perceived.

By the age of $4\frac{1}{2}$ he could produce vocally only versions of *no* and *yes*, but his head and body movements appeared to indicate, to his mother, good speech comprehension and from that age she started systematically to teach him, using these movements as responses to spoken questions.

Although he was taught to read in this fashion, his verbal comprehension of his mother's speech was the start of his intellectual development, just as for a normal child. Unlike the normal child, however, he was not able to use speech response, and although at the age of 5 he was able to run an electric train with his right foot using a control made by his father, (he is markedly right-footed), normal body development and manipulative ability were completely absent.

His formal education from his mother stopped when he was in his tenth year; although he was helped by his father in elementary mathematics, his subsequent education was derived primarily from books and BBC radio transmissions; and from the age of 13, BBC television. He first started listening regularly to the radio at the age of 7, and by that time he was regularly in the company of children of his own age—although he was unable to go to school. His communication with other people was severely limited and only his own parents were able to believe that any real communication with him was possible or that he had an intellectual ability superior to that of a young child. Even his parents were unaware of the extent of his language development. This situation persisted, and his self-education steadily progressed, until he was 30, when the Spastics Society in the United Kingdom enabled him to try one of the new typewriters and it was modified to incorporate a foot control.

The subsequent result completely vindicated his parents' belief and showed not only how good a general knowledge he had but that he had also managed to develop a useful degree of mathematical competence, largely unaided. This ability sprang, of course, entirely from his early tuition by his mother, and it is extremely important to note that the teaching involved, in considerable measure, the verbal presentation of information. His ability to read derived from his ability to comprehend speech.

At present, the most widespread hypothesis concerning the development of the ability to perceive speech involves, as a crucial postulate, the idea that the process of decoding the acoustic stimuli of speech is directly dependent on the mediation of the neural mechanisms that are basic to its production (Liberman, Cooper, Shankweiler, & Studdert-Kennedy, 1967). This viewpoint has been developed in order to effect an economy in our explanation of the processing that is basic to the use of speech. First, production and perception can share common procedures and involve the use of largely identical neural facilities; and, second, the complexities of acoustic form are mapped onto the possible simplicities of neural command. This point of view has important implications for any explanation of the development of speech, and language, ability in the child and it has profound consequences—since it has been implicit in the approach adopted for centuries past—in remedial speech training and in the teaching of foreign speech skills.

If it is necessary to decode speech by making reference to the means available for its production, at whatever level, then the very young child must infer the neural commands that he would employ in order to produce a presented speech sequence. He will do this with moderate accuracy when he is only partly skilled in speaking and—although the errors he makes do not entirely support this view—this could explain the imperfection of his speech comprehension. However, when the baby is first exposed to speech it will not be possible for him to interpret its implicit motor—neural form unless he has an innate mechanism capable of effecting at least some of the required acoustic-to-motor command transformations. We would expect that the child's ability to produce speech would always be greater than his ability to perceive it. In ordinary experience (Sheridan, 1968), this is not so. The child can perceive better than he can produce, and although he may consistently produce acceptable sound sequences in babbling he will not necessarily employ them in the words that are then at his command. As far as the development of speech ability is concerned, the "motor theory" contains, then, an essential paradox, and it does not seem possible to reconcile it with the ordinary facts of speech development. However, there is a further difficulty. For the speech perceptual system to function in a practical fashion, it must be able to operate readily on inputs from widely different sources. For large or small vocal tracts and high- or low-larynx frequency some sort of perceptual normalization must take place, which transforms the many acoustic forms into the few phonetic categories. This normalization must precede any putative motor command inference but its nature may make it quite unnecessary (Fourcin, 1972). The complexity of normalization, in bringing a multiplicity of inputs within the compass of a single set of categorization possibilities, may make all other operations of lesser significance at this first level of operation. Normalization will be readily performed as the complexity of the representation of the speech input is reduced, and it will be at its simplest when it has to operate with the perceptual features themselves. This can easily be accomplished if we operate in terms of speech patterns derived directly from the acoustic level without reference to the means of production. It is not readily achieved if the normalization involves vocal-tract inference as the basis from which a subsequent simplification in terms of motor commands is to be made.

If we accept that processing that does not require direct reference to production is important in the perception of speech, then it is worth considering what role this perceptual ability may have in the establishment of the motor patterns of speech activity itself. The perceptual mechanism that is capable of being applied to assess the patterns of speech sounds produced externally to the listener, could equally well be applied in an assessment of the listener's own speech output, and an auditory pattern feedback situation would then result in which the detailed means of production would be subservient to the overriding requirement of generating an acoustic output of the target pattern form (Fourcin, A. J. 1975). Once the motor control sequences are learned, the speaker would be able to generate speech outputs rather in the way that speech by rule is generated from a computer when only formant, rather than vocal tract, information is used as the basis of the programming. For the normal person, development of auditory speech ability will be reinforced by exposure to his own speech patterns, and it is perhaps reasonable to hope that for the disabled person, whether in speaking or listening, an exposure to the essential elements of the patterns of speech may be of corresponding help in developing his speaking or listening skill (Parker, Ann, 1974). What is really important in the present context, however, is that the recognition and linguistic use of the patterns of speech are not necessarily dependent on an expressive speech ability.

References

Fourcin, A. J. Perceptual mechanisms at the first level of speech processing. In A. Rigault (Ed.), *Proceedings, 7th International Congress of Phonetic Sciences*, Montreal, 1971, The Hague: Mouton, 1972. Pp. 48–62.

Fourcin, A. J. Speech perception in the absence of speech productive ability. In N. O'Connor (Ed.), *Language, cognitive deficits and retardation*. London: Butterworth, 1975. Pp. 33–43.

Lenneberg, E. H. Understanding language without ability to speak: a case report. *Journal of Abnormal and Social Psychology*, 1962, *65*, 419–425.

Liberman, A. M., Cooper, F. S., Shankweiler, D. P., & Studdert-Kennedy, M. Perception of the speech code. *Psychological Review*, 1967, *74*, 431.

Parker, Ann. The laryngograph. *RNID Hearing*, 1974, *29* (No. 9), 256–261.

Sheridan, M. D. *The developmental progress of infants and young children*. Ministry of Health Report No. 102. London: Stationery Office, 1968.

15. Mental Subnormality and Language Development

Joanna Ryan

This chapter is concerned with the effects of low intelligence on language development. Various methodological difficulties involved in investigating the subnormal by means of comparison with normal groups are discussed, with reference to the question of whether there is any special language handicap associated with mental subnormality. Most of the evidence suggests essentially similar language development in subnormal children and normal ones. The differences that are found are related to other features of subnormality.

Introduction: Comparison of Normal and Subnormal

Mental subnormality in a heterogeneous condition, both medically and behaviorally. It includes a very great range of ability. For most classification purposes, an IQ of 70 is used to distinguish the subnormal from the normal. There are many problems about the basis of such a classification, especially at the borderline; the present chapter, however, concerns the severely subnormal, where there is usually little doubt about the condition.

Some subnormal people never acquire language, and at present we do not know why. Most of the nonspeaking subnormal appear to live in institutions, rather than in the community, and in general tend to be those with the lowest IQ scores (Sheehan, Martyn, & Kilburn, 1968). Some never acquire the nonverbal skills that most 18-month-old infants possess and that may be considered necessary antecedents to language development. Others do develop further; in such cases it is possible that the failure to acquire language is a function of their relatively great chronological age, and of associated changes in the plasticity of the nervous system. Nothing, however, is known about this in the subnormal.

Most subnormal children, even those with very low IQ scores, do learn to speak and understand language to some degree. This apparent independence of intelligence level has been taken by Chomsky (1968) as an illustration of the species-specificity of language. However, it has also often been claimed that the subnormal are particularly handicapped with regard to language. Subnormal children do pass through the various "stages" of language development at much greater chrnological ages than do normal children. This is one of the defining characteristics of mental subnormality and is of considerable diagnostic significance. The questions of interest do not concern this but the further issue of whether there is any special relationship between language and mental subnormality. Does language development lag behind other areas of development to such an extent that it constitutes a special defect, over and above the general handicap? Does lack of intelligence particularly affect language learning?

Such questions are more difficult to answer than would appear at first sight. What is implied is not some relatively specific language disorder, such as childhood aphasia, where the discrepancy between verbal and nonverbal development is very obvious and where the language disorder is not a function of low intelligence. Rather, what is implied is a slightly greater difficulty with language compared to other areas of behavior, as a result of low intelligence. Such questions assume the existence of norms of development with which the subnormal can be compared, and this is where difficulties arise.

Most tests that provide such norms of development have been standardized on populations of higher IQ. As with cultural and racial comparisons, problems of interpretation arise when normative tests are applied to groups that differ from the standardization population in some way. Any apparent "defects" that are identified amongst the subnormal using such comparison methods are thus relative to norms of normal development. We do not know what the norms of subnormal development are. Further, we do not know enough about the lives of subnormal children to identify apparent lags, relative to normal development, as real defects for them—however the latter may be defined. Most investigations of the subnormal compare them with groups of higher IQ, matched not for chronological age but for "mental age." The point of this is to obtain groups who are at roughly equivalent development stages, and then to investigate the ways in which they differ. The validity of such comparisons depends not only on the concept of mental age, which can be criticized on many grounds, but also on the assumption that it is sufficient to match only for this. This assumption is certainly not true, as argued elsewhere (Ryan, 1973a). The lives of subnormal children differ from those of normal ones in many important ways that are relevant to their cognitive skills. It is not possible to control experimentally for being subnormal and for all that this entails as regards motivation and social and educational experience.

Using such comparison methods, subnormal children do indeed appear to be inferior on most tasks that either directly assess their verbal abilities or involve language (Bryant, 1970; Jordan, 1967; Lyle, 1961; Ryan, unpublished). However, they also perform worse on a great variety of other tasks that do not involve language, such as reaction time, attention, and visual discrimination. Zigler (1967) provides a brief account of the variety of "defects," allegedly characteristic of the subnormal, that have been identified in this way. In the majority of experiments using mental age matching, and on a variety of different tasks, the subnormal are found either to be equal or inferior to the normal comparison group; they are seldom found to be superior. This should lead one to ask how it is that the subnormal perform as well as they do on the IQ test used in the initial matching procedure, and to suspect some artifact in this that favors them (Ryan, 1973b). It also implies that language is not in any way special in its identification as a "defect" associated with mental subnormality, since so many other aspects of behavior have been similarly identified.

These difficulties in making adequately controlled and meaningful comparisons between the subnormal and the normal imply that the original question, concerning a relative difficulty with language, is not an answerable one. However, there are still some substantial questions to be asked that may illuminate the effect, if any, of lack of intelligence on language development. Does language development show all the same features that have been described for normal children, and are the same variables associated with it in similar ways? In particular, do subnormal children show evidence of rule-governed behavior, or do they, because of their limited abilities, learn only specific imitated responses? How can any differences that are found be related to other features of subnormality, and is there any systematic relationship to the various known pathologies associated with subnormality?

In what follows, evidence bearing on these questions will be considered that is drawn from the available literature and from continuing as yet unpublished study of my own. Briefly, this study compared 16 children with Down's syndrome (mongolism), 15 other subnormal children of various pathologies, and 13 children of average intelligence. The subnormal children lived at home and attended day schools; their chronological ages were between 5- and 9-years old, their Stanford-Binet mental ages between $2\frac{1}{2}$ and $3\frac{1}{2}$. The normal children attended nursery school and were aged between 2 and $3\frac{1}{2}$ years. Extensive recordings were made of their "spontaneous" speech during play, and a variety of different tests were carried out. The procedures were repeated at a later date to assess developmental changes.

Language Development in the Subnormal

There are several studies that suggest similar development for subnormal and normal children in several aspects of syntax, morphology, and semantics. Lenneberg, Nichols, and Rosenberger (1964) found that children with Down's syndrome passed through all the "milestones" in the usual order, with the relationship of language development to motor development roughly preserved, at least in the younger children. They also found that performance on various sentence repetition tasks did not differ in any way from that of normal children; they made similar kinds of mistakes and reconstructions based on their grammatical understanding and did not show an unusual amount of blind parroting. Lackner (1968) in a very detailed study of five subnormal children also found no evidence that their grammatical abilities were in any way different from those of normal children. The phrase structures of transformational rules he wrote for their spontaneous speech were subsets of adult grammar and generated structures that were comprehensible to normal children. Further, the subnormal children, like normal ones, were unable to repeat correctly sentences they could not understand. They also spontaneously corrected incomplete sentences presented to them. Graham and Graham's (1971) analysis of the speech of five subnormal children has produced similar results. Here the changes they found with greater mental age, in the rules necessary to describe the speech, are very similar to the changes Menyuk (1969) found with increasing chronological age in normal children. In my present study, some of the children were compared on the basis of the mean utterance length (MUL) of their speech; this was to provide a rough matching for complexity of language. Thus matched, no differences were found between the groups as regards the proportion of complete sentences (noun phrase + verb phrase) in their speech, of incomplete ones, or of clichés and "ready-made" utterances (see Lyons, 1968, for a definition of "ready-made"). No differences were found in the range and variety of verb transformations used. Similar errors of omission, of substitution, and of overgeneralization of the various inflections were made in all groups, although the range of individual variation within groups was very great in this respect. Other errors, such as inversion of word order and omission of auxiliaries occurred in all groups. It should be noted that in order to obtain children with a similar MUL, subnormal children of greater mental age than the normal children had to be selected from the whole sample. The reason for this will become apparent below.

A training experiment by Bartel (1970) using Berko techniques showed that subnormal children could generalize what they had learned about the morphology of specific items to new items. Dever and Gardner (1970) found similar patterns of error between subnormal and normal groups using the Berko test.

Word-association tasks also show few differences among children matched for mental age. For example, Semmel Barritt, Bennett, and Perfetti (1968) found similar proportions of syntagmatic and paradigmatic associations in noninstitutionalized subnormal and normal children. The institutionalized subnormal, matched for mental age, however, showed a higher proportion of syntagmatic associations. Vocabulary counts mostly show striking similarities. Mein (1961) found similar mental age trends as regards the proportions of nouns and verbs. Beier, Starkweather, and Lambert (1969), comparing institutionalized subnormal and younger normal children, found that in both cases the same number of words accounted for 50 % of their speech, and that the actual words used were mostly the same. O'Connor and Hermelin (1963) showed that semantic generalization was similar in both subnormal adults and young normal children.

It can be concluded from these studies that there is no essential difference in the organization of grammatical and semantic knowledge between subnormal and normal children. Furthermore, there is no evidence that subnormal children use radically different strategies in learning language. This conclusion should be qualified by several considerations. First, it cannot be said that we know exactly how normal children learn language; what is clear is that both very specific forms and also abstract rules, are learned. It appears from Cazden's (1968) work that general rules are formulated by the child on the basis of restricted imitated forms, and that the rules are applied in progressively wider contexts. Second, the extent of individual variation is very great with respect to some aspects of language development (Brown, Cazden, & Bellugi, 1969), and there are reasons to suppose that it will be even greater among groups of subnormal children (Ryan, 1973a). At present, we do not know how to interpret such variation. Third, it is pertinent to ask whether any other finding might have been expected, given how basic some of the features mentioned above are to the nature and structure of language. A consideration of the differences that have been found will place the similarities in a clearer perspective.

Most surveys of the institutionalized subnormal show an extremely high incidence of articulation and voice disorders (Jordan, 1967; Spradlin, 1963). The estimates, however, vary greatly between studies. There are many fewer studies of the noninstitutionalized subnormal, but they also show a high incidence of articulation defects, though somewhat less than among the institutionalized subnormal. Lyle (1961), for example, found subnormal children to be inferior in the discrimination and reproduction of speech sounds, compared to a normal group matched for mental age. In the present study, the effective intelligibility of the subnormal groups was slightly lower than that of the normal group, even matched for MUL rather than for mental age. Such articulation difficulties may be related to the high incidence of major and minor CNS impairments often found among the subnormal. For example, Birch, Belmont, Belmont, and Taft (1967) found that half of a large unselected sample of high-grade subnormal children had some kind of CNS (central nervous system) impairment. The proportion is likely to be greater with lower grade groups. In the present study, a modified version of Garfield, Benton, and MacQueen's (1966) motor impersistence test showed very large differences between subnormal and normal groups. The possibility of mildly imparied hearing must also be considered, particularly with Down's syndrome (Fulton & Lloyd, 1968). Lastly, the role of adults in maintaining defective articulation by a reluctance to correct subnormal children is probably important.

Apart from articulation, both Lyle's (1961) study and the present one suggest a differential patterning, on various verbal tests, between subnormal and normal groups. In both studies when compared on the basis of mental age with normal children, the subnormal children were inferior on tests involving grammatical abilities, and on measures of grammatical complexity of speech. However, on extensive tests of their single-word vocabulary, both recognition and naming, they were equal to or better than the normal children. In the present study this was true only for a noun vocabulary, not for tests involving prepositions, at which the subnormal were worse. These findings could be interpreted as a function of the subnormal children's greater chronological age and slower development. A subnormal child will spend a longer time at the one-word stage, leading to a greater accumulation of vocabulary items before the beginnings of syntax than is possible for a faster-developing child. Alternatively, or additionally, this differential patterning may reflect the relative simplicity of learning single words, compared to combining them into structured sequences. Further, it may be a function of how adults talk to subnormal children, emphasizing names for objects rather than the more complex aspects of language. There are a few studies (cited in Spradlin, 1963) that suggest that adults do adjust the complexity of their language when speaking to low-grade children, in such a way as to provide less linguistic information. It should be noted, in view of that finding, that the use of IQ tests that contain extensive vocabulary tests as a basis for mental age matching will inevitably result in inferior performance on the part of the subnormal on any test of their syntactic knowledge—as is frequently found.

Further differences between the groups in the present study were found when the scores on all the various verbal tests and the measures of the complexity of spontaneous speech were intercorrelated. Of 45 possible correlations, 18 were statistically significant for the normal group, 4 for the Down's syndrome group, and 2 for the other subnormal group. This implies that there is much more consistency within the normal group as regards the relative difficulty of the different tests than in the subnormal groups. Greater variability both between and within subjects is a common finding among the subnormal and is not restricted to language (e.g., Baumeister, 1968). It may well be related to the diverse causes and etiologies involved, and also to the consequences of being subnormal, as suggested in Ryan (1972a).

The question of whether the usual associations between language development and other factors also hold true for the subnormal was investigated in the present study by looking at social-class correlations. Of nine possible correlations of social class with verbal scores, six were significant for the normal group, one for the Down's syndrome group, and two for the other subnormal group. Carr (1970), in a study of the general development of infants with Down's syndrome, also failed to find the usual social-class effects, suggesting again that the present finding is not peculiar to language. One interpretation of these findings is that the usual patterns of parental expectations and behavior are altered by the presence of a subnormal child. This question is a complex one, about which there is at present no empirical evidence. However, there are grounds for supposing that the more usual modes of interaction are disrupted, and that subnormal children, considered as a group, experience rather extreme forms of care.

To sum up so far, most of the differences that have been found between subnormal and normal groups do not concern the structure of syntactic or semantic knowledge and therefore are not inconsistent with the similarities described earlier. The differences described can mostly be attributed to aspects of subnormality that are likely, or are known, to affect other areas of behavior, as well as language. It is therefore unlikely that language development is especially vulnerable to low intelligence. Now that differences between subnormal and normal have been considered, the question arises of whether there are systematic behavioral differences within the subnormal population, corresponding to the various diagnostic and etiological subgroups. This is a confused issue, partly because the known causes of subnormality are both numerous and very diverse, as are the conditions often associated with it (e.g., epilepsy, cerebral palsy) and partly because, even in severe subnormality, the majority of cases cannot be given any diagnosis. There has been relatively little research on differences between the various subgroups, and most of it has used spurious categories, such as "organic" and "cultural—familial" (Ryan, 1971). Such research has been quite inconsistent in its findings (Clausen, 1966). At present, we certainly cannot conclude, as Ellis (1969) does, that etiological heterogeneity can be ignored, because the relevant evidence is not available.

Work with the Down's syndrome subgroup is more promising because of their relative frequency and early diagnosis. The evidence is fairly consistent in suggesting a higher incidence of articulatory and voice defects in the Down's syndrome subnormal than in others (Evans & Hampson, 1968). This may be due to their frequently impaired hearing, or to poor control of the speech musculature, or both. The evidence is much less consistent as regards other aspects of language. Lyle (1960) found children with Down's syndrome to be inferior to other subnormal children as regards word definition and complexity of spontaneous speech, but equal as regards vocabulary. The difference were greater for the institutionalized sample than for the day-school one. Mein (1961), looking at developmental trends in vocabulary, found the Down's syndrome subnormal to be slightly behind others. However, Evans and Hampson (1968), in their review of the literature, conclude that there is no particular association between Down's syndrome and language difficulties. The present study substantiates this conclusion. On all the various measures the similarities between the two subnormal groups were more striking than the differences. What few differences there were, in favor of the group of mixed pathologies, were small and mostly not significant. These inconsistencies in the findings may be due to the fact that the comparison groups against which the Down's syndrome subnormal are assessed are usually unspecified in their composition and must vary greatly as regards etiology between studies.

Finally, what are the practical implications of these considerations? We have seen that when using existing normative tests it is impossible to tell whether the subnormal are particularly handicapped with respect to language or not. The findings that they are inferior to normal children on many verbal tasks may well be an artifact of the matching procedures. Language stimulation and remediation programs of various kinds are becoming increasingly fashionable, but the basis on which they are instigated is not always clear. Whether or not the subnormal are especially handicapped with regard to language, there are other, wider considerations that might indicate the need for special language programs, similar to the grounds for "special" education generally. There is some evidence to suggest that subnormal children learn best in highly structured situations, and that they have a limited ability to learn "spontaneously" from a so-called "stimulating" environment, where many different features have to be sorted out (Clarke & Clarke, 1972). Language, *par excellence*, is something that is learned spontaneously by the normal child, without explicit instruction, from a complex and often confusing input. Furthermore, it is also probable that the subnormal child effectively creates a less helpful and rich environment for himself than that experienced by a normal child. Though we have no direct evidence for this, it is likely to be much harder for the mother of a relatively unresponsive subnormal child to keep up over many years the kind of active informative dialogue that most mothers engage in with their children. Such general considerations, though they do not imply a special handicap, might be grounds for instigating a language program.

References

Bartel, N. R. The development of morphology in retarded children. *Education and Training of the Mentally Retarded*, 1970, *5*, 164—168.

Baumeister, A. A. Behavioral inadequacy and variability of performance. *American Journal of Mental Deficiency*, 1968, *73*, 477—483.

Beier, E. G., Starkweather, J. A., & Lambert, M. J. Vocabulary usage of mentally retarded children. *American Journal of Mental Deficiency*, 1969, *73*, 927—934.

Birch, M. G., Belmont, L., Belmont, I. & Taft, L. Brain damage and intelligence in educable mentally subnormal children. *Journal of Nervous and Mental Disease*, 1967, *144*, 247—257.

Brown, R., Cazden, C. B., & Bellugi, U. The child's grammar from I to III. In J. P. Hill (Ed.), *Minnesota symposium on child psychology*. Minneapolis: Univ. of Minnesota Press, 1969.

Bryant, P. E. Language and learning in severely subnormal and normal children. In B. W. Richards (Ed.), *Mental subnormality*. London: Pitman, 1970.

Carr, J. Mental and motor development in young mongol children. *Journal of Mental Deficiency Research*, 1970, *14*, 205—220.

Cazden, C. B. The acquisition of noun and verb inflections. *Child Development*, 1968, *39*, 433—448.

Chomsky, N. *Language and mind*. New York: Harcourt, 1968.

Clarke, A. D. B., & Clarke, A. M. What are the problems? In A. D. B. Clarke, (Ed.), *Mental retardation and behavioral research*. London: Churchill, Livingstone, 1972.

Clausen, J. *Ability structure and subgroups in mental retardation*. London: Macmillan, 1966.

Dever, R. B., & Gardner, W. I. Performance of normal and retarded boys in Berko's test of morphology. *Language and Speech*, 1970, *13*, 162—181.

Ellis, N. R. A behavioral research strategy in mental retardation; defense and critique. *American Journal of Mental Deficiency*, 1969, *73*, 557—566.

Evans, D., & Hampson, M. The language of mongols. *British Journal of Disorders of Communication*, 1968, *3*, 171—181.

Fulton, R. T., & Lloyd, L. L. Hearing impairment in a population of children with Down's syndrome. *American Journal of Mental Deficiency*, 1968, *73*, 298—302.

Garfield, J. C., Benton, A. L., & MacQueen, J. C. Motor impersistence in brain-damaged and cultural-familial defectives. *Journal of Nervous and Mental Disease*, 1966, *142*, 434—440.

Graham, J. T., & Graham, L. W. Language behavior of the mentally retarded: syntactic characteristics. *American Journal of Mental Deficiency*, 1971, 75, 623–629.

Jordan, T. E. Language and mental retardation. In R. L. Shiefelbusch, R. H. Copeland, & J. O. Smith (Eds.), *Language and mental retardation*. New York: Holt, 1967.

Lackner, J. R. A developmental study of language behavior in retarded children. *Neuropsychologia*, 1968, 6, 301–320.

Lenneberg, E. H., Nichols, I. A., & Rosenberger, E. F. Primitive stages of language development in mongolism. *Research Publications, Association for Research in Nervous and Mental Disease*, 1964, 42,

Lyle, J. G. The effect of an institution environment upon the verbal development of imbecile children. II. Speech and language. *Journal of Mental Deficiency Research*, 1960, 4, 1–13.

Lyle, J. G. A comparison of the language of normal and imbecile children. *Journal of Mental Deficiency Research*, 1961, 5, 40–51.

Lyons, J. *Introduction to theoretical linguistics*. London & New York: Cambridge Univ. Press, 1968.

Mein, R. A study of the oral vocabularies of severly subnormal patients. *Journal of Mental Deficiency Research*, 1961, 5, 52–62.

Menyuk, P. *Sentences children use*. Cambridge, Mass.: MIT Press, 1969.

O'Connor, N., & Hermelin, B. *Speech and thought in severe subnormality*. Oxford: Pergamon, 1963.

Ryan, J. F. Classification and behaviour in mental subnormality: Some implications for research. In Primrose, D. A. (Ed.), *Proceedings, 2nd Congress I.A.S.S.M.D.*, 1971, 155–160.

Ryan, J. F. Scientific research and individual variation. In A. D. B. Clarke (Ed.), *Mental retardation and behavioural research*. London: Churchill, Livingstone, 1973.(a)

Ryan, J. F. When is an apparent deficit a real defect?—Language assessment in the subnormal. In P. Mittler (Ed.), *Psychological assessment of the mentally handicapped*. London: Churchill, Livingstone, 1973.(b)

Semmel, M. I., Barritt, L. S., Bennett, S. W. & Perfetti, C. A. A grammatical analysis of word associations of educable mentally retarded and normal children. *American Journal of Deficiency*, 1968, 72, 567–576.

Sheehan, J., Martyn, M. M., & Kilburn, K. L. Speech disorders in retardation. *American Journal of Mental Deficiency*, 1968, 73, 251–256.

Spradlin, J. E. Language and communication of mental defectives. In N. R. Ellis (Ed.), *Handbook of mental deficiency*. New York: McGraw-Hill, 1963.

Zigler, E. Familial mental retardation: a continuing dilemma. *Science*, 1967, 155, 292–298.

16. Language Development in Malnourished Children

Antonio B. Lefèvre

This is a study of the effect of severe multiple insults, particularly protein malnutrition, on the normal course of development in children, particularly language development. Four groups were compared: (1) a control group of 50 healthy children; (2) fifty well-nourished but socially deprived children raised in an asylum for foundlings; (3) twenty children hospitalized for severe and chronic protein deficiency; and (4) fifteen children hospitalized for severe conditions other than malnutrition whose social background was identical with that of the malnourished children. Work-up included developmental assessment, neurological examination, skull X-rays, pneumoencephalography, EEG, clinical laboratory tests, and anthropometry. When compared with Group 1, Group 2 was primarily deficient in language development, whereas Group 3 was deficient in all aspects of development; however, when Group 3 was compared with either Group 2 or Group 4, the language deficit was not statistically larger than the other deficits. Nevertheless, when each malnourished child was examined individually, it was found that nutritional rehabilitation had less of an effect on catch-up in the language area than on catch-up in other areas of human development. Theoretical and methodological problems are discussed.

Language Development and Social Class

Innumerable aspects of language acquisition have been studied over the years, from the by-now classical work of McCarthy (1935) to the recent publications by

I wish to thank Dr. Jose Maria Marlet for his contribution in the statistical analyses.

Ingram (1969) and McGrady (1971). Extensive and thorough surveys of the literature have been made by these authors, in an attempt to distinguish those factors
that are capable of interference with the normal acquisition of communication
by the spoken word. One should recall that such factors may manifest themselves
in two ways: (a) by slowing down the arrival at the various milestones of language
acquisition, and (b) by causing a regression to earlier stages; the latter happens
when the causative factor begins to act after a delay, thus degrading the given
function, which had apparently been on the way toward proper development. It
is true that the distinction between these two is of more theoretical than practical
interest, since the families concerned are usually not equipped to furnish adequate
information with regard to the dynamic processes involved; even the specialist
who follows the gradual establishment of one or the other of these clinical pictures
does not have the sufficiently objective particulars needed to discern the necessary
details. The pathogenic agent may be transient, interrupting for a certain period a
continuing process of acquisition, and thus leading to a regression—which, in
turn, may also be transient, being followed by a wave of further acquisition, during
which the function re-establishes itself. The characteristic aspects of this evolution-
ary process are usually more apparent when the pathogenic agent acts in a more
acute fashion. The dysphasias due to cerebrocranial traumatization or to the
rupture of vascular malformations, for instance, allow us to evaluate both the
degree of language development attained premorbidly and the damage incurred
by the pathology, as well as the various stages of language re-acquisition.

In contrast, language disturbances due to adverse environmental conditions
present enormous difficulties for correct evaluation. The situation is complicated,
first of all, by the varied nature of the factors involved; further, these factors may
be active for variable periods of time and at varying intensities, producing clinical
manifestations that must be analyzed in terms of a gradient of severity.

In the economically advanced countries, adverse environmental factors are usually tied to the cultural level of the family, to marital problems, to chronic or intermittent deprivation of affection or stimulation, or to "socio-economic" factors.
The latter have a particular connotation in the economically well-developed
countries that must be clarified here in order to understand the research reported
in this paper.

The survey by McCarthy (1935) calls attention to various viewpoints, beginning
with a statement attributed to Degerando that "the child of rich parents understands more words and fewer actions." This rather old-fashioned and subtle point
is the product of an epoch in which socioeconomic differences were characterized
with less realism than they are today. In more recent times, as discussed by Mc-
Carthy, at the beginning of this century, Stern maintained categorically that there
was an 8 month difference in language development between children from the
"educated class" and children from the "working class" (*sic*), an observation
resulting from the administration of verbal tests to children of lower and higher
social classes. Still more recently, Markey (also cited in McCarthy, 1935), basing
himself on vocabulary tests, reached the conclusion that children of educated
families without economic problems exceeded those of poor families by a ratio of 2

to 1, not only in terms of general precocity, but also in terms of the exactness with which they interpreted the test words. McCarthy herself compared the language development of two groups of children whose parents had "higher" and "lower" occupations. She again demonstrated the same fact, this time analyzed in greater detail; she not only observed that the children from the "higher" group had a larger vocabulary at their disposal; she also noted that their construction of phrases was much more advanced. The "lower" group used a greater number of nouns in proportion to other parts of speech, which is considered to be an index of a lower degree of maturation. The difference between the two groups became more accentuated with advancing chronological age, always in favor of the "higher" group.

There appears to be no doubt that children of a higher socioeconomic level develop earlier and better verbal communication than poor children, and that cultural factors are responsible for this difference. Certain sophisticated details explain the individual differences within the socioeconomic groups: the age of the people surrounding the child; the occurrence of frequent trips, which offer opportunities for wider experiences; the number of siblings, and the order of the subject's birth among his siblings. These are important factors. Bilingualism has also received attention from students of language, and is frequently associated with socioeconomic status. The children of immigrants, for example, suffer not only from the possible damaging handicap of bilingualism, but from poverty and problems of adaptation to their new country.

In recent work by McGrady (1971), four causes of language disturbances are analyzed: sensory deprivation, deprivation of experience, emotional disorganization, and neurological disfunction. These various factors, of course, may interact, thus causing new characteristic pathologies; they deserve special attention.

When "deprivation of experience" is being considered, it is of interest to examine the condition of the child in an institution; in the opinion of Casler (cited in McGrady, 1971), deprivation of experience may manifest itself as early as 6 months of age, when affective reaction normally begins to appear. Institutionalized children have poor language development, primarily due to a lack of proper stimulation.

McGrady has studied language retardation in connection with mental deficiency due to various causes and in connection with neurological dysfunction. We must also remember what may happen when minimal cerebral dysfunction occurs: the language areas may be affected or traumatized; the "organic character" of language disorders is, however, in many cases poorly documented. McGrady discusses the role of "maturational lag" and of real cerebral lesions and their respective influences upon the development of language capacity.

Poverty and Malnutrition in Developing Countries

Language deficits are cumulative, according to McGrady, which explains the fact that the differences between upper- and lower-class children become more apparent as the children grow older. At this point, it is proper to raise the question of reversibility of the damage. This question has not been properly answered, but McGrady judges that since language is the fundamental prerequisite for the development of intellectual concepts and many other cognitive processes, the child who is behind in his language development begins school with a handicap that will cause an educational lag throughout his academic years.

In the economically advanced countries there is, thus, a well-established line of research that directs itself to discovering how cultural deprivation, emotional abnormalities, and acquired diseases may affect the process of language acquisition. A collection of articles such as "The Child Who Does Not Talk" (Renfrew & Murphy, 1964) should be subtitled "In the Economically Advanced Countries."

In the developing countries, a different focus is in place, since it is impossible, except under special circumstances, to study the action of isolated factors upon language development. It is clear, of course, that in a country such as Brazil there are some regions where research done in richer countries can be replicated; areas of higher development do exist, and within them groups comparable to those studied in the United Kingdom or the United States. It was possible, for example, for us to make a comparison between children from a middle-class environment and children living in an asylum, in an attempt to discover the importance of environmental stimulation for language development.

The great difficulty encountered in the poor countries— and our research is a good demonstration of this—is to evaluate the influence of an isolated factor such as malnutrition upon psychomotor development and especially upon language. When one examines extremely poor children, such as those who were the subjects of our major research, it is impossible to distinguish which of the many and various deprivations they suffer is responsible for which developmental lag. As a point of departure, we can state that such children suffer not only from protein and vitamin deficiencies, but from hygenic inadequacies, from stimulus deprivation, and from severely limited opportunities for play. The cultural resources at the disposal of these children, who live in the very poorest areas, are negligible, and the little that is available must be divided up among many; the parents are always busy trying desperately to make a living, when they are not sick themselves.

As one may see, we are in quite a different world from the world described at the beginning of this chapter, in which, for instance, one could discuss the role of traveling upon language development (Drever's work, cited in McCarthy's [1935] excellent survey). In fact, there is bitter irony in talking of the effect of travels made by the family on the language development of the child. In the developing countries, it is common that poor families lead a nomadic life; their "travels" are invariably accompanied by a host of deprivations, since these miserable people are in a ceaseless and exhausting quest for conditions of minimum survival. Weighing my words with great care, and with no intent of shocking my reader by a comparison that may perhaps seem tasteless, I may say that the malnourished children in the developing countries could be looked at in the same way as we look at the deliberately malnourished dogs subjected to experimental work by Platt and Stewart (1968). When the offspring of malnourished parents receive a diet low in protein, their anomalies are more accentuated than those observed in equally malnourished children of normally nourished parents. The families who live under conditions of chronic malnutrition give birth to defective children, whose handicaps become even more serious with the deficient nourishment on which they subsist.

We must insist that the problem of malnutrition in the developing countries is not identical with that in Europe. Yudkin and Yudkin (1968) maintain that there are 2 million children in the United Kingdom living in poverty; they preface this statement by others such as "the effects of early severe and prolonged malnutrition are still under discussion [since we must remember that] malnutrition of children is not planned by parents in a careful way and studied in order to incorporate the results in a scientific dissertation on the relationship between diet and longevity." We understand the doubts expressed by the Yudkins, since the poverty in the United Kingdom, the effects of which are "still under discussion," cannot be compared to the poverty of a family of 8 persons who "live" on a monthly budget of less than 20 dollars, as we have been able to verify in at least one of our cases. The clinical cases we have studied are the children of the miserable families who live in the poverty-stricken surroundings of São Paulo; these children have congenital handicaps, the result of intrauterine malnutrition, and a chronic condition of postnatal malnutrition, particularly intense after weaning, at the beginning of the second year of life. The poverty to which we refer is a daily problem, chronic, invariable, and merciless. Its effects have to be different from those cited by the British authors.

Methods and Procedures

We used the Gesell scale of development in a study of various groups of children in the city of São Paulo. In the preliminary investigation (Lefèvre, Altenheim, & Penna, 1953), a comparison between two groups of children without nutritional problems was undertaken.

GROUP 1

This group consisted of 50 normal children from fairly varied family backgrounds; 34 came from the middle or lower class and were examined in an ambulatory well-baby clinic; the parents of 16 were in the medical professions. No socioeconomic breakdown was undertaken; the children all lived with their own families, they had no nutritional problems, and they enjoyed good health.

GROUP 2

The second group, also of 50 children, lived in an asylum whose population was drawn from rejected children, orphans, and children from maladjusted families with low economical resources. The asylum was maintained through public charity. Seventy-five children lived in this institution; they were looked after by seven rather overworked aides, who were either illiterate or just semiliterate. Their play opportunities were limited to one slide, one sandbox, and a few broken toys. Obviously, their environmental stimulation was negligible; their nutrition, however, though inferior in quantity and quality to that of Group 1, at least reached the required minimum, so that there was no problem of chronic malnutrition with these children. Nor did they have neurological diseases or other physical handicaps.

The objective of this first investigation was to compare the development, as shown by Gesell tests, of these two groups of children, who differed so substantially in terms of the degree of stimulation they received, Group 1 being given the usual unplanned but acceptable kind, Group 2 being neglected in this respect. We hoped thus to discover the role of environmental stimulation in the development of normal children who had no chronic, clinical problems of nutrition. There was no attempt to establish a standard with absolute values for comparison with any subsequent groups to be studied.

GROUP 3

A second investigation was undertaken with a group of 20 malnourished children. They were subdivided into two groups: the first consisted of five infants whose ages, at the beginning of the study, were limited to from 5 to 14 months, and who presented with a serious clinical malnutrition; the second subgroup consisted of fifteen older children, from 13 to 88 months at the onset of the study, presenting with a serious protein deficiency. These 20 children were admitted to the Department of Pediatrics (Children's Hospital, Medical Faculty, University of São Paulo) because of conditions that their families had not related to their chronic malnutrition. None of these children had had seizures or neurological disease, and their early history indicated that none had suffered perinatal insults likely to affect the nervous system. Children with perinatal trauma, neonatal jaundice, or convulsions were excluded from this study.

The children were evaluated in terms of biochemistry, anthropometry, general development, and neurological status. Most of the patients (17) were seen 3 times. The first examination occurred close to the time of their admission to the hospital, immediately after the acute problems that had brought them in had been corrected clinically (the most common symptoms were severe diarrhea and acute dehydration); the second examination was made about 2 months after admission, and the third about 4 months later. The third examination was omitted in one of the children, and two children were studied only at the time of admission. The children were under the direct supervision of the physicians responsible for the program in the period between the first and second examinations; in the next period they were in a convalescent unit of the hospital.

The biochemical examination consisted of assessments of hemoglobin, cholesterol, fasting blood sugar, and protein electrophoresis. Growth was assessed by weight, height, and bone age. The general development was ascertained by Gesell tests if the children were less than 3-years old; in the two elder children (aged 67 and 88 months), the Terman Merrill and Goodenough tests were used. The neurological status was determined by clinical neurological examination, cranial X-rays, pneumoencephalograms, electroencephalograms, and examination of cerebrospinal fluid. Details of the clinical picture of these children have been reported previously (Marcondes, Lefèvre, & Machado, 1969; Marcondes et al., 1970). We must here focus on the neurological development, with special emphasis on language. One case, with 49 months, has been excluded from the study.

GROUP 4

Finally, a fourth group, of 15 children, was studied; these patients had no chronic nutritional problems, but were seen in the Department of Pediatrics for conditions similar to those affecting the undernourished children, with whom they shared the same social background. These children were also studied clinically and by means of the Gesell scales, and thus served as a control group for the undernourished children.

Results

Let us examine the results of the various investigations made by means of the Gesell developmental scales (Gesell & Amatruda, 1941). From the outset, it is necessary to point out that this test was used because its clinical value had already been proved. Recall that there is no well-established standard for the development of the Brazilian child. Thus we decided to use the Gesell test for Group 1, which may be considered as our general control group—50 normal children free of chronic nutritional problems and suffering no stimulus deprivation. A first comparison was made with the 50 institutionalized children of Group 2. (We previously had compared children younger than 18 months and older children to see whether the nervous system is more susceptible to the environment at one age than another. The F value (Scheffe test) in all the tests of significance in all comparisons between these various age groups was always below the standard level of confidence; the highest value was $F = 1.94$. Because of this lack of a statistically significant difference, we grouped all ages together in our analysis.)

The comparison of Groups 1 and 2 (see Table 16—1), which differed fundamentally in the degree of stimulation they received, reveals a statistically significant difference only in the development of language and in personal-social development. In other words, children suffer from the effects of stimulus deprivation to a higher degree in some developmental areas than in others. The highest degree, according to this study, is in the area of language development; it could hardly have been otherwise. The institutionalized children rarely communicate with one another, and only rarely hear spoken language; it is thus natural that

TABLE 16–1 COMPARISON OF THE DEVELOPMENT OF THE CONTROL GROUP WITH A GROUP OF INSTITUTIONALIZED CHILDREN

Developmental area	Group 1 (control group) average scores	Group 2 (institutionalized children) average scores	F values (Scheffe test)
Motor	119.76	90.94	3.72 (ns)
Adaptive	116.34	91.08	3.33 (ns)
Personal-social	121.02	87.14	4.27*
Language	120.20	81.58	4.79*

*p $\geq$ 0.05 (Scheffe's F = 3.82).

they differ from the control group in this respect. Their low averages in the area of personal-social development are also easily explained if we consider the shortage of personnel in the institution and the resulting lack of social interchange over any but the absolute necessities.

The area of adaptive development, which Knobloch and Pasamanick (1963) considered to be the most relevant to the development of intelligence, also shows a difference between the two groups; this difference, however, does not reach statistical significance. This suggests that the institutionalized children did not differ from the control group because of a constitutional lack of intelligence, but rather in that aspect of intelligence that is dependent upon the transmission of ideas and thoughts by words spoken by the people surrounding the growing child.

A comparison was also made between Group 1 and Group 3 (see Table 16–2, p. 287), the severely malnourished children. The averages of development in the various categories were obtained from the final examination given the Group 3 children, 6 months after hospital admission. (It did not seem reasonable to base the comparisons on the earlier examinations; the children at that time presented with clinical conditions so dramatically low that assessment of their development would have made the mistake of confounding the influence of momentary or transient conditions with that of more chronic ones.)

Before presenting the results of this comparison, it is necessary to give a quick summary of the most important clinical and neurological findings for Group 3 (see, for further details, Marcondes *et al.*, 1969, 1970).

The five children of 14 months of age or less were all malnourished during the first year of life. Although the period of severe malnutrition was shorter than in the older children, the insult occurred during a period of intensive growth of the nervous system, which may thus have been irreversibly compromised (Dobbing, 1968). Four of these patients had well-documented cases of marasmus; the other was in a transitional state between marasmus and kwashiorkor. All were seriously

TABLE 16-2   COMPARISON OF THE DEVELOPMENT OF THE CONTROL GROUP WITH A GROUP OF MALNOURISHED CHILDREN

Developmental area	Group 1 (control group) average scores	Group 3 (malnourished children) average scores	F values (Scheffe test)
Motor	119.76	70.62	6.35*
Adaptive	116.34	72.12	5.83*
Personal-social	121.02	65.81	6.95*
Language	120.20	61.75	7.24*

*$p \geq 0.05$ (Scheffe's $F = 3.82$).

deficient in weight and stature, which improved with treatment but did not catch up to the normal standard. The neurological examination at the time of their admission also showed marked psychomotor retardation, marked hypotonia, hypoactivity, preservation of reflexes characteristic of earlier periods, and microcephaly. At the third examination, the neurological abnormalities had disappeared in three of the patients. Of the other two, one was now presenting with focal signs that had not been evident at the time of the first examination. The psychomotor development in all five continued to be retarded, as will be seen presently. The pneumoencephalogram was abnormal at the time of the first examination, with diffuse cortical atrophy in all cases, and also, in one case, with subcortical atrophy. When the clinical conditions had improved and the blood chemistry had been corrected, a follow-up pneumoencephalogram done on four of the children still showed diffuse cortical atrophy in three. Electroencephalograms were recorded for all five children at the beginning and at the end of the observation period. One of the records showed an abnormality suggestive of an irritative focus in the left temporal region, a fact of particular interest because this patient had release phenomena (in H. Jackson's sense) on the right side.

The older children of Group 3 presented with a typical picture of protein malnutrition (kwashiorkor). There was a wider age range in this subgroup: nine children were from 12- to 23-months old, three from 24 to 35 months, and three older than 36 months. Just as in the subgroup of the younger children, they all presented with marked weight and height deficits at the time of their first examination. At the time of their last examination, the average for the group as a whole, though improved, was still short of the norm. The following were the most outstanding findings in their neurological examination. (1) All had microcephaly. (2) Diffuse cerebral damage was observed in 12 cases, characterized either by poorly developed or absence of speech, or by motor immaturity, abnormal muscle tonus, ataxic stance and gait, abnormal deep tendon reflexes or superficial reflexes;

the diffuse cerebral damage was marked and symmetrical in seven cases, moderate in two, with clinical evidence of asymmetry in three. (3) In four cases, the peripheral nervous system was compromised. From their medical history we note that two patients failed to show these neurological signs at the time of discharge, even though their psychomotor development was still retarded. The cranial circumference increased appreciably during the 6 months of treatment. That is, the increases were larger than those to be expected in children of the same age under normal conditions; however, in none of the cases did the circumference reach normal values by the time of discharge. The pneumoencephalogram was normal in only one case during the first examination, being equivocal in one other. In all the other cases, cortical and/or subcortical atrophy was observed. In three of the twelve cases in which a pneumoencephalogram was done at the time of discharge, abnormalities had persisted. The electroencephalogram was essentially noncontributory, even though six EEGs were read as abnormal at the beginning of the observation period; five of these had become normalized by the time of the last examination. It is important to point out that in several cases with clinical signs of marked cerebral damage, the EEG was entirely within normal limits.

As already mentioned, the Gesell test was administered three times to children in Group 3; the comparisons of these children to those of Groups 1 and 2, to be discussed presently, are based on the findings at the third examination. Since there was no significant difference between the children with marasmus and the children with kwashiorkor, the averages constitute those of the pooled data from these two subgroups. It is true that with this procedure we lost the opportunity of comparing the effects of malnutrition incurred during the first year of life with those incurred by the older children. There are some interesting suggestions in this respect that may be found in our earlier publications (Marcondes *et al.*, 1969, 1970). However, in the present study the number of patients in the marasmus group is too small to permit statistical evaluation.

Inspection of Table 16–2 and its comparison with Table 16–1 shows the dramatic slowness of development in the children of Group 3. As already mentioned, these averages constitute the development of the 17 children after their clinical problems had been corrected and their chemistries had reached more acceptable levels. We are dealing here with the chronic sequelae of malnutrition, although, unfortunately we do not have the follow-up data by which to judge how permanent the situation is. There was general developmental retardation, and as in Group 2, the personal-social development of these children and their language development suffered most. The insult produced by malnutrition augments the effects of the lack of stimulation received by these desperately poor children, because intelligence is severely affected in the undernourished. This is well shown in figures by the high F value of the Scheffe test of significance (Table 16–2). Notice that the value of 4.79 for language in Table 16–1 (comparison of Groups 1 and 2) is here increased to the value of 7.24 (comparison of Groups 1 and 3).

We are here at the heart of our problem. We have attempted to see whether stimulus deprivation is capable of retarding development independently from the effects of malnutrition, and to discover what the interaction would be between the two handicaps: Would malnutrition aggravate the situation created by stimulus deprivation? The figures of Table 16—1 and 2 are most suggestive.

Group 3 is apparently more affected than Group 2 in all areas of development (Table 16—3), although the differences between the two groups are not statistically significant by the Scheffe criterion. A simple inspection of the *F* values in isolation may be misleading, however. The difference in the average score for language, for instance, between Groups 2 and 3 is so small, not because Group 3 is free from language problems, but because language development in Group 2 had already suffered severely.

A comparison was also made between the results obtained from Group 3, the undernourished children, and Group 4, the relatively well-nourished children from the same social background as Group 3 (Table 16—4). From this comparison we hoped to find out what effect malnutrition alone would have on the development of children from an exceedingly deprived social environment. The figures in Table 16—4, although not statistically significant, indicate that malnutrition as an isolated factor aggravates the developmental deficit in all areas, and particularly in language.

In another attempt to discover the role of nutrition alone, the results of Group 3 were compared with the pooled averages from Groups 1, 2, and 4 (Table 16—5). In this tabulation, we used the *F* values already obtained in the earlier comparisons, and thus pitted the results of our study of malnourished children against those of a heterogeneous group of children, none of them malnourished. In this comparison, whose results were significant, we see that the handicap suffered by Group 3 in all areas of development was further augmented in the development of language and in personal-social development. This form of comparison is interesting, in that it dramatizes the effects of malnutrition; however, one must remember that Groups 1, 2, and 4 comprised 115 children; Group 3 had only 17.

TABLE 16-3   COMPARISON OF THE DEVELOPMENT OF INSTITUTIONALIZED CHILDREN WITH MALNOURISHED CHILDREN

Developmental area	Group 2 (institutionalized children) average scores	Group 3 (malnourished children) average scores	F values (Scheffe test)
Motor	90.94	70.62	2.62 (ns)
Adaptive	91.08	72.12	2.50 (ns)
Personal-social	87.14	65.81	2.69 (ns)
Language	81.58	61.75	2.46 (ns)

p $\geq$ 0.05 (Scheffe's F = 3.82).

**TABLE 16–4   COMPARISON OF THE DEVELOPMENT OF
MALNOURISHED CHILDREN WITH WELL–NOURISHED,
HOSPITALIZED CHILDREN FROM THE SAME SOCIAL
ENVIRONMENT**

Development area	Group 3 (malnourished children) average scores	Group 4 (well-nourished, hospitalized children) average scores	F values (Scheffe test)
Motor	70.62	85.27	1.89 (ns)
Adaptive	72.12	91.53	2.56 (ns)
Personal-social	65.81	86.73	2.63 (ns)
Language	61.75	87.33	3.17 (ns)

p $\geq$ 0.05 *(Scheffe's F = 3.82).*

**TABLE 16–5   COMPARISON OF THE RESULTS FOR GROUP
3 (MALNOURISHED CHILDREN) WITH THE POOLED
RESULTS FOR GROUPS 1, 2, AND 4 (CONTROL GROUP,
INSTITUTIONALIZED GROUP, WELL-NOURISHED GROUP
FROM SAME SOCIAL ENVIRONMENT AS GROUP 3).**

	Motor development F value	Adaptive development F value	Personal-social development F value	Language development F value
Group 3 × Groups 1, 2, 4 (pooled data)	5.08*	4.84*	5.80*	5.64*

p $\geq$ 0.05 *(Scheffe's F = 3.82).*

Discussion

We have already mentioned the great difficulties that we encountered in making comparisons of the kind reported in this paper; perhaps the greatest of these was the total absence of standards for language development in Brazil. To overcome this difficulty, we first had to select and study control groups that had not suffered malnutrition. Gesell and Amatruda (1941) had already called attention to the poor language development in institutionalized children living, as it were, in "islands of isolation" with respect to verbal communication. These authors studied many factors responsible for the developmental lags in language, but they did not study malnutrition—because, in their own words, "It is not our purpose to discuss abuses [p. 283]." The literature apparently relevant to our problem does not help us much. We have already referred to the disparity between that which is considered poor or deficient in the advanced countries and the conditions in Latin America. Birch (1967), for example, calls our attention to the absence of research on the influence of malnutrition on the health and education of children in unfavorable socioeconomic conditions. As an illustration of such conditions, he cites families whose *weekly* budget varies from 36 to 43 (in U.S. curency). With such a budget, says Birch, it is impossible to supply the necessary nourishment to families with seven and eight members. Such a budget in Brazil (where, it must be remembered, the cost of living is only slightly lower than in the United States) would imply that we were dealing with well-fed people living under excellent conditions. The *monthly* budget for the families in our Group 3 runs as low as $20 for a family of eight!

In this discussion, we shall limit ourselves to an analysis of the findings for Group 3. It is vitally important that these children and their families be studied by means of various psychological and sociological criteria; such research is being planned. Under no circumstances can we use the findings cited in the literature, nor can we adhere to the various interpretations there. Even the very thorough recent publication by Talbot and Howell (1971), which appears to deal with the same problems raised here (particularly the effects of nutritional deficiencies on social factors, on learning ability, and on the general behavior of the child), does not apply. Their patients have nothing in common with those in our Group 3, whose living conditions are infrahuman. In Gesell's terms, we are clearly dealing with nothing but "abuse," in terms both of social deprivation and nutritional deficiencies.

Unfortunately, we did not have the means to follow up the development of our malnourished children, as was done by Barrera (1963); only a few cases were followed after discharge from the hospital. All we can attempt here, therefore, is to give a general evaluation of what was actually observed on our patients in the 6 months that we studied them.

It is not easy to distinguish between the area of personal-social development and that of language development. As Barrera has described, in the succession of stages in which the central nervous system is compromised, there is, from the beginning, an intense apathy, which keeps the child alienated from social contacts; it is thus impossible to say exactly what is specific to language development. There is an enormous impoverishment of expression, which is constant through all the various stages of recuperation, even though it becomes somewhat attenuated with clinical improvement.

It seems to us that in the area of language development the child reacts in a manner similar to that which we have described in our study of acquired aphasia in childhood (Lefèvre, 1950), and which has recently been called to attention by Geschwind (1971). The central nervous system of the child has a peculiar reaction to acute or chronic insults: a restriction of verbal communication. This restriction, which was quite clear in the stimulus-deprived institutionalized children, presents itself even more dramatically among the malnourished. Early on, the child's crying noises are weak and poorly articulated, and there is an impoverishment of mimic expression. These children may use gestures to express their needs. To the extent that the clinical picture and the chemistry improves, the verbal communication also improves, but it always remains below the expected norms.

Table 16—6 shows the evolution of language in each of the 17 children of Group 3, from the time of their admission to the hospital to their discharge. There was large individual variation. In some cases (1, 4, 5, 10), language rehabilitation had not yet reached the 50% mark at the time of clinical recovery. Others showed more favorable catch-up. However, even those patients who made better progress were still not within normal limits at the end of the observation period.

It is important to point out that there was no correlation between failure of language development and other neurological findings (for details, see Marcondes *et al.*, 1969, 1970). Patient 4 is a case in point: although his language development was still retarded by the time of the third examination, the results of his neurological examination had become normal—there were no focal signs, the tonus was unremarkable, and reflexes were within normal limits. The pneumoencephalogram, however, which had shown marked diffuse cortical atrophy at the first examination, continued to be abnormal at the time of the third. Patient 10, who at a chronological age of 29 months had a language development, according to Gesell, of 12 months at the time of the third examination, also had an unremarkable neurological examination at that time. In this case, the pneumoencephalogram improved with the neurological normalization, and the signs of discrete cortical and subcortical atrophy apparent in the first examination had disappeared in the third. The psychomotor development, according to the Gesell scale, had reached the 21-month level at the time of the first examination, whereas language development at that time was still on the 9-month level.

What may be concluded from these and similar studies? Woodward and Stern (1963) investigated the development of severely subnormal children with etiologies other than malnutrition; they called attention to the disparity observed between motor and language development, the latter being much more affected than the former. The work of these English authors is of special interest, since their analysis was made in terms of Piaget's concepts. In the same spirit, Hunt (1961) also studied development; he attributed to Gesell the notion that development is predetermined and therefore may be studied without bothering to evaluate the interaction between the environment and maturation, in contrast to the beliefs of Piaget.

It is not our intention to establish a doctrine based on the few cases we have studied. As mentioned at the outset, our observations are based on material that is extremely difficult to interpret; the children are suffering severely and are not very inclined to collaborate; further, the examiner who approaches them may not have the courage to perturb them during what are, perhaps, the first moments of comfort they have enjoyed. Moreover, the pathological process consists of such complex dynamics that we find it impossible to untangle the threads: an exogenous unfavorable factor (malnutrition) acts upon a function (language) that is in the

TABLE 16–6 COMPARISON BETWEEN CHRONOLOGICAL AGE AND AGE IN TERMS OF LANGUAGE DEVELOPMENT, AS MEASURED BY THE GESELL SCALE, IN 17 MALNOURISHED CHILDREN (GROUP 3)

Case	Chronological age (months, days)		Age in terms of language development (months)	Case	Chronological age (months)	Age in terms of language development (months)
1	4 m	15 d	1 m		22 m	9 m
	6 m	2 d	2 m	10	24 m	12 m
	9 m		3 m		29 m	12 m
2	6 m	25 d	4–5 m		14 m	7 m
	8 m	11 d	5–6 m	11	16 m	15 m
	11 m	5 d	9 m		20 m	15 m
3	11 m		5–6 m		26 m	15 m
	13 m		5–6 m	12	28 m	15 m
	15 m	15 d	11 m		31 m	18 m
4	6 m	23 d	2 m		24 m	24 m
	8 m	10 d	3 m	13	26 m	24 m
	11 m	10 d	5 m		—	—
5	14 m		4 m		18 m	7 m
	15 m	26 d	7 m	14	20 m	13 m
	18 m	19 d	8 m		24 m	18 m
6	14 m		5 m		31 m	15 m
	16 m		13 m	15	33 m	21 m
	21 m		15 m		36 m	30 m
7	23 m		5 m		20 m	6 m
	25 m		5 m	16	22 m	12 m
	30 m		18 m		25 m	13 m
8	22 m		8 m		15 m	3 m
	24 m		11 m	17	17 m	7 m
	29 m		15 m		20 m	15 m
9	13 m		6 m			
	15 m		13 m			
	19 m		13 m			

process of organization. As a consequence, the function regresses, clashing with the wave of organizational development. At this point, one begins to treat the child, attempting to nullify the exogenous handicap; one thereby induces a new wave of development, which mingles with the previous ones but—and this is the important point—which may encounter more or less of a barrier due to possible (perhaps fixed) lesions caused by the malnutrition. The capacity for recuperation or reorganization, as Piaget might say, depends on the interaction between the various elements mentioned and the severity of the acquired lesion.

The events may be similar to those already alluded to in children with acquired aphasia (Lefèvre, 1950; Lefèvre & Wanderley, 1969). The impoverishment of spontaneous speech and the reduction in utterances even when elicited, together with the preservation of comprehension (which is only rarely affected), are characteristics of acquired aphasia in children. On the whole, this clinical picture is similar to that found in the undernourished child. The capacity for recuperation, as in the case of acquired aphasias for other reasons, depends on the intensity of the pathogenic factors and on the degree of reversibility of the cerebral lesions incurred. We are proposing this as a hypothesis to be further tested by means of more detailed studies and a larger array of cases.

References

Barrera, M. G. *Estudios sobre alteraciones del crescimiento y del desarrollo psicomotor del sindrome pluricarencial (kwashiorkor).* Caracas: Grafos, 1963.

Birch, H. G. Health and education of socially disadvantaged children. Paper presented at a conference on Bio-Social Factors in the Development and Learning of Disadvantaged Children, Syracuse, New York, April 1967.

Dobbing, J. Permanent retardation of brain growth related to the timing of early undernutrition. *Memoria, 12th Congreso Internacional Pediatria,* 1968, *1*, 105—106.

Geschwind, N. Fundamentos neurológicos del lenguaje. In H. R. Myklebust (Ed.), *Transtornos del aprendizaje.* (Span. trans. by S. P. Moreno) Barcelona: Científico-Médico, 1971.

Gesell, A., & Amatruda, C. S. *Developmental diagnosis.* New York: Hoeber, 1941.

Hunt, J. M. *Intelligence and experience.* New York: Ronald Press, 1961.

Ingram, T. T. S. Developmental disorders of speech. In P. J. Vinken & G. W. Bruyn (Eds.) *Disorders of speech, perception and symbolic behavior. Handbook of Clinical Neurology.* Vol. IV. Amsterdam: North-Holland Publ., 1969.

Knobloch, H., & Pasamanick, R. Predicting intellectual potential in infancy. *American Journal of Diseases of Children,* 1963, *106*, 43—51.

Lefèvre, A. B. Contribuição para o estudo da psicopatologia da afasia em crianças. *Arquivos de Neuro-Psiquiatra,* 1950, *8*, 345—393.

Lefèvre, A. B., Altenheim, D., & Penna, H. A. Estudo comparativo do desenvolvimento psicomotor, pelo metodo de Gesell, entre crianças asiladas e criancas mantidas em ambiente familiar. *Pediatria Prática,* 1953, *26*, 214—242.

Lefèvre, A. B., & Wanderley, E. Afasia adquirida na infancia. *Arquivos de Neuro-Psiquiatria,* 1969, *27*, 89—96.

McCarthy, D. Desarrollo del lenguaje. In C. Murchinson (Ed.), *Manual de psicologia del niño.* (Span. transl. by L. O. Duran & A. Brook) Barcelona: F. Seix, 1935.

McGrady, H. J. Patologia del lenguaje y transtornos del aprendizaje. In H. R. Myklebust (Ed.), *Transtornos del aprendizaje*. (Span. transl. by P. S. Moreno) Barcelona: Científico-Médica, 1971.

Marcondes, E., Lefèvre, A. B., & Machado, D. V. M. Desenvolvimento neuro-psicomotor da criança desnutrida. I. Má nutrição protêica. *Revista Brasileira de Psiquiatria*, 1969, *3*, 173—219.

Marcondes, E., Lefèvre, A. B., Spina-França, A., Setian, N., Valente, M. I., Barros, N. G., et al. Desenvolvimento neuropsicomotor da criança desnutrida. II. Subnutrição. *Arquivos de Neuro-Psiquiatria*, 1970, *28*, 221—234.

Platt, B. S., & Stewart, R. J. C. Effects of protein-caloric deficiency in dogs: Reproduction, growth and behaviour. *Developmental Medicine and Child Neurology*, 1968, *10*, 3—23.

Renfrew, C., & Murphy, K. (Eds.) *The child who does not talk*. Clinics in Developmental Medicine No. 13. London: Heinemann, 1964.

Talbot, N. B., & Howell, M. C. Social and behavioral causes and consequences of disease among children. In N. B. Talbot, J. Kagan, & L. Eisenberg (Eds.), *Behavioral science in pediatric medicine*. Philadelphia: Saunders, 1971.

Woodward, M., & Stern, D. J. Developmental patterns of severely subnormal children. *Brit. Journal of Educational Psychology*, 1963, *33*, 10—21.

Yudkin, S., & Yudkin, G. Poverty and child development. *Developmental Medicine and Child Neurology*, 1968, *10*, 569—579.

17. Postural System, Corporal Potentiality, and Language

J. B. de Quirós / O. Schrager

We stress the importance of posture, equilibrium, and motor coordination as the basis for the acquisition of many skills, including speech. Normally, the integration of these neuro-motor activities must become "automatized" (needing no conscious control) before higher integrative functions including language can develop. Hemispheric specialization is instrumental in this process: The right hemisphere is said to be responsible for motor integration, while the left hemisphere becomes "freed" from this responsibility during the course of development and is thus available for various cognitive activities, especially language. We shall discuss the empirical basis of our thesis and its importance for diagnosis and management in clinical language disorders.

Terminology

The goal of this chapter is to review some investigations that we carried out on the relation between the development of children's posture and their learning capacities, including within the latter the earlier stages of language acquisition. Before the presentation of the main subject, it is essential to define a number of terms as used in this chapter, specifically *posture, position, attitude, equilibrium, postural system, corporal potentiality*, and *language*.

Posture is the reflex activity of the body in relation to space. Muscles, limbs, or the whole body intervene in posture through reflexes (e.g., flexed or extended tonic postures). Since any posture implies tonic or intersegmentary modifications, relations between different parts of the body, as well as those between the whole body and the spatial environment, are undoubtedly established during rest as well as during movement. Young infants have control over posture before they can maintain and control equilibrium. That is to say, the body reacts in a reflex manner in response to multiple environmental stimuli.

When an organism displays a posture that is characteristic of the species (e.g., *sitting* in dogs), it is preferable to speak of *position*. Each species has its own characteristic positions, which in vertebrates are chiefly related to the horizontal plane (standing, prone, supine, position, etc.).[1]

On the other hand, *attitude* is related to reflexes (of some intentionality) that lead to the return to a species-specific position. The decerebrate animal does not have attitude reflexes, but the thalamic animal does. There are also certain prominent aspects of an animal's characteristic posture that show inner states or that express purpose or wishes; these aspects are also called "attitudes" (open, anxious, enraged, etc.).

Equilibrium is the interplay between various forces, particularly gravity, and the motor power of the skeletal muscles; an organism has achieved equilibrium when he can maintain and control posture, position, and attitude. If equilibrium is slightly disturbed, the only failures seen will be failures in attitude (as in Romberg's test or other tests that introduce strange attitudes for the species). As equilibrium is more disturbed, position also may be impaired, and so more voluntary control will be needed. As equilibrium needs more voluntary control, internalization of new information (coming from outside the body) becomes more and more difficult. It is well known that equilibrium organizes itself through the integration of input from (1) deep sensitivity, (2) labyrinthine function, and (3) vision, the cerebellum being the principal coordinator of this information. In young blind or deaf children (when the latter also have vestibular damage, as frequently happens), there are attitude disturbances; and position impairments are sometimes also present—chiefly those that relate to dynamic positions: feet-drag, motor awkwardness, and so on, which are not directly related to the sensory deficiency but to equilibrium.

Only after equilibrium is reached is it possible to proceed to the development of motor skills and those skills necessary for the survival of the species and the internalization of a great amount of external information—that is what we call *useful equilibrium*, i.e, the position that allows the processes of natural learning.

But the use of instruments or objects, the learning of nonconditioned language, the possibility of developing creativeness, and the capacity for high-level learning require something more than useful equilibrium. They need the noninterference of the afferences related to the body itself. These considerations lead us to the notion of *corporal potentiality*. Human beings, after establishing a "body scheme" (and its allied consequences, body image representation, body concept, etc.), must displace the body's hierarchy (or supremacy) in order to allow symbolic development and to introduce language as an instrument, thus making abstraction possible. As we

---

[1] Posture and position are considered synonymous by some medical writers. The word *position* is also used for the placement of a patient (e.g., painless position) or to make examinations or medical maneuvers easier (e.g, knee–chest position, Trandelenburg position).

shall see, to obtain these results, human awareness must set aside many stimuli supplied by the body. The information from these stimuli is not at all eliminated, but *potentially* continues on the basis of automatic mechanisms of posture and position. The development of such corporal potentiality clearly indicates that a great number of high mental skills can be used for purposes other than the control of the body itself. This implies the use of central nervous structures in human cultural learning, which is far removed from the natural world of instincts and survival.

Corporal potentiality is established upon a conjunction of anatomical-functional structures, which on the whole we recognize as constituting the postural system. Peripheral receptors and exteroceptive, proprioceptive, vestibular, auditory, and visual pathways, cerebellum, reticular formation, gray nuclei of the brain stem and the cerebral base, cortical areas and their afferent and efferent pathways or projections, must be counted among these structures. On that basis, we define *postural system* as the conjunction of anatomical-functional structures, series of parts, organs, or apparatus, positions that allow a definite and useful activity or that enable learning (Quiros, 1965, 1967, 1972; Schrager, 1971).

Postural systems are common to man and animals alike; on the other hand, corporal potentiality implies a function of the postural system that is specifically human; it allows the definite symbolic orientation of one of the cerebral hemispheres (as it is more and more liberated from somatic information) and the cerebral laterality of our species.

Language is defined not as a function but as a complex phenomenon, which uses signs and symbols both within and between persons. It is established on the basis of central neural possibilities, and develops through appropriate psychosocial-cultural interactions. Language in its proper sense is the possibility of symbolic communication. This possibility surpasses the world of animal instincts. Anatomical-functional structures and environmental influences that take part in human language are not yet precisely known, but it is clear enough that the postural system facilitiates the acquisition of the fundamental "instruments" (like language or mathematical thought) that intervene in human learning processes (Quiros and Götter, 1963; Quiros, Schrager, & Tormakh, 1971).

Some Studies of Postural Disturbance, Corporal Potentiality, and Learning

Our intention here is to summarize some of the research on posture, equilibrium, and learning that we have been doing since 1958. We started out by studying what happens when the postural system fails. Deep sensitivity and vestibular function act together in young children; we may call this integration "proprio-ception." In accordance with the theory described above, we thought that research on the relationship between posture and language acquisition must be done on the basis of neurolabyrinthine examinations. Within the latter were included especially tests of infants' postural reflexes and vestibular tests (caloric rotatory).

The first series of experiments was performed in the Children's Hospital of Buenos Aires; the second at the Centenario Hospital (Rosario); the third series in different schools for both normal and exceptional children, as well as in an "experimental" school; at present, the fourth series is under way at the Medical Center of Phoniatric and Audiological Research, Buenos Aires. The total number of children examined was 1902, with different distributions of age and diagnosis for each series, according to the aim of the particular study. This figure does not include numerous cases that have not yet been processed statistically.

FIRST SERIES OF EXPERIMENTS

The goal was to obtain a research methodology for the study of postural disturbances of newborn babies. (For relevant literature up to 1958, see Andre-Thomas, 1955; Andre-Thomas & Ajuriaguerra, 1948; Andre-Thomas & Saint-Anne Dargasses, 1952; Barany, 1906; Kleijn, 1923; Landau, 1925; Magnus, 1924, 1926; Magnus & de Kleijn, 1924; Moro, 1920; Rademaker, 1926, 1935; Schaltenbrand, 1925; Zador, 1938; etc.).

We studied children from 1 day to 2-years old, using different procedures of examination (Hald, 1909; Ruttin, 1910; Alexander, 1911; Barany, 1918; Mygind, 1919; Minkowski, 1921; Thornval, 1920; Vesselle, 1925; Lorente de No, 1926; Voss, 1927; Galebsky, 1927; Arnaud, 1938; Di Giorgio & Castelli-Borgiotti, 1938; Tronconi & Bollettino, 1938; 1941; Tronconi, 1953; Lawrence & Feind, 1953; Giordano & Barbiero, 1953; Bieber, 1954; Esente, 1958; etc.).

Neurological and labyrinthine data of our research were submitted to statistical methodology and computation. Our overall conclusions are presented in the "Discussion" section. (For details of these studies see Quiros, Coriat, & Benasayag, 1961; Quiros, 1967; Quiros, Cowes, Götter, Schrager, & Tormakh, 1969; cf. Rius, 1964, 1965.)

SECOND SERIES OF EXPERIMENTS

Here we established the existence of a syndrome the main characteristics of which were: (1) vestibular areflexia to caloric stimulation; (2) delay of motor development; (3) walking instability; and (4) speech delay (Quiros, 1967). Subsequent to our work we found a description of Precechtel (1925) that mentioned some of these same symptoms. Precechtel referred to these symptoms as typical of the congenital defect of the otolithical apparatus. We feel that the syndrome is frequently also found to be associated with different brain conditions (organic or psychic) and with deafness (Quiros, 1969a, b; Quiros *et al.*, 1971). In these cases possibilities of speech acquisition and development are still further reduced (Quiros, *et al.*, 1971; Rosenblüt, Goldstein, & Landau, 1960; Colbert, Koegler, & Markham, 1959). Some other similar syndromes, as well as the so-called "infantile aphasias," may easily be confused with the above-mentioned condition (Quiros, 1969a, b; Worster-Drought & Allen, 1929/30; Ley, 1929, 1930; Launay *et al.*, 1949).

THIRD SERIES OF EXPERIMENTS

Groups of normal, deaf, mentally retarded, and slow-learning children were studied from the point of view of posture and learning abilities (including speech). At first, the conclusion of this investigation was "Children with learning disabilities give responses to the vestibular caloric test that may be comparable to normal ones." (More or less simultaneously, a similar experiment was carried out in Montreal by Mc Hugh [1962], who reached similar conclusions.) However, we later learned that this conclusion was premature; unfortunately, we studied a rather mixed group of language-impaired children. Learning disabilities in the group of mentally retarded children, for instance, are usually due to the mental retardation itself, and there is no reason for this group to reveal more cases of vestibular disturbance than a group of normal children. That is why in 1963 we repeated the investigation of this condition in school children. The choice of children was made now on the basis of other criteria: learning disability *without apparently justifiable cause*. In this study, our initial working hypothesis was confirmed: 52 children out of 63 fully-tested cases had abnormal vestibular responses with caloric stimulation. In the other cases, it was eventually possible to demonstrate the presence of other factors that might cause the disturbance (Quiros, 1967).

Postural disturbance at primary school is characterized by restlessness (which we differentiate from hyperactivity), motor awkwardness in reading and writing, dysgraphia, and loss of interest in school learning, among other symptoms. (For a description of this condition, see Quiros, 1967, 1968). The condition is frequently confused with other learning disabilities, particularly "developmental specific dyslexia" (Quiros, 1971).

FOURTH SERIES OF EXPERIMENTS

It is definitely known now that children born with postural disturbances suffer delays in the development of motor skills, as well as in many other learning capacities (including language). At present, we are investigating the possibility of genetic factors in postural disturbances; pedigrees have been published of families with vestibular areflexia (Schrager & Braier, 1972). In other investigations we are making statistical assessments of neurological, proprioceptive, and vestibular data, together with the data from the neuro-labyrinthine examination.

Discussion

"SYMBOLIC" AND "POSTURAL" CEREBRAL HEMISPHERES

The human being has evidently "sacrificed" a great deal of corporal and spatial information in order to "assign" one of his cerebral hemispheres to symbolic performance. We all know that dominant hemisphere damage (chiefly in certain areas) produces in adults the complex syndromes designated by the generic name of "aphasia." Lesion of the same areas in the nondominant hemisphere produces a very different clinical picture, in which body scheme and spatial relation disturbances are the outstanding symptoms. This clinical picture received the name of "apractognosia" (Hecaen, Penfield, Bertrand, & Malmo, 1956).

Pathology in adults shows that functions of each cerebral hemisphere are basically different. Also, pathology in the adult is different from pathology in young children. Young children do not have cerebral dominance, and initially their processes of learning are somewhat comparable to animal learning. Later a symbolic value is assigned to one of the infantile cerebral hemispheres. This allows language development and the acquisition of reading and writing and "reading–writing" (lectoescritura), which really are also stages of language development.

It is impossible to speak about a proper language development without admitting the existence of a complete dominance of one cerebral zone over the other zones. On the other hand, when body spatial information predominates over symbolic work, the progress and developmental possibilities of the latter are seriously disturbed.

In regard to learning processes, a clear diffentiation between the work of the human brain and that of higher animals can therefore be admitted, on the basis of a "symbolic" hemisphere and a "postural" or "corporal" hemisphere. In order to be able to dedicate itself to symbolic skills, the symbolic hemisphere transfers to the nondominant hemisphere information coming from the body and/or its spatial relationships. Undoubtedly this phenomenon must have important implications for body laterality. When unusual or very strong corporal-spatial information arrives at the higher levels, the symbolic hemisphere must necessarily dedicate itself to process this information. In such circumstances, symbolic processes will be displaced or superceded by urgent vital needs. In cybernetical terms, it could be said that if the available circuits for a lower program cannot process the information, thus requiring the interaction of other circuits ordinarily used for a higher program, these "higher" circuits will fail to execute their own functions. That is why language will not develop properly if the postural "program" is not yet established. This is why we consider that in the acquisition of human learning, examination of postural systems and corporal potentiality are of great significance.

Corporal potentiality was defined some years ago (Quiros, 1965) as the possibility that human beings have to "exclude" the body in order to allow processes of higher learning. That is to say, to allow processes of elaboration, transformation, and inclusion (symbolization) of the information received. Body "exclusion" is the consequence of the inhibition of the "minor" hemisphere by the dominant one. This notion has particular relevance to language learning and to one of its derivatives, reading–writing (lectoescritura), which is an exclusively human type of learning. Both postural system and corporal potentiality examinations are, according to our criteria, the only methods that allow a relatively simple clinical approach to language pathology, within the whole framework of biological factors that make the human type of learning possible.

At present it is still difficult to study any one of the biological foundations of language. Lenneberg (1967) mentions the very rapid weight increase of the brain, the interconnection of cells, the dendrogenetic maturity, the hypothetical molecular changes within cells, the chemical and electrophysiological changes that accompany those structural modifications, as the main maturational factors of the human brain that may, perhaps, control the ontogenetic emergence of language. Certainly none of these factors can be checked directly by the present clinical procedures. It is essential to realize that all these factors, before determining language acquisition, intervene in the establishment of hemisphere dominance and corporal potentiality. Both of these phenomena can now be studied clinically, and the methods and procedures of such studies are constantly being perfected. Naturally we are still far from a well-developed semeiological procedure, and the research possibilities in this field are therefore wide open.

POSTURAL INTERFERENCE AND LANGUAGE LEARNING

As stated above, language internalization is obtained on the basis of the exclusion from the level of conscious awareness of a great amount of body information (or external information transmitted through the body). We have also mentioned that the postural system allows the incorporation of basic processes of learning, which in appropriate situations can reach language acquisition.

The postural system must be carefully studied in order to interpret many symptoms that usually appear in language pathology. This is not the place to reproduce different papers we have previously written on this theme (Quiros *et al.*, 1969, 1971, 1972; Schrager & Cowes, 1968). But attention must be called to some facts within the anatomical-functional complexity of the postural system. All the nervous structures that directly or indirectly contribute to it work as "sensory-motor" or "motor sensory" circuits, with real feedback mechanisms. In the postural system there are spinal low-levels ("readiness level"), which basically act through Sherrington's stretch reflex and Laporte and Lloyd's anti-stretch reflex; there are brain stem and cerebellar levels, which also take part in afferent and efferent circuits with the spine; there are thalamic and strio-pallidal levels; and there are cortical levels. All these levels can facilitate or make difficult the appearance of language. As early as 1957 we proposed that all the central nervous structures (including the spine) directly or indirectly intervene in language acquisition through sensory-motor circuits of permanent interaction (Quiros & Ruiz Moreno, 1957; Quiros & Götter, 1963; Schrager, 1971). The stronger the corporal information and the body requirements, the more remarkable will be the delay in language acquisition. We insist on the fact that language acquisition is a learning process. Every system able to learn must have acting and informing possibilities through proper amplification and inhibition, in regard to the received stimuli. For instance, if the constituent elements of the speech message and the environmental noises cannot be simultaneously amplified and inhibited, respectively, learning of speech becomes impossible. This simultaneous amplification and inhibition of an oral message is also obtained when there are no corporal interferences or exigencies.

If handicaps are great, high levels of the central nervous system ("high programs") will be needed in order to maintain the postural system in "action." The higher the level of the central nervous system used to maintain the "service" of the body, the greater will be the difficulty in concentrating the higher skills on learning processes. Therefore, internalization of language will be very difficult when such handicaps are present.

The interference of the postural hemisphere with the symbolic work of the dominant hemisphere can be avoided by various normal or abnormal circumstances:

1. Reaching postures and positions that allow the proper development of corporal potentiality. This can be obtained when body interferences such as afferent inputs (due to corporal disturbances), pain, tiredness, etc., are not present.
2. Under certain situations of great environmental or tensional pressure.
3. Inducing activities in the nondominant hemisphere (for example: putting it at the command of servo-mechanisms of automatic movements).

In regard to the third point, it is a well-known fact that many times, particularly when fatigue is present or during intellectual emergencies, better concentration and symbolization are achieved when automatic walking is initiated. This makes it possible for the postural hemisphere to keep "busy," thus making the work of the symbolic or dominant hemisphere easier. When intellectual work must continue, and symptoms of physical and/or psychic tiredness appear, drowsiness included, the production of pain, or walking, or other motor activities can keep the individual awake and allow him to continue work. Conversely, if the individual adopts a comfortable position when tired, sleep overcomes him. However, the same position at times of mental alertness would allow him to continue efficient intellectual work. The opposite case is also true: During dangers of life, many body afferences are absolutely excluded, and the "life emergency services" (vision, hearing, locomotor apparatus, sometimes quick thinking—all of them based on neuro-endocrine reactions) are brought into action. In emergencies of life, the postural "program" predominates. In social or intellectual emergencies, the action belongs to the symbolic "program."

Symptoms showing the proper symbolic hemisphere dominance will not be considered here. We only call attention to the fact that in language pathology a lack of adequate dominance of the symbolic hemisphere is revealed through echolalic or perseverative speech, or through stereotypic writing. When these symptoms are transitional, they can be due to tiredness or body interferences. But if they are constant, they show the existence of disturbed hemispheric symbolization.

Conclusions and Summary

1. Equilibrium means not only the possibility of reaching standing position or walking, but a real sequence of successive acquisitions of postures, positions, and attitudes.

2. Normally developed animals and young children acquire many learning processes through useful equilibrium.

3. Nevertheless, without the development of corporal potentiality, acquisition of real language cannot be reached. Corporal potentiality is defined as the human possibility to "exclude" the body in order to allow processes of higher learning (symbolic processes).

4. From posture to useful equilibrium, all body achievements depend on the postural system. Appropriate and normal language development requires not only a proper postural system, but corporal potentiality.

5. Language is built upon nonspecific neurological structures. The whole central nervous system takes part (directly or indirectly) in the phenomenon recognized as "language." In humans there is a symbolic cerebral hemisphere and a postural hemisphere. A definition of language can be summarized as the possibility of symbolic communication.

6. Without the "exclusion" of much body information and responsibility for body functions from the higher levels of the central nervous system, symbolic communication cannot be accomplished.

7. Several investigations on newborn and young children were carried out against the background of the above ideas. After establishing a methodology for postural examination, different groups of children were assessed. A clear conclusion could be reached from these studies: Young children with noncompensated postural disturbances show delay in both motor and symbolic acquirements.

8. At present, we consider postural examinations (corporal potentiality, hemispheric dominance, body laterality, etc.) to be of great importance for the correct diagnosis, prognosis, and treatment of several conditions related to communication and language pathologies.

9. These examinations are clinically feasible; therefore, they have an advantage over other types of biological examinations (also relevant to language), which are, so far, clinically unpractical.

10. On the basis of these ideas, various projects are under development, which are designed to obtain a basis for better interpretation of the symptoms revealed by different syndromes of language pathology. We believe that in this way, clinical and medical examinations will be improved, diagnosis will be more accurate, and rehabilitation more successful.

References

Alexander, Die Reflexeiregberrkeit des Ohrlabyrints am menschlichen Neugeborenen. *Zeitschrift Für Psychologie*, 1911, *2*, 153.

Andre-Thomas. L'equilibre et la fonction labyrinthique chez le nouveau-ne et le nourrisson. *Encephale* 1955, *44*, 97—137.

Andre-Thomas & Ajuriaguerra, J. de *L'Axe Corporel.* Paris: Masson, 1948.

Andre-Thomas & Saint-Anne Dargassies. *Etudes neurologiques sur le nouveau-ne et le jeune nourrisson.* Paris: Masson, 1952.

Arnaud, G. *Le labyrinthe membraneux posterieur du nouveau-ne*. Paris: Librairie Felix Alcan, 1938.

Barany, R. Ueber die vom Ohrlabyrinth ausgelöste gegenrollung der Augen bei Normalhörenden, Ohrenkranken und Taubstummen. *Archiv. fur Klinische und Experimentelle Ohren-, Nasen-, und Kehlheilk Kopffheilkunde* 1906, *68*, 1—30.

Barany, R. Ueber einige Augen und Halsmus Kehlreflexe bei Neugeborenen. *Acta O. L.* 1918, *1* : 97.

Bieber, G. Ricerche sul determinismo del reflesso di aggrappamento nel neonato. *Rivista di Clinice Pediatrica* 1954, *54*, 401—419.

Colbert, G., Koegler, R. R., & Markham, C. H. Vestibular dysfunction in childhood schizophrenia. *Archives of General Psychiatry* 1959, *1*, 62—600; 79—617.

Di Giorgio, A. M., & Castelli-Borgiotti, C. Sul graduale instaurarsi nel'uomo, della corrispondenza fra il piano dell'orbita in cui si manifesta il nistagmo oculare da eccitamento rotatorio, ecc. *Archivio di Fisiologia* 1938, *38*, 117—185.

Esente, I. *Physiologie de la Vision chez le Premature et le Nourrisson Normal*. Paris: G. Doin, 1958.

Galebsky, A. Vestibular nystagmus in new-born infants. *Acta O. L.* 1927, *11*, 409—423.

Giordano, G. G., & Barbiero, C. H. Contributo allo studio delle reazione posturali nel bambino. *Acta Neurologica* 1953, *8*, 229.

Hald, T. Om Diagnosen Labyrint destruktion. Uger Kr. I. Loeger (quoted by Arnaud, 1938).

Hécaen, H., Penfield, W., Bertrand, C. & Malmo, R. The syndrome of apractognosia due to lesions of minor cerebral hemisphere. *A.M.A. Archives Neurology and Psychology* 1956, *75*, 400—434.

Kleijn, A. de. Experimental physiology of the labyrinth. *Journal of Laryngology and Otology* 1923, 646.

Landau, A. Ueber motorische Besonderheiten des zweiten Lebehnshalbjahres. *Monatsschrift fur Kinderheilkunde*, 1925, *29*, 555.

Launay, C., Borel-Maisonny, S., Duchene, H., & Diatkine, R. Les troubles du langage chez l'enfant *Semaine des Hopitaux de Paris* 1949, *25*, 3732—3737.

Lawrence, M. M., & Feind, C. R. Vestibular response to rotation in newborn infants. *Pediatrics* 1953, *12*, 300—306.

Lenneberg, E. H. *Biological Foundations of Language*. New York: Wiley, 1967.

Ley, J. Un cas d'audimutite idiopathique. Aphasie congenitale chez des jumeaux monozygotes. *Encephale* 1929, *24*, 121—165.

Ley, J. Les troubles de developpement du langage. *Journal Belge de Neurologie Psychiatrique*, 1930, *30*, 415—457.

Lorente de No. On the tonic labyrinth reflexes of the eyes. *Acta O. L.* 1926, *9*, 162—176.

McHugh, H. Auditory and vestibular disorders in children. *Laryngoscope* 1962, *72*, 555—565.

Magnus, R. *Korperstellung*. Berlin: Springer, 1924.

Magnus, R. Some results of studies in the physiology of posture. *Lancet* 1926; *211*, 535—536; 585—588.

Magnus, R., & Kleijn, A. de. Experimentelle physiologie des vestibulapparates. *Handb. Neurol. Ohres* 1924, *1*, 465.

Minkowski, M. Ueber Bewegungen und Reflexe des menschlichen Foetus während der ersten Hälfte seiner Entwicklung. *Schweizer Archiv fur Neurologie und Psychiatrie* 1921, *8*, 148—152.

Moro, E. Zur persistenz des Umklammerungsreflexes bei Kindern mit zerebralen Entwicklungshemmungen. *Munchener medizinische Wochenschrift* 1920, *67*, 360.

Mygind, S. H. Den vestibulere Kindreflex. *Ugeskrift fur Laeger* 1919, 1205.

Precechtel, A. Contribution a l'etude de la fonction statique dans la periode foetale et dans la premiere periode de la vie extrauterine; syndrome typique du defaut congenitale de l'appareille otolithique. *Acta O. L.* 1925, *7*, 206—226.

Quiros, J. B. de. Examen vestibular del lactante. XII Jornadas de O. R. L. de Valparaiso, Chile, October 12, 1965.

Quiros, J. B. de. Vestibular-proprioceptive integration: Its influence on learning and speech in children. In *Aportaciones de la Psicologia a la Investigacion Transcultural. Mem. X. Cong. Soc. Interamer. Psicol.* Mexico, Trillas, 1967.

Quiros, J. B. de. Diagnostico diferencial de los sindromes vestibulares en el nino pequeno y de las mal llamadas "afasias infantiles." *Fonoaudiologica* 1968, *14*, 86—102.

Quiros, J. B. de. Disturbances in the language of a child: The child who does not speak. *Clinical Proceedings of Children's Hospital* (Washington, D.C.) 1969a, *25*, 192—205.

Quiros, J. B. de. Les aphasies infantiles: un probleme diagnostic. *Reeduc. Orthophon.* 1969b, 7, 243—254.

Quiros, J. B. de. El diagnostico diferencial de la dislexia especifica. *Fonoaudiologica* 1971, *17*, 117—123

Quiros, J. B. de. Ceguera y psicomotricidad. *Revista Argentina Tiflologia* 1972, *1*, 34—54.

Quiros, J. B. de., Coriat, L. F., & Benasayag, L. Hacia el encuentro del esquema corporal a traves de las respuestas neurologicas vestibulares. *Fonoaudiologica* 1961, 7, 27—55.

Quiros, J. B. de., Cowes, L., Götter, R., Schrager, O., & Tormakh, E. *Los Grandes Problemas del Lenguaje Infantil.* Buenos Aires, CEMIFA, 1969.

Quiros, J. B. de., and Götter, R. *El Lenguaje en el Nino.* Buenos Aires, CEMIFA, 1963.

Quiros, J. B. de., and Ruiz Moreno, G. Bases neurologicas de la foniatria. *Revista de la Asociación Med. Argentina,* 1957, *71,* 101—108.

Quiros, J. B. de., Schrager, O., & Tormakh, E. Aprendizajes y terapias del lenguaje. *Actas XV Cong. Internac. Logopedia Foniatria,* Buenos Aires, 1971.

Quiros, J. B. de., *et al. Las Llamadas Afasias Infantiles.* Buenos Aires, CEMIFA, 1971.

Quiros, J. B. de., *et al. Lenguaje, Psicomotricidad y Aprendizaje.* Buenos Aires, CEMIFA, 1971.

Rademaker, G. G. J. *Die Bedeutung der roten Kerne und des Ubrigen Mittelhirnes L. Muskeltonus, Korperstellung und Labyrinthereflexe.* Berlin: Springer, 1926.

Rademaker, G. G. J. *Reaction Labyrinthique et Equilibre.* Paris: Masson, 1935.

Rius, M. Exploracion del VIII par craneal en el nino recien nacido y en el lactante pequeno. Su importancia y su tenica. *Anales de Uruguay* 1964, *34,* 65—100.

Rius, M. El examen vestibular y su expresion grafica. *Otorrinolaringología Uruguay* 1965, *35,* 29—34.

Rosenblüt, B., Goldstein, R., & Landau, W. N. Vestibular responses of some deaf and aphasic children. *Annals of Otology, Rhinology, and Laryngology* 1960, *69,* 747—755.

Ruttin. Disk. i Oest. ot Gerellsch. *Monatsschrift fur Ohrenheilkunde* 1910, 225.

Schaltenbrand, G. Normale Bewegungs, und Haltungs-und Lagereaktionen bei Kindern. *Deutsche Zeitschrift fur Nervenhheilkunde* 1925, *37,* 29—59.

Schrager, O. L. El sistema postural y sus relaciones con las llamadas afasias infantiles. In J. B. de Quiros, J. B. de., *et al. Lenguaje, Psicomotricidad y Aprendizaje.* Buenos Aires, CEMIFA, 1971.

Schrager, O. L., & Braier, J. L. Perturbaciones en el aprendizaje y la motricidad por aberraciones cromosomicas y enfermedades geneticas. In J. B. de Quiros *et al.* (Eds.), *Lenguaje, Psicomotricidad y Aprendizaje,* Buenos Aires, CEMIFA, 1972.

Schrager, O. L., & Cowes, L. Exploracion vestibular en el nino pequeno. *Fonoaudiologica* 1968, *14,* 51—70.

Tronconi, V. Importanza dello studio della reazioni e contrareazioni di adattamento stattico con riguardo allo sviluppo psico-motorio umano. *Archivio di Psicologia Neurologia e Psichiatria* 1953, *14,* 639—649.

Tronconi, V., & Bollettino, A. Contributo allo studio della reazioni di equilibrio nel bambino. *Bollettino della Societa Medico-Chirurgica* (Pavia), 1938.

Tronconi, V., & Bollettino, A. Le riazioni di adattamento stattico nella inversione del movimento. *Bollettino della Societa Medico-Chirurgica* (Pavia), 1941.

Vesselle, P. *Otite du nourrisson.* Paris Thesis, Faculte de Medecine, Paris, 1925.

Voss, O. Geburtstrauma und Gehörorgan. *Acta O. L.* 1927, *11,* 73—108.

Worster-Drought, C. Speech disorders in children. *Developmental Medicine and Child Neurology,* 1968, *10,* 427—440.

Worster-Drought, C. & Allen, J. M. Congenital auditory imperception. *Journal of Neurology and Psychopathology* 1929—1930, *9,* 192—208; 289—309; 193—236.

Zador, J. *Les Reactions d'Equilibre chez l'Homme.* Paris: Masson, 1938.

IV. Reading and Writing

The topic of this last section has long been dealt with by linguists and psychologists as if it were an odd appendix to psycholinguistics proper. It is precisely reading and writing, however, that constitute the bulk of all practical problems in the language and communication field. It is only in recent years that modern scientific developments have been brought to bear upon the problems besetting the acquisition of reading and writing. The chapter by Frank Smith in particular brings us up to date in this matter. The pathological, acquired disorders of reading and writing have also been subjected to new analysis, as described by Critchley and Weigl, respectively. Read's chapter is a good demonstration of how a fairly familiar phenomenon may be subjected to entirely new and original investigation, yielding important new insights into the mechanisms of the acquisition of reading and writing. Philips's chapter is unique in that it combines observations in the areas of anthropology, sociology, and linguistics in order to reach some eminently practical conclusions.

18. Preconditions for the Development of Writing in the Child

J. de Ajuriaguerra / M. Auzias

In this chapter the conditions for the acquisition and development of handwriting are discussed in the light of many different aspects: motor organization; psychomotor and praxic organization required for writing; speed; hold of the tool; and tonicity. We shall analyze the "directional conventions" view of the spatial constraints of writing. Also discussed are stages in mastery of the graphic space by the child; the most usual tools; methods of learning and handwriting scales; writing disorders that may develop in some children, their causes, and relevant re-education methods. Finally, teaching suggestions drawn from experimental investigations and practice in re-education are given.

The Nature of Writing

We must first determine the place of writing in the human sciences. When studying writing in the context of communication systems, one notices with J. Derrida (1967) that more antagonism than cooperation is expressed when the history of writing and language science meet on the same ground. This author demonstrates, on the basis of an in-depth analysis, to what extent such diverse authors as J. J. Rousseau, F. de Saussure, Jakobson, Halle, and Levi-Strauss tend to depreciate writing on the grounds of its being external, arbitrary, instrumental, auxiliary, parasitical. It is also accused of lack of authenticity, of misrepresentation, of being harmful and inconsistent. Again, writing is considered static, tyrannical, deceptive, a mechanization of language and a loss of the living idiom.

On a more lyrical note, Voltaire remarks that writing is the painting of the voice; the more it resembles it, the better it is. It is true that writing lacks melody, intonation, the tempo of speech, and its spontaneity. When writing attempts to substitute accents for accent, it is but a hollow sham, remarked Derrida. In some cases, however, poetry tries to overcome the absence of accent.

We are in agreement with Alarcos Llorach (1968) when he points out that the elements that make up writing are graphic signs with a structure analogous to that of linguistic signs; in other words, there are two constituents, the *signans* and the *signatum*. Both of these communication media, speech and writing, share the same *signatum*—human experience in general. It would be useful to undertake a systematic "graphematic" study of the communication function of graphic elements and the problems of their material expression. It is not our intention to take on all of these problems in this chapter. For this we refer the reader to the article by Alarcos Llorach (1968) and to the works collected by the Centre International de Synthèse (1963) under the heading, *L'Écriture et la Psychologie des Peuples*.

We do not intend to define the value of written language here, but to study the framework in which writing as such is situated and how it comes about.

In writing, whether transposition or not, the hand that speaks gives pleasure to the child, for whom it is a "discovery" and a means of representing something within himself. It is speech and motion. "The tyranny of letters," as de Saussure (1916) said? Not necessarily. It is rather mastery of a tool and a new method of handling language. Although its inert forms may restrict the liberty of language, to the child they represent mastery of a new mode of expression. Writing does not become a constraint until certain school requirements make their appearance. Of all manual skills, writing allows the child the least liberty, while affording him the greatest satisfaction, because it can provide an indelible trace of what language can express. Writing is graphic representation using conventional, systematic, recognizable signs. It is linear. In Cohen's words (1958), it consists of a visual and durable representation of language, which makes it transportable and conservable. The essential requirement of writing is that it should be transmissible. It is vehicular. In our society, writing is to be seen and read (although in braille, touch replaces sight).

All modes of representation or transcription of language i.e., braille, deaf/mute sign language, as well as writing are physical gestures conveying meaning. According to Alarcos Llorach (1968), the normal and primary manifestation of language is phonic, while writing (graphic representation) is its secondary manifestation; from the linguistic point of view, it cannot be studied alone, but only in relation to the former.

In the ontogenesis of the child, writing comes after speech. A conventional, codified activity, writing is an acquired accomplishment. It is not a gift. It is within our reach once a certain level of intellectual, motor, and affective development has been attained. It is language and movement, but it is restricted by the context in which it takes place, by its rigorous graphic figuration, and the rules of spelling governing transcription of the language. Serving society in line with certain norms, the modes of graphic expression, despite their variability, remain fairly stable in the overall organization of their planning and as a result of the equivalence of writing instruments. The social framework imposes limits on us to ensure that the signs retain their value as a form of general communication.

Every normal individual, given a certain level of development, has the ability to write. But this potential, which depends on the completeness and maturation of several systems, cannot become effective except by learning. As Leischner (1957) states, the systems in question are not the same for the different levels of writing. In *copying*, sight and perception of the form of the visual symbols are foremost, as are the faculties of motor innervation required for execution. In *dictation*, verbal understanding of the text transmitted orally by another and transcription into graphic symbols are essential. In *spontaneous writing*, it is necessary to set down in symbolic form material formulated by the internal language, and a choice must be made from among the forms of speech and the graphic symbols that society has made available to us. What is required, therefore, is the transcription of verbal formulations into meaningful graphic formulations. Furthermore, in the last two instances, a knowledge of spelling must continuously inform the graphic transcription.

Writing is praxia and language. It only becomes possible when a certain level of motor control has been attained, a fine coordination of movements in space. It is a gnosopraxia, both when copying and when performing the other graphic activities—the anticipatory image, preformed action, and optical to-and-fro motions combine in its execution.

In our society, writing follows a measurable course, since it is controlled partly by organofunctional maturation factors, partly by a graduated process of learning. Consequently, and despite its arbitrary nature, writing develops in the child in accordance with laws that can be compared with those of overall psychophysiological development.

On the other hand, like motor control in general and any expressive activity, writing has a personal style intimately bound up with individual characteristics, and this opens up differential psychophysiological horizons.

Writing is not only a permanent method of recording our ideas and memories; in our society it is also a method of exchange, a medium of communication between ourselves and others. For this reason the child must, within the bounds of his personal ability, meet certain requirements imposed by society with regard to legibility and speed.

Although the aesthetics of writing may have changed with the times and the canons varied with the teachers, one element has been constant: the *layout*, which gives writing its "verbal melody" and value as an ordered narrative. It is this, rather than the aesthetic qualities, that modulate this silent way of expression.

Legibility is determined by both the shape of the letters and their ligature, and by the oganization of the sequence of letters.

Speed is one of the requirements of the modern world; typists are chosen in accordance with speed scales, and shorthand was invented to compensate for the slowness of handwriting.

These three types of requirements are to a certain extent contradictory and cannot be reconciled except by suitable teaching methods. According to the child's ability, these methods will take into account the shape of the letters, the ligatures, the tools. The first steps in learning are decisive, since each child comes to writing with his own inherent organization, his motor ability, his faculties of structuration, orientation, and verbal representation, writing being an ordered figuration with a meaning. With this in mind, and on the level of pedagogies in general, learning writing should be approached as a school subject that is shaped by the data here described, data that it confirms at the same time, the hand being no more than the instrument of a broader frame of reference.

The Motor, Psychomotor, and Praxic Organization in Writing

Calling for skilled handling of the writing tool, graphic activity cannot take place without the activation of certain muscles, which, first, maintain the writing position with some force, and second, allow flexibility in the sequence of movements on a flat surface. In writing, as in any effector activity, the muscular activity is controlled by the organization of various anatomico–physiological systems. This organization develops with time; it is to a great extent the result of maturation, but it can only be completely understood and studied in *functional performance*.

In fact, one is in the presence of ideokinesthetic activity patterns (Paillard, 1960), of which the form and meaning are dependent on the task performed; in writing, an activity that engages the whole individual, these patterns are as much "gnoso-praxic" and psychological as they are motor.

The strictly physiological point of view will not be tackled here; we have gone into it elsewhere (Ajuriaguerra, Auzias, Coumes, Denner, Lavondes, Perron, & Stambak, 1964, Vol. 1), and a great many experimental works exist that are devoted to a study of the mechanics of the inscriptive movement considered as the model of a deliberate gesture of extreme refinement (e.g., Essing, 1965; Luthe, 1953; Michel, 1971).

To achieve writing on a small scale, the hand must be capable of fine prehension; furthermore, it must adopt a specific position (in half-supination when a pencil is used), which must be maintained with some force for a fairly extended period of time. Various synergies and coordinations must be put into operation to perform the graphic movement; they develop during the prewriting stage (Lurçat, 1968); the child improves them gradually with practice. The movements, general to start with, have to become precise; the movements of the fingers must gain in refinement and be differentiated from the movements of the wrist and arm, be capable of slight braking while the body learns to keep still to facilitate the complex distal movement. These elementary motor conditions are achieved around the age of six, but at a minimum. The exercise and development of these motor and praxic abilities will enable the movements to become *organized* and gradually to become smooth, quick, supple, economical, and automatic (Ajuriaguerra *et al.*, 1964, Vol. 1; Freeman, 1954).

To illustrate certain aspects of graphic motor behavior, we shall consider three problems: the hold on the tool, the speed of writing, the regulation of tonicity.

Prehension of a Writing Instrument

The position of the fingers on the tool varies with the tool used (pencil, brush), convention, and more or less conscious imitation. These different factors contribute to an accepted so-called "standard" hold (for a given tool), while the manner of proceeding of individual adults more or less conforms to this norm, depending on various individual factors.

In children, the position changes with age. For example, a pencil is first gripped by the whole hand before the age of 1. Prehension thereafter gradually becomes more distal, until the ends of the thumb and the index finger are opposite one another near the instrument's point. After 6 years of age, another change occurs: the flexion of the fingers decreases. Sometimes unusual, defective types of prehension occur. They are related either to tension stemming from widely differing origins (too fine a tool, awkwardness, psychic tension about writing), or to gnoso-praxic difficulties: difficulties in awareness, representation, and use of parts of the body, particularly the fingers. Lastly, a particular hold may be the mark of an ostentatious attitude intended to attract attention. From this simple example, it is clear that the graphomotor organization is also psychomotor and praxic.

Speed of Writing

Handwriting scales have been designed to measure children's writing speed Ajuriaguerra *et al.*, 1964, Vol. 1; Bang, 1959; Cormeau-Velghe, Destrait, Toussaint & Bidaine, 1970; Harris, 1960, pp. 622—624), as well as speed of execution of other activities. They show that speed of movement increases with age and depends on maturation factors, especially in the young child. But other factors influence speed of writing. Daily learning and practice contribute to the *organization of graphic movements*. We have studied the organization of writing gestures when performing a "horizontal" sequence. Between 5 and 6 years of age, the action is *discontinuous*, the hand being almost parallel with the line and the paper held straight. Inscriptive movements alternate with the progression of the hand along the line. During the stages that we were able to describe precisely, this infantile progression is replaced by a well-coordinated, *continuous*, and economic progression. The elbow tends to remain in one place (between ages 12 and 14), serving as a pivot for the forearm (Callewaert, 1954), while the hand rests below the line and the sheet of paper is tilted, thus liberating the graphic field. Various improvements in graphic action occur simultaneously with this new organization, particularly an increase in speed.

Still other factors influence writing speed. It can be impeded (1) by synkinetic (Ajuriaguerra & Stambak, 1955) and tonic elements, (2) by spelling difficulties, and (3) by specific emotional attitudes toward writing (as at the outset of infantile cramp, to which we shall refer later).

Tonic Regulation

The writing activity is not related only to brachial and manual mobility. The maintenance of immobility of the central pillar formed by the body axis is all the more necessary as the movements become more delicate and distal. For the forearm to slide easily and smoothly over the table, the body axis must remain motionless, but as Wallon (1928) remarked, in a "very active state of immobility" with imperceptible compensatory reactions. This function of postural regulation, which develops with acquisition of the walking ability, improves with writing. Between five and seven years of age, the child's torso tends to lean sideways, drawn by the distal movement of the arm and hand advancing along the line. Toward the age of 9, the distal movements are better compensated and are more independent of the trunk, which remains still.

With individual variations that may be considerable, tonicity brings about changes in posture (upright position of the torso between ages 5 and 14), changes in support (gradual elimination of trunk leaning on the table and lightening of the hand), stability of the hand (the constant position in half-supination is acquired between seven and eight years), and elasticity of the shoulder, wrist, and fingers.

Force and pressure are important tonic factors that affect graphic motor control (Essing, 1965; Harris & Rarick, 1959; Luthe, 1953). It is essential for the child to learn, with practice, to use and distribute his own strength (in accordance with his age and tonic typology) in such a way as to limit his energy output. Sometimes it is necessary to help him do this. Experience gained in re-education has demonstrated that the child can improve his writing skill by learning to make a better use of his strength and by correcting unsuitable tonic reactions (Ajuriaguerra *et al.*, 1964, Vol. 2).

Tonic regulation in its various aspects governs the entire writing activity and therefore plays an essential role in handwriting. Serious or even slight defects in tonicity and a lack of strength impede motor control, the support function, and prehension of the implement. On the one hand, good tonicity facilitates writing, and, on the other, is evidence of a positive adaptive response to the situation. Any emotional reaction of displeasure can at the physical level produce *paratonic* reactions (exaggerated tonic reactions that impede movements) because of the close relation between tonicity and affectivity—relations that are established in early childhood (Ajuriaguerra, 1970; Wallon, 1949).

Spatial Constraints on Writing

The writing act is a meaningful graphic movement inscribed on a flat, two-dimensional space. Control over this space, which is always sharply defined, demands of the writer a continuous effort of anticipation. Furthermore, whether writing on a blackboard or on a sheet of paper, one always writes in a *space of representation* that is in relation to the points of reference of the writer's body. The support facing the writer has a top and a bottom, as well as a right and a left side separated by an imaginary median, the vertical projection of the body's axis. For the writer these spatial references to some extent ultimately become qualities inherent in the support, regardless of its position on the table.

Writing takes place in this particular space in accordance with various conventions relating to the shape of the letters and directions to be used, conventions that vary from place to place in the world. Here we shall consider the *directional* conventions, since they are a factor common to many forms of writing and make it possible to take a detached view of the infinite variety of characters used in the world. For a study of these characters we refer the reader to various works (Centre International de Synthèse, 1963; Cohen, 1958; Diringer, 1948; International Conference on Public Education, 1948). It would be advisable to supplement these studies with a survey updating the list of written languages used at present, since in our own day, as in the course of history, some die, others are born (Houis, 1971), and those that live, evolve. There are countless reasons for the birth of written languages and their evolution (Centre International de Synthèse, 1963). One is the need to bring writing within reach of children and also of illiterate adults (a need felt by many countries).

The directional conventions of writing are related to the following considerations:

1. *The direction of the development of the line*: the first large unit on a written page is broken down into smaller units consisting of graphic signs (words in phonographic scripts using consonantal or alphabetical representation; ideographs or groups of ideographs in ideographic forms of writing).

2. *The sequential production of minimum units of words*: letters in an alphabetical system, groups of strokes in the elements of an ideogram in an ideographic system (letters and strokes do not serve the same purpose) (Alarcos Llorach, 1968; Alleton, 1970).

Regardless of which method of graphic representation of language is adopted, the hand has to delineate the minimum units in accordance with certain codified directions and in a given order; these units, juxtaposed or connected, are grouped in words, which are aligned according to certain directions that are also codified.

Most types of writing follow a horizontal development of the line (or a horizontal progression of the line), the first line being parallel to the upper edge of the paper, each of the following lines being situated below the preceding line (progression on the page thus being vertical, from top to bottom). Horizontal development is characterized by the fact that the characters are placed side by side, as for example, the personages in the well-known pictograms of the Cuna Indians of Panama (Cohen, 1958). Horizontal development can be done systematically from left to right, as in Roman script (Western Europe, North and South America, etc.), in modern Greek writing, Cyrillic script, Indian writing, and so forth; or from right to left, as in Hebrew and Arabic script. There are also boustrophedon inscriptions, as in ancient Greek writing, in which the lines run alternately from right to left and from left to right, and there is the particular arrangement of signs varying from line to line in the ancient writing discovered on the Easter Island tablets (Centre International de Synthèse, 1963; Cohen, 1958). In Arabic, as in Hebrew script, written from right to left, numbers (Arabic numerals) are written from left to right, in the opposite direction to the writing. Children must therefore learn to allow the necessary space to write down a number in mid-sentence. After the number is set down, the writing continues from right to left. In Hebrew script, two systems of numerical notation exist simultaneously and are learned by children: Arabic numerals and the ancient Hebrew system using certain letters of the alphabet (direction R—L), of which the principle is analogous to that used in upper case Roman numerals.

In the types of writing used in China, Japan, and Korea, the development of the line (or rather column) was until recently vertical, from top to bottom. Progression on the page was from right to left, each column being placed to the left of the preceding one. In vertical Chinese writing, the characters are placed one below the other (like figures standing one below the other), an arrangement followed in ancient Egypt for monumental hieroglyphics (Centre International de Synthèse, 1963).

At the present time in China, as in Japan, horizontal development, starting in the top left-hand corner of the page, is tending to become institutionalized (Alleton, 1970), which does not change the orientation of the characters; they are placed side by side instead of one under the other. This new arrangement is used in printed publications and is taught at school, while the traditional (vertical) system continues to be used, for example for any type of monumental writing (posters) or for some personal uses (wishes, dedications). Vertical writing, and use of the brush and Indian ink, lend the text a certain emphasis derived from the cultural and sentimental value attached to them.

The *ductus* or direction of the stroke of the small units (letters, strokes) is also codified. This codification is far from arbitrary. It derives from usage that has fashioned writing through the centuries. The ductus of each letter is designed to facilitate the cursive development of a word and, where connected script is concerned, to facilitate the ligatures (connections between letters), which tend to follow the direction of the development of the line established by convention. Where a technical problem of ligature arises (e.g., connections with *a, d, g, q, o, c* in Roman script), codification seeks to solve the problem, codification that can vary from one method to another (the American Palmer-type ligatures, or the continental-type lift of the pen). Sometimes the organization of motor control and the laterality of the child lead him to produce types of ductus contrary to normal usage. Generally speaking, since the microspace of a letter at the beginning of the learning process renders perception of its form and development a little difficult, large writing on the blackboard is frequently used to facilitate learning. The same principle is applied to adults in literacy courses (*Guides practiques pour l'éducation extra-scolaire*, 1960–1966).

The study of the genesis of writing (Gobineau & Perron, 1954) shows that the child first writes discontinuously; gradually he learns to connect several latters; later he transforms the calligraphy learned into a personal style of writing with new ligatures adapted to it. Some forms of writing are separate by tradition (Arabic and particularly Hebrew), but adult writers also introduce personal ligatures here and there.

Similarly, in cursive Chinese writing, some strokes are connected (Alleton, 1970). It should be remembered that in this writing the various strokes in one ideograph must not only follow certain directions; they must also follow a strict order of succession (they are numbered in the school children's exercise books). Learning the order of succession is facilitated by certain general rules. This order and the ductus of strokes must therefore be carried out by the children for each character they learn (some of which have been simplified since 1958)—in other words, 1000–2000 of the most common characters. This way of writing may seem extraordinarily difficult to users of alphabetic scripts, which all in all have about 30 forms of letters to learn (60 including capital letters). But, in fact, although it takes longer to learn Chinese writing than alphabetic script (Gray, 1958), there is no doubt that the children do finally master this system of writing, and even the still more complicated Japanese system.

But are alphabetic scripts really easier to write? Actually, the intellectual and perceptomotor activity of the alphabetic writer is, if we think about it, just as complex. Any form of writing calls for *anticipation* of the spatiotemporal development of small units in accordance with the development of the narrative and the method of representing language. A sequence of graphemes must correspond to a sequence of phonemes, which is achieved through a graphomotor rhythm and internal formulation of narrative proper to writing, a medium of expression that ultimately acquires a certain autonomy in relation to the spoken language (Alarcos Llorach, 1968).

Matters are still relatively simple—in phonographic systems—when the laws of correspondence between graphemes and phonemes are themselves fairly simple. But the difficulty of certain written languages can be considerably increased by the polyvalence of graphemes and the polygraphy of phonemes, as in French and even more so in English, where the writing system is quasi-semiographic (Alarcos Llorach, 1968, p. 562). One could even go so far as to say that these scripts are at least as complex as ideographic or semiographic writing, because they continue to be taught as phonographic writings—which they basically are, according to the system of representation of language adopted—and because continuous reference to the *signatum* is as necessary as it is in Chinese writing to transcribe the correct sign and correct spelling.

Difficulties inherent in various scripts do not therefore stem exclusively from their particular spatial constraints. However, the child must pass certain stages, on the level of representation of space, to arrange the layout and development on the page of the writing he has to learn.

Stages in the mastery of graphic space by the child have been thoroughly studied by many writers (Lurçat, 1968; Piaget & Inhelder, 1948; Vereecken, 1961). This skill develops through the first spontaneous strokes which gradually take the form of symbolic representations. It is the simultaneous production of units of graphy and their meaning that enable the child to relate himself to the space on the sheet.

The writing movement develops before the definite representation of landmarks in space (top, bottom, right, left). If the child sees others about him drawing and is given the necessary tools, he will start to scribble between the ages of two and three. The origin of such scribbling is primarily a straightforward motor impulse stimulated by the need to imitate. The first strokes (continuous, then discontinuous: circular marks, curves, descending lines, then lateral) are directly goverened by the maturation of the motor processes and the role played by the body axis, which acts as an axis of symmetry and affects the direction of the strokes.

The child acts, then considers the result of his efforts. If the adult is encouraging, he takes pleasure in some repetition. Between the ages of three and four, he tries to make the strokes more precise and to vary them (a closed circular stroke, lines in various directions, isolated loops, then the execution of the square) while coordination improves between the movement of the hand and the eyes, which began to develop with the first sensory motor activities. At the same time, a new and very important synthesis occurs: the child interprets the drawing after it is completed. He gives a meaning to as yet indefinite lines: "It's a bird." Some coincidence of form is possible between the graphic marks and the ideographic interpretation, but one is not determined by the other (Wallon, cited in Lurçat, 1970—1971). A new step forward is made when the child anticipates what he is going to draw ("I will draw a tree"). There is a transition from spontaneous (or semideliberate) movements to movements controlled by the intention to depict (Wallon, cited in Lurçat, 1970—1971).

Between the ages of 4 and 6, the drawing becomes richer and more precise. A pleasurable activity for the child, who enjoys handling color, and a basic educational activity, as has frequently been stressed, drawing plays an important role in the development of the symbolic functions and the affective life of the child. At the same time, drawing enables the child gradually to relate to the space on the sheet of paper. In exploring this space with the point of his tool and placing on it his houses and little men, he builds up landmarks as a result of the confrontation of his movements, the limits of the sheet, and his drawings on it. The top and the bottom acquire a meaning.

During this period, the child also assimilates certain topological relations

(Piaget & Inhelder, 1948) from experience: internal—external relationships, inter-section, and order. He learns to recognize in himself and on the sheet of paper the right- and the left-hand side, which will be related to the top and the bottom. The acquisition of all these relations necessary to writing and reading will, toward the age of 6, enable him to learn the written language. But well before the age of 6, before he can copy a sentence, the child shows an interest in writing provided he sees it going on around him. Next to the figurative drawings, little signs appear (miniature sketchy curves, or small enclosed figures, or lines placed next to the drawings, or wavy lines like lines of writing); the child will then say that he is writing. In fact, it is no more than an imitation of writing (Wallon, 1952). But this imitation already reveals an intuition of abstract symbolic configuration; when the time comes to learn to write, this will be an advantage.

In the representative drawings and later in the early stages of writing, the moving hand and the eyes that anticipate and guide it together define an external space and identify a before and after, a top and bottom, and so on, on the sheet of paper. Through movement, space has been defined. Then the child can juggle within the system of coordinates that he has organized, go in one direction or another if necessary, depending on the conventions of the writing that he learns. On the other hand, he will be unable to draw characters or learn their order of succession according to a continuous direction if maturation at the level of practice and knowledge is not sufficiently advanced; in other words, before the system of spatial reference is constituted or if it is still uncertain.

The Tools

The graphic tools used in the course of history have been many and have played an important role in the evolution of forms of writing (Centre International de Synthèse, 1963).

Here we shall deal with a few aspects of the graphic tools most commonly used at the present time (Alleton, 1970; International Conference on Public Education, 1948): pencil and ball point pen the most common, fountain pen, felt pen, chalk, and still occasionally a brush or quill dipped in ink.

The instrument used by each individual may be determined by tradition, by changes in technique, by personal or national economic requirements, by teaching conventions, and lastly by personal needs and tastes. Quite frequently, several tools are variously used as much for the interest and visual pleasure afforded by variety of color and thickness of line as for the need to adapt the tool to the type of writing required or to its recipient.

Modern teaching methods call for instruments that facilitate the learning of writing and avoid contraction of muscles (Auzias, 1970; Dottrens, 1966; Gray, 1958). Soft chalk (for writing on the board) and soft lead pencil, of necessity used by developing countries, are, in the opinion of many, the instruments best suited to the hand of the young child (Gray, 1958). It is recommended that the pencil be fairly thick, particularly in infant schools (to facilitate the grasp) and that it should also be used at the beginning of primary school, as for example in certain English-speaking countries; the pen with a metal nib is considered particularly unsuitable (Dottrens, 1966; Gray, 1958).

When the time comes to write in ink, which gives writing some relief and makes it more lasting, a ball point pen is usually preferred, sometimes a fountain pen. In some countries, a pen dipped in ink is still used (Gray, 1958), because of its "magic" qualities; these are derived from the cultural, moral, and aesthetic values associated with the art of the calligrapher who used to produce the beautiful lettering in poetic and occasionally sacred texts. The gifts of men have been "projected" into the tool. They are still: if writing is poor and the hand contracted, it is hoped that frequent changes of tool will bring about a cure, a significant act in one who has developed "writer's cramp."

Depending on the country, the price of a fountain pen is quite high, or moderate, or inexpensive, as in the People's Republic of China where it has replaced the bruch in school and in daily life (Alleton, 1970), although the brush is still frequently used for posters and announcements. In Japan, children learn at the same time to write with a brush and a ballpoint pen. Dedications and wishes are produced with the brush in vertical columns, the brush technique being frequently combined with vertical writing.

The typewriter, more and more used by adults, is also made available to children, especially handicapped children (with motor defects, and the blind). Various facilities have been developed for these children (Brachold, 1966a; Tardieu, 1972). We were able to observe that the multiple techniques for transmission and recording (handwriting, braille, typewriting, tape-recording) used by the same child (very near-sighted) provide an opening on the word, a means of adaptation, and therefore of balance.

But the machine cannot solve all problems for handicapped children, any more than it can for anyone else. It has freed man from the effort of achieving legibility and to some extent from planning layout, but not from the need to formulate the text to be written (a major difficulty for some children with language problems) or from the intervention of the hand, whether handling a tool or tapping the keys. A sound recording dictated by one person can be transcribed by another, who is an extension of that person and on whom that person depends. Furthermore, the more elaborate the machine, the less it is available to the great number; also, as a rule the more elaborate it is, the more cumbersome—there is not yet a pocket computer. Moreover, the real problem of the survival of literature—or its decline, predicted at various times—does not reside in its instruments, which are nevertheless essential. The continuance or disappearance of writing, whether handwriting or some quite other form, will depend on the requirements of society.

Methods of Learning to Write and Scales of Writing

Every normal individual, after reaching a certain stage of development, has the capacity to write. But this potential, which depends on the completeness and the maturation of various systems, cannot become effective without apprenticeship.

We do not intend to review the learning methods used today. For this we refer the reader to various works (Ajuriaguerra & Auzias, 1960; Bang, 1959; Gray, 1958; Rudolf, 1973) and to current UNESCO publications relating to functional literacy programs for adults.

We would merely say that the methods of teaching writing vary greatly and are based on a certain conception of it. For synthetic methods that tend to emphasize penmanship (the oldest), writing is an art of exact imitation of set forms. These methods have been criticized on various grounds, in particular for being tedious, requiring complicated forms that are slow to execute, with the down and up-strokes made by pressure exerted on a metal pen (and not by traction, as was the case with the reed pen or the goose quill, a more functional method). All the same, the synthetic methods have certain positive aspects: forms learned one by one, with their particular ductus (direction of stroke), and the simultaneous learning of reading and writing.

Subsequent methods have tended to adapt writing to the child (simplified forms, ligatures adapted to these forms, tools easy to handle, uniform thickness of strokes), and above all, to restore to writing all its value as language, while stressing its meaning (global methods), its role of expression, and of communication (Freeman, 1954; Freinet, 1956). Still other methods have stressed motor and linguistic preparation for writing (in kindergarten), and writing as motion, or its dynamic and cursive aspects (American and Canadian methods).

But some of these, the global methods for example, of which the positive feature was to emphasize the content of writing with the help of illustration by drawing, had a tendency to reduce the grapheme-phoneme correspondence of written signs (although they dealt with writing as a form of phonographic representation) and did not teach the ductus of letters—which does facilitate the production of precise forms and the cursive movement. Although a child who has no impediments can easily adapt himself to global methods, there is a danger for those who confuse certain phonemes, ill-distinguish the parts of a sentence, or have difficulty in relating to the graphic space.

At the present time, mixed methods are frequently used (Gray, 1958). They tend to retain the positive aspects of earlier methods: learning the letters separately with their phonic value, letters that are soon connected into meaningful words that are deciphered during the reading lesson. As soon as possible, the child himself constructs a short sentence that he writes (whereas in calligraphic writing methods the text was given) and illustrates with a drawing or painting. This dynamic aspect of the method, which provokes a positive attitude to learning in the child, is the most outstanding feature of modern methods compared with earlier ones. They eliminate passivity and boredom and develop in the child a liking for expression, which is the best stimulus to writing. The most valid methods of functional literacy also seek to integrate learning of the written language with the needs and interests of the learners and attempt to make literacy an instrument of genuine education and not of "domestication."

In most countries, writing is taught at 6 years of age, sometimes 7 (International

Conference on Public Education, 1948; *Statistical yearbook*, 1970), which corresponds to the necessary level of maturation for learning the written language. But the maturity of some children can vary quite sharply from the average. A minority of countries introduce writing at the age of 5 in kindergarten, but such early learning is not suitable for most children (Auzias, 1970).

The letters used vary with the method. Sometimes connected cursive letters are taught from the beginning, sometimes separate script is preferred (similar to the letters in primers) (Gray, 1958), the transition to cursive writing being introduce later (Harris, 1960). The advantages and disadvantages of both systems have led to much discussion. Findings of an experiment (Bang, 1959) show that retention of separate script throughout the school years impedes speed.

Writing Scales

Many authors have made a point of building up handwriting scales (Ajuriaguerra *et al.*, 1964 Vol. 1; Bang, 1959; Fernandez-Huerta, 1950; Freeman, 1954; Gobineau & Perron, 1954; Gray, 1958). These make it possible to identify the growth levels of forms of writing and of graphic motor processes. All these studies on the genesis of writing and stages in its development have made it possible to discern more clearly the child's capability at each age: a child of 6 does not write like a child of 9 or 12 years of age. These works have therefore provided the teacher with points of reference. They have also made it possible to study writing disabilities more precisely (Ajuriaguerra *et al.*, 1964; Auzias, 1970) and have contributed to the development of re-education methods. These methods have also influenced the teaching of writing in school since the longitudinal method of observing dysgraphia in children has furthered understanding of the mechanics of writing disabilities and led to the institution of techniques that make it possible to prevent them.

Writing scales are therefore reflections of the child's writing, supported by experimental research. Historically, they constitute a new phenomenon in the evolution of writing.

Handwriting Difficulties

Learning to write can follow a fairly smooth pattern through various normal stages, including the mastery of difficulties inherent in any learning process. It can, on the other hand, be impeded either by defective teaching conditions or inadequate methods, or by the child's own problems.

Left-handers first attracted the attention of teachers, psychologists, and doctors (Auzias, 1970, pp. 101–110; Clark, 1957). We do not regard left-handedness as a disorder or an anomaly (with the exception of some special cases) (Auzias, 1973), but left-handers do pose a problem for teachers, because their laterality is not always clearly determined and because of their specific graphic behavior patterns.

In practice, three types of problems arise with these children: choice of hand (Ajuriaguerra *et al.*, 1964; Freeman, 1954), teaching methods (Cole, 1939; Hildreth, 1947), and sometimes mirror writing (Ajuriaguerra, Diatkine, & Gobineau, 1956; Critchley, 1927).

Nowadays tolerance towards left-handers tends almost everywhere to replace the former intolerance, but the old anxiety about writing with the "wrong" hand still exists. In fact, although the writing difficulties of left-handed children may be caused by motor disorders or defects in spatial orientation, most frequently they are the result of teaching deficiencies. Left-handers' writing problems can be reduced or even eliminated if parents and teachers are adquately supplied with information that will limit anxiety reactions and define techniques to be used to facilitate the learning of writing for these children.

Left-handers are not the only children with writing problems. Some children, regardless of their laterality, suffer from genuine handicaps that can be the result of motor, praxic, tensional, or affective difficulties or the result of ignorance of the language. If these difficulties are severe, or even slight, they can be aggravated by unpleasant circumstances (emotional trauma, crowded classes that do not allow the teacher enough time to pay individual attention to such and such a child) and lead to genuine troubles in the development of writing, or dysgraphia. Moreover, functional troubles may develop that cannot be attributed to a neurological or intellectual defect. Such troubles are distinguished from simple learning difficulties by the initial very strong resistance to the teaching efforts of parents and teachers and the consequent need for strictly therapeutic treatment.

These troubles may take different clinical forms that are defined by a certain semiology and certain etiology. On the etiological plane, it is possible to distinguish troubles that derive from (a) disorders of motor organization (motor debility, slight disturbances of balance and of the kinesthetic and tonic organization, instability); (b) somatospatial disorders—disorders in the organization of gesture and space (difficulties in awareness, representation and use of the body; difficulties in spatial orientation); (c) difficulties in learning language and reading that lead to difficulties in graphic expression of the language; (d) behavior disorders—anxiety, nervousness, inhibition, and other manifestations of uneasiness that are reflected in one form or another in the writing (Ajuriaguerra, *et al.*, 1964; Olivaux, 1971).

Sometimes various causes of disturbances are combined in the same child and lead to polymorphic disorders, among them the onset of infantile cramp which is similar to writer's cramp in the adult. Symptoms of this syndrome are more or less intense awkwardness, paratonia, catastrophic reactions when faced with the writing activity, and conflicting attitudes (related to the self-concept), sometimes also associated with problems of laterality and difficulties in handling the written language. The most obvious signs of the onset of cramp are a very severe contraction of the whole arm (particularly in the proximal and distal areas), forced halts in the course of writing, painful and neuroautonomic phenomena (sweating), and a definite dislike of writing.

The semiology of the various writing disabilities (on the level of graphic forms and graphic motor processes: position, kinesthetic development, tonicity, etc.), can be related to their origin; for example, there are specific graphic signs of awkwardness, of spatial disorientation, of tension, inhibition, obsessional tendencies, and so forth. Each type of disability has its own unique and particular form related to the factors involved, to the more or less widespread organization of the disorder and its evolution, to the particular coloration given by the child's age (a primary factor), and to the forms of compensation adopted by the child.

Re-education methods have been developed to treat the problems described here, including some of the specific problems of handicapped children (Ajuriaguerra *et al.*, 1964, Vol. 2; Brachold, 1966a,b; Olivaux, 1971; Tardieu, 1972). Our re-education methods have demonstrated that it is no use dealing with the graphic symptoms as such, writing difficulties being no more than the magnifying glass of various problems. A change must be brought about in the whole complex of which the symptom is part. Although re-education methods and techniques (general relaxation, picto- and scriptographic techniques, etc.) must be familiar to the re-educator, he must not apply them rigidly but rather must mold them, vary them, adapt them to the case of each child, while handling the special relationship between the child and the re-educator, which is an integral part of a dynamic re-education process.

Experience of functional disorders of writing and various data described in this article would point to the advisability of instituting pedagogical measures of all kinds, both practical and psychological, at the time of learning the written language, so as to eliminate certain hazards that can hinder the child and to create an open and genuinely educative situation: preparatory exercises, tools easy to handle, simple forms clearly taught, a calm class atmosphere, opportunity for the child to compose the texts he writes, and elimination of improper or punitive exercises in the written language. Writing should be experienced by the child not as an alienating yoke, but as a language and a praxis available to him in order to plan, construct, and create.

References

Ajuriaguerra, J. de. *Manuel de psychiatrie de l'enfant.* Paris: Masson, 1970.

Ajuriaguerra, J. de, & Auzias, M. Méthodes et techniques d'apprentissage de l'écriture. *Psychiatrie de l'Enfant,* 1960, *3,* 609—718.

Ajuriaguerra, J. de, Auzias, M., Coumes, F., Denner, A, Lavondes, M., Perron, R., & Stambak, M. *L'écriture de l'enfant* (2 volumes; Vol. 1, *L'évolution de l'écriture et ses difficultés,* and Vol. 2, *La rééducation de l'écriture*). Neuchatel & Paris: Delachaux & Niestlé, 1964.

Ajuriaguerra, J. de, & Gobineau, H. de. L'écriture en miroir. *Semaine des Hopitaux,* 1956, *32,* 80—86.

Ajuriaguerra, J. de & Stambak, M. L'évolution des syncinés ies chez l'enfant. *La Presse Médicale,* 1955, *39,* 817—819.

Alarcos Llorach, E. Les représentations graphiques du langage. In *Le langage.* Paris: Editions Gallimard, 1968.

Alleton, V. *L'écriture chinoise.* Paris: Presses Universitaires de France, 1970.

Auzias, M. *Les troubles de l'écriture chez l'enfant.* Neuchâtel: Delachaux & Niestlé, 1970.

Auzias, M. La vitesse d'écriture chez les enfants qui écrivent de la main gauche. Revue de neuropsychiatrie infantile, 1973, *21*, 10–11, 667–686.

Bang, V. *Evolution de l'écriture de l'enfant à l'adulte; Étude expériméntale.* Neuchâtel: Delachaux & Niestlé, 1959.

Brachold, H. *Einschulung Schwergeschädigter Armloser, Armbehinderter Kinder.* Stuttgart: Ernst Klett, 1966. (a)

Brachold, H. Synthetischer oder ganzheitlicher Schreibunterricht? *Praxis der Kinderpsychologie und Kinderpsychiatrie,* 1966, *15*, 308–315. (b)

Callewaert, H. 1954. *Graphologie et physiologie de l'écriture.* Louvain: Nauwelaerts, 1954.

Centre International de Synthèse. *L'écriture et la psychologie des peuples.* Paris: Armand Colin, 1963.

Clark, M. *Left-handedness.* London: Univ. of London Press, 1957.

Cohen, M. *La grande invention de l'écriture et son évolution.* Paris: Imprimerie Nationale, 1958.

Cole, L. Instruction in penmanship for left-handed children. *Elementary School Journal,* Feb. 1939, 436–448.

Cormeau-Velghe, M., Destrait, V., Toussaint, J. & Bidaine E. Normes de vitesse d'écriture: étude statistique de 1844 écoliers belges de 6 à 13 ans. *Psychologica Belgica,* 1970, *X-2,* 247–263.

Critchley, M. *Mirror writing.* London: Kegan Paul, 1927.

Derrida, J. *De la grammatologie.* Paris: Editions de Minuit, 1967.

Diringer, D. *The alphabet: A key to the history of mankind.* New York: Philosophical Library, 1948.

Dottrens, R. *Au seuil de la culture; Méthode globale et écriture script.* Paris: Editions Scarabee, 1966.

Essing, V. W. Untersuchungen über Veränderungen der Schreibmotorik im Grundschulalter. *Human Development,* 1965, *8,* 194–221.

Fernandez-Huerta, J. *Escritura didactica y escala grafica.* Madrid: Consejo Superior de Investigaciones Cientificas, Inst. San José de Calasanz de Pédagogia, 1950.

Freeman, F. N. *Teaching handwriting.* Washington, D.C.: Amer. Educ. Res. Ass., 1954.

Freinet, C. *les méthodes naturelles dans la pédagogie moderne.* Paris: Bourrelier, 1955.

Gobineau, H. de, & Perron, R. *Génétique de l'écriture et étude de la personnalité,* Neuchatel & Paris: Delachaux & Niestlé, 1954.

Gray, W. S. *The teaching of reading and writing; An international survey.* Paris: Unesco, 1958. (2nd ed., 1969.)

Guides pratiques pour l'éducation extra-scolaire. Paris: Unesco, 1960–1966.

Harris, T. L. Handwriting. In C. W. Harris (Ed.), *Encyclopedia of education research.* New York: MacMillan, 1960.

Harris, T. L., & Rarick, G. L. The relationship between handwriting pressure and legibility of handwriting in children and adolescents. *Journal of Experimental Education,* 1959, *28,* 65–84.

Hildreth, G. *Learning the three R's.* Minneapolis: Educ. Publ., 1947.

Houis, M. *Anthropologie linguistique de l'Afrique noire.* Paris: Presses Universitaires de France, 1971.

International Conference on Public Education, XIth, Geneva. *The teaching of handwriting.* Publ. No. 103. Geneva & Paris: International Bureau of Education/Unesco, 1948.

Leischner, A. *Di Störungen der Schriftsprache.* Stuttgart: Thieme, 1957.

Lurçat, L. *Etude de l'acte graphique.* Paris et La Haye: Monton, 1974.

Lurçat, L. Genèse de l'idéogramme; graphisme et langage. *Bulletin de Psychologie,* (Paris) 1970–1971, 16/18, 932–947.

Luthe, W. Der Elektroscriptograph. *Psychologische Forschung,* 1953, *24,* 194–214.

Michel, F. Étude expérimentale de la vitesse du geste graphique. *Neuropsychologia,* 1971, *9,* 1–13.

Olivaux, R. *Désordres et rééducation de l'écriture.* Paris: Editions ESF, 1971.

Paillard, J. The patterning of skilled movements. In Hw. Magoun (Ed.), *Handbook of physiology,* Section I: Neurophysiology, Vol. 3. Washington, D.C.: Amer. Physiol. Soc., 1960.

Piaget, J., & Inhelder, B. *La représentation de l'espace chez l'enfant.* Paris: Presses Universitaires de France, 1948.

Rudolf, H. *Schreiberziehung und Schriftpsychologie.* Bielefeld: Pfeffer, 1973 (preface by O. Lockowandt).

Saussure, F. de. *Cours de linguistique générale*. Lausanne: Payot, 1916 (17th ed., Paris, Payot, 1972.
Statistical yearbook. Paris: Unesco, 1970.
Tardieu, G. Education thérapeutique de l'habileté. *Les feuillets de l'infirmité motrice cérébale*. Paris
(33 rue Blanche): Ass. Nat. Infirm. Motrice Cérébraux, 1972.
Vereechen, P. *Spatial development; Constructive praxia from birth to the age of seven*. Groningen: Wolters,
1961.
Wallon, H. La maladresse. *Journal de Psychologie Normale et Pathologique*, 1928, *25*, 61—78. Also in
Enfance, 1959, *3/4*, 264—276.
Wallon, H. *Les origines du caractère*. Paris: Presses Universitaires de France, 1949.

19. Lessons to Be Learned from the Preschool Orthographer

Charles Read

Certain preschool children print messages, employing an orthography that is partly of their own invention. They represent English words with the standard alphabet, and are thus compelled to classify distinct phones in some way. They do so according to articulatory features, making judgments of similarity that are quite different from those that most parents or teachers might make. In particular, the children collapse certain phonetic and even phonemic distinctions according to an apparent hierarchy of features, which may constitute a tacit but consistent notion of significant phonetic variation. Some preliminary studies have examined the performance of other preschool and primary-grade children and have found some judgments similar to those underlying the preschool orthography. These judgments are different from those reflected in either phonemic or standard spelling; insofar as they turn out to be general, they will help to define the task of learning to read and write.

Preschool Orthographers

Imagine, if you will, that you have just received the following message from an acquaintance:

HOW R YOU   WAN YOU GAD I CHANS SAND IS OL I LADR. AD DOW GT ANE CHRIBLS

Along with this message is a drawing of a fish-like figure amidst wiggly blue lines. The caption reads:

FES SOWEMEG EN WOODR[1]

Your correspondent is nearly 4-years old. The message is representative of those constructed by some preschool children, using spellings that are partly of their own invention. Although this behavior is relatively rare, at least in American culture, it is common enough that I have been able to identify more than 20 children, who have provided a substantial corpus. It is possible to compare the spellings invented by different children and to ask what the spellings reveal about the children's phonological judgments.

The most striking conclusion is that aside from minor variations, all of the children appear to have invented similar spellings, which reflect certain judgments of English sounds and their representation. These judgments differ in important ways from those that are embodied in standard English spelling and those that would be made by literate adults.

The circumstances of this invented spelling varied somewhat from child to child, of course, but there are certain common characteristics. Each child learned the conventional names of the letters of the alphabet at a relatively early age, sometimes as early as 2 years, 6 months. By questioning and observing adults, they also learned a general orthographic principle. They seem to have inferred that letters represent sounds, and that at least one of the sounds represented by a letter is usually contained in the name of that letter. Most of the children played with lettered blocks or some other movable-alphabet toy, and each of them began at about this point to spell simple words, usually between the ages of 3 and $4\frac{1}{2}$.[2] Later the children mastered the use of pencil and paper (or their equivalents, such as crayon and wallpaper), with which they produced the more lasting representations that I have studied.

The writings are usually sentences or phrases that constitute a message, so it is possible to use both context and spelling to identify with some certainty the words that were intended. Some are letters addressed to parents, relatives, or friends; others are titles on a child's drawings; still others are stories, poems, protests to parents, and other expressions of various sorts. Their functional utility is dubious; frequently the addressee, if there was one, could not read the message. Sometimes, at the early stages, the writer himself could not read what he had written, after a day or two had passed. Clearly, some children began to write before they could read, in the usual sense. In that respect, this is a case of production preceding comprehension.

[1] The message reads *How are you? When you get a chance, send us all a letter. And don't get any troubles.* The caption says *Fish swimming in water*, naturally. The spellings are representative in that they include one or two learned spellings (YOU) and at least one "mistake," relative to the child's orthography, along with the characteristic invented spellings.

[2] For one mother's description of the beginning of this activity, see Carol Chomsky (1971).

For the parents, the spelling was sometimes a puzzle. It was often clear from spelling or context what the child had written, but the spelling was usually bizarre by comparison with standard spelling. With the exception of two linguists, the parents did not recognize that the spelling is systematic and that it has a reasonable phonetic basis. Nevertheless, the parents all treated the spelling as a surprising but acceptable activity of the child. They provided the materials, they answered the child's questions, but otherwise they neither actively encouraged nor discouraged it. They may have had tacit doubts about the disastrous spelling "habits" that the child seemed to be developing, but they did not make unsolicited comparisons between the child's spelling and the standard variety. The one characteristic that the various parents had in common, and that may have been a necessary condition for the spelling to develop, was this tolerance of spellings that are incorrect by adult criteria.

For his part, the child occasionally asked, for instance, "How do you spell [θə]?" and he adopted the standard spelling of some words, but on the whole, he constructed his own spelling, apparently on the basis of what the words sounded like to him and his knowledge of the letter names. One problem confronting the child who attempts to spell on this basis is of a familiar sort: There are not enough letters to represent distinctly the various phones that the child can distinguish. This is certainly true if the child wishes to represent the phonemes of his dialect of English; we will see evidence that a phonemic representation is not exactly what the children aim for, but the alphabetic problem remains.

Basically, the children spell consonants with letters whose names contain consonantal segments, and vowels with letters whose names contain only vowels and glides. Thus a, e, i, o, u, and y represent vowels and glides exclusively, and the remaining letters represent consonants exclusively. The letter names provide only partial help, of course. There are quite direct clues to the representation of /p, t, k, b, d, f, v, s, z, ǰ, m, n, r/ and /l/ in the names of the corresponding letters, and /č/ occurs in the name of h. The names of the remaining letters, c, g, q, w, and x, provide no additional information, since the consonants they contain are already accounted for. The children use c, g, and occasionally w in ways that will be illustrated below, and they rarely use q and x. Thus the letter names leave the child with no direct suggestion for representing /θ, ð, š, ž, g, η/ and /h/. The vowels of English are much less well provided for by the letter names, but the children devise rather ingenious spellings for them, as we will see.

In attempting to solve this problem, a child has four choices: he could give up systematic spelling, leaving out puzzling sounds or inserting any letter at all; he could make up new symbols, creating a phonetic alphabet of his own; he could ask for the adult spelling; or he could relate sounds on some basis, using known spellings for more than one sound. It is this last choice that is both typical and revealing.

The young spellers did not choose letters randomly or invent additional symbols. They were quite independent of the adult system in some ways, but they seemed to accept the alphabet as a condition of the problem. They did get information from adults, usually when they asked for specific spellings. Many of them evidently learned from adults the digraphic spellings of [θ], [ð], and [č], for example. Various words appear in standard spelling for any particular child, although often they occur along with obviously invented spellings of the same words. Copied or dictated spellings reveal nothing about the child's own judgments, of course. When a standard spelling occurs, I ordinarily have no way of knowing whether it was adopted or invented, so I will base no conclusions on it.

In general, the children invented their own spellings by relating the sounds as they heard them to the letter names that they knew. The interesting results differ sharply from standard spelling and are therefore unlikely to have been learned from adults. They are consistent and have plausible phonetic bases; in short, they reflect the children's own judgments of phonological relationships. Furthermore, the various pre school spellers made the same judgments, in general. I do not know to what extent this conclusion can be generalized to other children, but its potential practical significance lies in the fact that the spellings appeared one to three years before the child entered school and continued in use until they were gradually replaced by standard spellings, usually as the child received formal instruction in reading and writing. In that respect the spellings represent judgments that a child may bring with him to school; this inference will be examined below.

Classification by Articulatory Features

VOWELS

When the children are compelled to group sounds together, spelling different ones with the same letter, they do so on the basis of similarities in articulation. Up to this point, I have referred to what the spellings represent as "sounds" or "phones," delaying the question of just what aspects of speech sounds the children choose to represent; in fact, they classify phones according to place and manner of articulation, especially place.

The children's representation of tense vowels constitutes a clear and unsurprising system. The names of the letters *a, e, i, o,* and *u* correspond quite directly to the tense vowels of *bait, beet, bite, boat,* and *beauty.* The children use these letters for such vowels, without the standard devices, such as doubling of vowel letters or final "silent" *e,* to indicate tenseness.

FAS	*face*	**LADE**	*lady*	**TIGR**	*tiger*	**BLO**	*blow*
DA	*day*	**EGLE**	*eagle*	**LIK**	*like*	**BOT**	*boat*
KAM	*came*	**FEL**	*feel*	**MI**	*my*	**JOK**	*joke*
FABUARE	*February)*			**UNITD**	*UNITED*		
CUNGRAJULASHINS	*congratulations*			**JANUARE**	*January*		

A more interesting question is how the children use these same letters to represent lax vowels, such as those of *bit*, *bet*, *bat*, and *pot*. They make this extension systematically, according to similarities in place of articulation. That is, the children spell, with the same letter, vowels that correspond phonetically except for tenseness. These pairs are as follows:

	tense	lax	tense	lax	tense	lax
Symbol[3]	[īy]	[i]	[ēy]	[e]	[āy]	[a]
Spelling	*beet*	*bit*	*bait*	*bet*	*line*	*phonic*

With these correspondences in mind, consider the following typical invented spellings:

SEP	*ship*	PAN	*pen*	BICS	*box*
FES	*fish*	FALL	*fell*	SCICHTAP	*Scotch tape*
EGLIOW	*igloo*	LAFFT	*left*	GIT	*got*
FLEPR	*Flipper*	ALRVATA	*elevator*	CLIK	*clock*

Such examples could be multiplied many times, for until the children learn standard spelling, these representations of the lax vowels are extremely regular. The [i] of *fish* is spelled E, the [e] of *fell* is spelled A, and the [a] of *Scotch* is spelled I, because the names of these letters, which are diphthongal, begin with the tense counterparts of the lax vowels the children want to represent. Evidently the children can recognize the phonetic similarity (in place of articulation) and ignore the difference in tenseness.

Standard spelling uses the same vowel letters but makes a quite different pairing, of course. The [āy] of *divine* is spelled with same letter as the [i] of *divinity*. If adults without phonetic training ventured any judgments of vowel relationships, they would presumably follow the pairings of standard orthography. Thus it seems reasonable to assume that the children created the spellings above; they could hardly have learned them from most adults.

Further evidence that the children spell on the basis of phonetic relationships appears rather late in their careers as preschool spellers. After they have learned the standard spelling of the lax vowels (usually together with learning to read standard orthography), some of the children make an interesting mistake. They occasionally spell a high or mid *tense* vowel with the letter they have recently learned to use for the phonetically corresponding *lax* form.

SIKE	*seek*	CEME	*came*
AIRFILD	*airfield*	PLEY	*play*
FRONTIR	*frontier*	TEBL	*table*

---

[3] The notation employed is that of N. Chomsky and Halle (1968), because it represents rather directly the relationships the children recognized. Note that in this system [i] corresponds to [I] and [e] to [ε].

It is as if, having learned that the spelling of lax vowels is not based on what they can hear in the letter names, the children attempt to save the phonetic correspondence between lax and tense forms, even at the expense of ignoring the obvious congruence between letter names and tense vowels that they began with. This error, as they are on the verge of learning the standard system, actually carries them away from it momentarily, overthrowing the best-practiced vowel spellings of all. This seems a plausible error only if a tacit recognition of the phonetic correspondences does underlie the invented spellings. It also suggests that the children's knowledge of such relationships may be a more important basis for their spellings than the establishment of "habits" through practice.

Finally, the children all spell the lax vowel of *bat* [æ] with an *A*; since this is the standard spelling, it may have been learned from adults. In any case, it has one interesting consequence; words like *bait*, *bet*, and *bat* all have the same spelling: *BAT*. Some homography is required by the use of five letters, one at a time, to spell more than five vowels, of course, but the children's specific choices of which phonetic relationships to represent (and which differences to ignore) are of theoretical interest, and their creation of a system with this degree of homography is also interesting. Evidently, they find this result acceptable enough that they neither introduce invented symbols nor give up spelling. To that degree at least, they do not adopt any form of the one phoneme, one spelling principle that has been much-discussed in connection with English spelling.[4]

CONSONANTS

Other evidence that the children spell according to a phonetic-feature analysis appears in the case of certain consonants. Consider first the following spellings:

AS CHRAY	*ash tray*	**CWNCHRE**	*country*
CHRIBLS	*troubles*	**JRADL**	*dreidel*
CHRIE	*try*	**JRAGIN**	*dragon*

As these examples suggest, the invented spellings of [t] and [d] when these occur before [r] are *CH* and *J*, respectively. The children involved had learned to spell [č] as *CH* and [ǰ] as *J* ordinarily, so it appears that they related [t] and [d] in this environment to [č] and [ǰ], respectively.

The phonetic basis is that before [r] in English, [t] and [d] are affricated; that is, they are released slowly with a resulting momentary turbulence. Thus the first segments of, say, *truck* and *tuck* are not identical. To a degree, the former is articulated in the manner of the palatal affricate [č]. A similar relationship holds

---

[4]For some discussion of the spellings of back rounded vowels and reduced vowels, see Read (1971). Although more complex, these also suggest that the children categorize according to phonetic similarities, including rounding as well as place of articulation. For further details of these and other matters, see Read (1975).

for [dr], as compared with [d] and [ǰ]. Evidently, the children perceive this affrication. Not knowing the standard spellings, they must choose between the known spelling for similar phones, namely *T/D* and *CH/J*. In this light, it is not surprising that they sometimes choose on the basis of the similarity in affrication, despite other similarities between [tr] and prevocalic [t].[5]

I have encountered several cases in which this same judgment appeared among children who did no preschool spelling, and I have conducted an experimental investigation with 135 children who had done no original spelling, seeking to determine their judgments of these affricates. The children were asked to indicate which words in a set of examples like *train*, *turkey* and *chicken* begin with the same sound as *truck*. There were 11 words in a set, so that the consistency of a child's judgments could be measured. The children supplied the words themselves by naming pictures, so that I, as tester, rarely had to give my own pronunciation. Of the 80 kindergarten children, many could not make consistent judgments, but of those who could do so, fully half chose words like *train* and *chicken*, rejecting *turkey*, *tie*, and the like. The 28 nursery-school children had even more difficulty making the required judgment consistently, a fact which suggests, not surprisingly, that the children who spelled spontaneously were better than others their age at making explicit phonological judgments. But again, most of the consistent nursery-school children chose the affricates and rejected the stops.

The 27 first-graders had encountered *tr-* words in their early reading, and most made the adult judgment. However, there were children even in this group who insisted on the similarity between [tr] and [č]. Four of them easily demonstrated (individually) their ability to read a set of words like *train*, *teddy bear*, and *chair*, and then asserted with great confidence that it is the first and last that begin with the same sound, even while they looked at the printed forms. Pointing to the standard spelling, I said, "But look, *train* and *teddy bear* begin with the same letter." "Oh yeah, but that's different," one of them assured me. Such observations as these indicate at least that the spontaneous spellers are not unique in their phonological judgments, although they may be somewhat unusual in their ability to make them explicit, and that the affrication of stops before [r] in English may be an important phonetic fact for young children.[6]

The fact that some children, particularly the preschool orthographers, are able to make a consistent judgment of these affricated [t]'s and [d]'s is more important than the fact that they represent the "wrong" phonetic feature, judging by standard spelling. They have yet to learn that standard spelling ignores most regular phonetic variation, such as the affrication in this case. Teachers of primary reading and spelling should be aware of both the principle and this instance of it. They should recognize that children may wish to represent in a quite appropriate

---

[5] In certain dialects of English, particularly British dialects, /t/ and /d/ before /r/ are in fact heavily affricated, so that the phonetic form of *try* is actually [črāy], in which case the spelling *CHRIE* would simply represent a correct phonetic judgment. I have interviewed both the children and their parents, but I have not found any whose speech has this characteristic.

[6] For more details of these tests, see Read (1975, Ch. 3).

manner certain phonetic characteristics that untrained adults are not aware of, and that the basis for this representation is the child's tacit *classification* of what he hears.

Another such abstract classification appears in the case of syllabic liquids and nasals. When [r], [l], [m], [n], or [ŋ] occur in an English word between two consonants (or at the end of a word after a consonant), they are syllabic. That is, the segment constitutes a sonority peak (a local maximum of loudness), and it is perceived as a syllable, as in the case of the [n] of *garden*, phonetically [gardn]. Adults, knowing that the peak of most syllables is a vowel and no doubt influenced by the standard spelling, judge such syllables to contain a vowel before the liquid or nasal. The preschool children virtually never represent such a vowel.

TIGR	*tiger*	**DIKTR**	*doctor*
SOGR	*sugar*	**OVR**	*over*
AFTR	*after*	**SMOLR**	*smaller*
LITL	*little*	**CANDL**	*candle*
WAGN	*wagon*	**OPN**	*open*

This spelling is particularly persistent; it appears even in words for which a child has otherwise learned aspects of standard spelling, such as the *I* and *T* of **LITL** or the *LY* in **SODNLY** (suddenly). Like the spellings of [tr] and [dr], it may turn up in school. On a spelling dictation exercise given to 47 first-graders, 21 of them produced all three of the following spellings:

    BRUTHR *brother*   **TABL** *table*   **FETHR** *feather*

These same first-graders produced other spellings consistent with the invented ones, but none as frequently as this one.

The interesting point is that the children apply this spelling to liquids and nasals quite consistently, and not to similar syllables containing other consonants. In syllables consisting of a reduced vowel and an obstruent (a nonnasal true consonant, which cannot be syllabic) the children represent the vowel[7] as in **CERIT** *carrot*, the second syllable of **SRKIS** *circus*, and many other examples. In other words, the invented spellings reveal not only a reasonably accurate representation of the phonetic facts, but also a classification in which liquids and nasals are treated differently from other consonants.

Such a classification must be embodied in an adequate system of phonetic features.[8] The fact that liquids and nasals can be syllabic is related to their similarity

---

[7]This vowel /ə/ is spelled *E* at the stage at which the children use *E* to represent [i]. Later, when the spelling of [i] develops to *I*, this vowel also becomes *I*. Here again, the children make a reasonable phonetic judgment, pairing [ə] or [i] with [i].

[8]See N. Chomsky and Halle (1968, pp. 353—355) for a discussion of a feature system that makes this distinction.

to vowels, namely that in their articulation there is a less radical obstruction of the flow of breath than in the articulation of true consonants (obstruents). Assuming that this distinction underlies the invented orthography, we see once again that a classification of English segments according to articulatory features may be part of the knowledge of the language that a child brings to school.

The continuation of these spellings longer than some others may be attributable to the fact that they are appropriate to the general principle of English spelling, that predictable and free phonetic variation is not represented. Since the syllabic quality of liquids and nasals is predictable from their context, the children's spellings already adhere to this principle. In this and a few other cases in which the child must learn to mark a redundant phonetic detail, the invented orthography is quite persistent. This persistence is precisely what one would expect if in learning standard orthography, a child is in fact learning a principle, as well as specific spellings.

Abstraction from Perceived Phonetic Detail

I have emphasized the children's ability to relate segments on the basis of similarities in their articulatory features. One must also consider the counterpart of that ability, namely that in order to spell, the children systematically ignore certain phonetic differences. In spelling an affricated [t] or [d] as the corresponding palatal affricate, the children are representing the similarity in affrication, but ignoring differences such as type of tongue contact. In spelling each lax vowel with the letter whose name contains its tense counterpart, they preserve place of articulation but ignore differences in tenseness and diphthongization. We may say that the children "abstract from" certain phonetic differences in spelling various segments alike.

In this respect, the preschool spellings are, of course, like every alphabetic orthography ever devised. No one would seriously propose a detailed phonetic transcription as a reasonable orthography; every orthography attempts to capture just *significant* variation, in some sense. It is one notion of "significant variation" that underlies the concept of the phoneme; it is quite another notion that forms the basis of standard English orthography, as some analyses have recently revealed;[9] and it is yet a third notion that underlies the invented spellings.

It is precisely this relationship to other orthographies that makes the invented spellings interesting. The number of symbols available compels the children to represent segments abstractly, but their choices indicate that they regard certain phonetic features as relatively more significant than others, in that they consistently represent certain similarities at the expense of others. One might propose—quite tentatively—an ordering of certain features in terms of their relative

[9]For a thorough examination, see Venezky (1970). For discussions within the framework of generative grammar, see Noam Chomsky (1970) and Chomsky and Halle (1968, pp. 54–55 et passim), For introductory treatments of the latter, see Carol Chomsky (1970) and O'Neil (1969).

prominence in children's judgments. For vowels, perhaps backness, height, and tenseness are so ordered, from most to least important. For consonants, stridency may be more important than type of tongue contact. From other evidence, it appears that the place-of-articulation features are more important than voicing or nasality for consonants.

One can then investigate whether there is any generality to this order, as revealed by other children and in other kinds of judgments. It contrasts with the order observed in frequent "sound substitutions," such as [t] for [θ], where children are least likely to preserve place of articulation (Menyuk, 1968). This comparison suggests that the abstract judgment involved in constructing an orthography is quite distinct from difficulties of production.

These inferences have both a theoretical and a potentially practical importance. On the theoretical side, we know rather little about the development of children's phonological judgments, as opposed to their production and perception. In addition to studying the development of phonological discriminations, as reviewed in Chapter 9 of this volume by C. A. Ferguson and O. K. Garnica, we need to study the development of phonological classifications, that is, children's ability to relate one phone to another and to recognize abstract similarities among discriminable segments. Such tacit classifications are, after all, typically the terms in which phonological rules are stated and presumably learned (Anisfeld, Barlow, & Frail, 1968; Messer, 1967). Insofar as the evidence presented here suggests that some preschool children treat, say, mid front vowels, affricates, and potentially syllabic segments as uniform categories for spelling purposes, we have evidence of tacit classifications. This development must be an important early step in the acquisition of a general English phonology.

On the practical side, we can compare the children's invented orthography with others, especially standard English orthography, in terms of the level at which it represents phonetic variation. Both are highly abstract, as is required by the alphabet and indeed by the concept of an orthography. But the difference is important: in general, standard orthography represents only lexical or morphophonemic variation, whereas the invented system represents those distinctions that are most significant according to an apparent hierarchy of phonetic features. This difference between the two systems may define a large and central part of what a child must learn in order to read and write.

As a final example of the ways in which preschool spelling reflects certain phonetic similarities and not others, consider the spellings of nasals. As was illustrated in connection with syllabics, [m] and [n] are spelled with the customary letters.

MARED	*married*	**NIT**	*night*
HOM	*home*	**WAN**	*when*

But for the velar nasal [ŋ] there is no clue in letter names; presumably the children must choose among *M*, *N*, and *G*, which they use to spell the voiced velar stop

[g], as in standard spelling.

GEVS *gives*   **EGLIOW** *igloo*

In fact, they choose *G*, so the *-ing* ending [iŋ], for example, is normally spelled *-EG* (at the age at which a child is spelling [i] as *E*). Thus the children again preserve place of articulation, relating the two voiced velars and ignoring the difference in nasality.

FEHEG	*fishing*	**GOWEG**	*going*
SOWEMEG	*swimming*	**COLAKTGE**	*collecting*

But when any of these nasals occurs before a stop, the children typically omit it from spelling:

BOPY	*bumpy*	**AD**	*and*	**WOTET**	*want it*
NUBRS	*numbers*	**ED**	*end*	**DOT**	*don't*
THOPY	*thumpy*	**MOSTR**	*monster*	**PLAT**	*plant*
HACC	*Hanks*				
THEKCE	*thinks*				
AGRE	*angry*				
SIC	*sink*				

written three times in my presence, along with a monologue on its nominal, transitive, and intransitive meanings.

FAC *Frank*   the [r] is also omitted
NOOIGLID *New England*

This treatment of preconsonantal nasals is quite consistent; it is the usual spelling for all the children up to about age 5, or until they begin to read standard orthography. Note that in the special case of the velar nasal, these rules give the same spelling for [ŋg] and [g]:*G*. Words which include [ŋg], such as *finger* and *longer*, are spelled **FEGR, LOGR**, etc., where the *G* evidently represents [g] and the nasal is not represented, judging from the children's spelling of other nasals and stops. Of course, more homography results from this practice. For instance, **BAT**, mentioned above, not only spells *bait*, *bet*, and *bat*, but also *bent*. (This example is not attested in the data, but quite parallel cases are, such as **SAT**, *sent*.) It is important to note that this spelling is not required by a lack of alphabetic characters; the children consistently use *M*, *N*, and *G* for the nasals in other contexts. Nor does it seem plausible that children do not hear the nasal, that is, that they do not discriminate *bet* from *bent*. Questioning preschool children about such minimal pairs indicates that $3\frac{1}{2}$-year-olds can make that discrimination (Read, 1970, pp. 134–136). In fact, this spelling remains characteristic of 5-year-olds and sometimes older children. It seems to be extraordinarily common in primary-grade spelling errors (Read, 1971, p. 19; Wilding, 1971).

There is more than one possible explanation for this phenomenon, but one is especially interesting. According to the spectrographic and kymographic evidence presented by Malécot (1960), nasals before stops have the effect of nasalizing preceding lax vowels. In fact, the nasals constitute phonetic segments only before voiced stops, as in *amble, candor,* and *anger.* Before voiceless stops, as in *ample, cantor,* and *anchor,* the nasality is realized as vowel nasalization only. This result holds in most dialects of English for [ʌ], [i], and [æ], especially the last. If these are the phonetic facts, then any consistent representation of preconsonantal nasals is an abstraction. As the examples indicate, the children do create a consistent representation, without the nasal. It may be that given the phonetic sequences [nasalized vowel + stop] and [nasalized vowel + nasal + stop], the children regard the nasalization as primarily a feature of the vowel. Evidently, this feature is one that need not be represented; indeed, assuming that [vocalic] is a more significant feature of vowels than [nasal] and assuming a principle of one letter per segment, it cannot be represented in a natural way. This interpretation begs for more investigation, but it seems clear at least that the nonrepresentation of prestop nasals is an abstraction from a phonetic contrast that the children do perceive.

Not only is the children's spelling abstracted from certain perceived phonetic and even phonemic differences, but it becomes more abstract, in the direction of standard spelling, during the preschool period. For instance, the preschoolers begin by representing past tense according to its phonetic form:

MARED	*married*	**HALPT**	*helped*
LAFFT	*left*	**HOP-T**	*hopped*

But before they go to school, they may adopt a *-D* spelling fairly regularly:

WALKD	*walked*	**STARTID**	*started*
PEKD	*peeked*	**ARIVD**	*arrived*

Each child from whom I have past-tense examples made this development; in fact, for one girl there is a month-by-month sequence in which this development occurred gradually from 5 years, 10 months to 6 years, 3 months. The general development and the choice of *-D* is no doubt prompted by adult examples—in that sense it is not spontaneous, but it is worth noting that the spellings are clearly not entirely copied or dictated. The interesting fact is that the children adopted this morphophonemic spelling at an age at which they continued to use other aspects of the invented orthography, especially the spellings of the syllabics and the preconsonantal nasals. One could make a similar argument for the spellings of plurals, which are always *-S* and *-IS*, never *-Z* or *-IZ*. The importance of these observations is that at the age at which they first receive formal instruction, children may be ready to make certain abstractions in spelling, and that some abstractions may be more acceptable than others. This possibility clearly deserves careful investigation.

Conclusion

In general, then, the preschool orthographers represent certain phonetic similarities and ignore others, making judgments according to principles quite different from those of standard orthography. Nor do the children spell phonemically. Given the limited alphabet, they relate one phone to another in terms of their constituent properties. They choose representations in terms of phonetic features such as nasality, syllabicity, backness, height, and affrication, and they treat certain of these relationships as more significant than others. In fact, these judgments appear not only where the alphabet requires a choice, as with vowels, but also where alternative spellings are available, as with the nasals and the syllabics.

Such children need not approach standard orthography as a matching of phonemes with spellings. They already recognize a system of phonetic properties and relations, and in terms of it, they create abstract spellings. What they do not know are certain more complex relations, such as those affected by Vowel Shift, and the principle that certain regular phonetic variations are not represented, such as the affrication of /t/ and /d/ before /r/. For them, one major aspect of learning to read and write in standard orthography is learning these principles.[10]

The fact that preschool children may make a tacit phonetic analysis bears specifically on the creation of a special teaching orthography. Any such orthography must be based on an assumption about what relationships children recognize. In fact, the virtually unchallenged assumption has been that a natural orthography for children is phonemic. One such assumption, based on Daniel Jones's (1962, Ch. 27) concept of the *diaphone*, clearly underlies the best-known pedagogical orthography, the Initial Teaching Alphabet,[11] although the ITA also includes certain compromises intended to ease the transition to standard orthography. The preschool invented orthography strongly suggests that the nature of the child's "experience of the spoken language," as Pitman puts it, is not to be taken for granted, if one wishes to create a well-motivated teaching orthography. One interesting possibility is that a phonemic orthography may be unnecessarily concrete in certain respects. It may also be that there is great individual variation in this matter; in any case, children's judgments must be investigated carefully.

It is possible, but I believe wrong, to disregard the evidence presented here as having been produced by exceptional children. In inventing the orthography and, in many cases, beginning to read early, these children were exceptional. Some of

---

[10]See the references of Footnote 9, page 337 for discussions of the principles underlying standard spelling.

[11]The precise assumption has rarely been stated explicitly in the ITA literature, but see Pitman and St. John (1969, pp. 41, 41n, and 123), for example.

them were unusually independent and creative in other ways. Their one clearly crucial ability was to make overt judgments of phonological relationships at an age at which most children do not do so. I know of no reason to attribute this ability to any global factor, such as general intelligence.

Most of the parents were successful middle-class professionals and academics; reading and writing were important adult activities in most homes. In each case, several factors coincided, especially the child's early learning of letter names and his interest in printed messages, along with the parents' willingness to accept the child's own spelling efforts. The prevalent belief that English orthography is essentially a set of unsystematic habits may suppress this willingness in many parents; this belief seems to me unfortunate, quite aside from its possible effect on preschool spelling. The parents provided just the information that any inexpert literate person could provide: the names of the letters and the answers to such questions as "How do you spell [čə]?" They did not coax or expect their children to spell; in fact, most were surprised. The children needed no encouragement; several of them produced messages in flurries of great abundance. Under certain circumstances preschool spelling, while exceptional, is not entirely rare. For example, although the practices in Montessori schools vary widely in this country, such schools are a good place to look for preschool orthographers.[12]

In the absence of any reason to connect individual and situational variables with the specific and uniform orthography the children created, these factors seem of marginal relevance. Despite individual differences in development, the fact remains that children may (and to some extent, must) make abstract inferences about the sound system of their language before they learn to read and write. It is then an interesting empirical question whether other children share the judgments of the preschool orthographers. Research is proceeding along lines parallel to the experimental and spelling-error studies mentioned above.

For instance, children's phonological judgments might appear also in their judgments or productions of rhymes. This possibility is particularly plausible, considering that rhyme and alliteration in various folk and literary traditions require, not phonemic identity of segments, but similarity in terms of distinctive features.[13] That is, off-rhymes are tolerated just in case the segments involved differ by certain features or certain numbers of features. Might children's judgments of rhymes be compared with those of the invented spelling? Two pilot studies of this question have had negative results. The studies involved the preconsonantal nasals, specifically the possibility that children would regard, say, *cap* as rhyming with *lamp* (along with *stamp*), ignoring the difference in vowel nasality, just as in invented spelling. With twenty-two 5- and 6-year olds, I found that those children

---

[12]For a description of spelling at age four, see Montessori (1964, pp. 282—283, 292—293, 296—297). Unlike the children described in this chapter, the pupils at the Casa dei Bambini were notable for their *low* socioeconomic status.

[13]See Scott (1971), Maher (1969), and Ryder (1963) for some observations on off-rhymes in various forms, including (Maher) Mother Goose.

who could consistently judge rhymes did not ignore the nasality. This result held also for their production of rhymes, they were much more likely to produce *bunk* than *buck* as a rhyme for *trunk*. Two conclusions may be drawn from these results. It seems that five-year-olds do hear the nasality, even when it is primarily a feature of the vowel, as was assumed in the analysis of the invented spellings. Second, the relevant difference between spelling and rhyming may be that in spelling the children were required to make an abstract judgment; that is, having no reasonable symbols to distinguish *VC* from *ṼNC* from *ṼC*, they were forced to generalize. In rhyming, however, there was no such requirement; the children could produce a precise counterpart of the given syllable, so that we cannot know what judgment of similarity they would make. Investigations of "forced-choice" situations, in which children are asked which of several alternative words rhymes best with a given word, provide relevant data; such situations are interesting precisely because they compare with spelling, both invented and learned. Some results appear in Read (1975).

Further corroborative evidence appears in a report by Josephine Wilding (1971), a Berkshire schoolmistress. She analyzed 2000 spelling and oral reading errors of 125 middle-class boys, ages 6—11, in an investigation of phonological development. The errors of these older children reflect the influence of standard orthography in relation to their dialects, as in the spellings **CERMENT** *cement* and **DUCY** *juicy*, where the child evidently overgeneralizes the insight that phonetic [ə] and [j] are often spelled -*er* and *d*- respectively. Furthermore, the "vowel alternations" that occur do not include the tense—lax correspondences found in the invented spellings. But other aspects of the invented spellings do appear, including the representation of affricate [t] and [d], as in **CHRI** *try*. Again, the children over-generalized their knowledge of standard spelling in such cases, as in **TRILDREN** *children* and **GRADRAL** *gradual*. Most notable is the nonrepresentation of nasals (67% of the errors involving nasals were orthographic "deletions"), which occurred especially with preconsonantal nasals, judging from the examples given. This error appeared at all the ages studied. In general, Wilding's observations suggest that the judgments reflected in invented spelling interact with a knowledge of standard spelling in older children.

An interesting possibility is that reading or spelling impairment in older children may reflect in part the persistence of judgments like those made in the preschool orthography. Emily Menzel (1971) has analyzed errors made by 36 students who had completed second or third grade (along with one each from the fourth, fifth, and sixth grades) and who had been recommended for a remedial reading program by their classroom teachers. Each child took the Gates—McKillop Reading Diagnostic Test (Gates & McKillop, 1962). Menzel analyzed the errors on Part VI—4, in which the child is asked to identify the vowel letter "that makes the sound in the middle" of a *CVC* nonce word. The child looks at the array, a e i o u, as the examiner pronounces a nonce word such as [keb]; then the child points to one of the letters. Menzel predicted that the children would choose on the basis of the letter names, with backness being a more important determinant than height, as in the invented spellings. Of 88 errors, 65% supported this hypothesis, 25% contradicted it, and 10% were ambiguous; had the errors been distributed evenly, the corresponding figures would have been 35%, 42.5%, and 22.5%. For [īy, i, ēy, e,] and [a], for each of which the preschool orthography suggests a particular error (*I, E, E, A,* and *I*), 55% of the errors were just those choices, whereas an even distribution would have produced 25%. As Menzel points out, there are several ways in which this preliminary study might be refined, in both test items and research design, and a second- or third-grade child's performance on this task is no doubt influenced by many factors. Nevertheless, the results suggest, as do Wilding's observations, that phonological judgments like those of the preschool orthography may influence spelling errors, even after two or more years of instruction. This possibility deserves to be investigated, along with the question of whether preschool children who have created no spelling system make the same judgments as the orthographers.

These questions bear on the understanding of language acquisition as well as on the teaching of reading and writing. We know that a child makes some judgments of phonological similarities and differences; he must do so in order to interpret speech, for example. We now see that we cannot assume that his judgments at age 5 are the same as those of adults or that they are strictly phonemic. Rather, we must ask what phonological analyses children make at various stages of development and what these analyses suggest about language acquisition. It is an interesting question, for example, to what degree the judgments reflected in preschool orthography are based on experience and to what degree they represent a universal hierarchy of the sort envisioned in Jakobson (1968). Detailed answers will be difficult to obtain, for children's phonological judgments are rarely explicit, as they are in invented spelling.

A child may come to school with an unconscious notion of phonological categories, in terms of a hierarchy of articulatory features that defines for him an ordering of more and less significant phonetic variation. In his first encounter with standard spelling, he may seek some systematic relationship to this analysis, rather than to unanalyzed phonemes. If so, the difference between these systems defines an important part of literacy instruction. Thus, examining children's phonological judgments may have practical significance. Until we understand them better, we can at least respect them and attempt to work with them, if only intuitively.

In the classroom, an informed teacher should recognize that seemingly bizarre spellings may represent reasonable phonological judgments. A child who wants to spell *truck* with a *ch-* will not be enlightened by being told that *ch* spells "chuh," as in *chicken.* He already knows that; in fact the relation between the first segments of *truck* and *chicken* is exactly what he wishes to represent. Similarly for the child who wishes to spell *pen* with an *a, plant* without an *n,* or *table* without an *e*; in each case, it may seem that the child has "mis-heard" some sound, but in fact he has not only heard accurately but has categorized segments according to their articulation. In such cases, we should say to a child that his judgment is reasonable, but that standard spelling represents rather different relations.

Standard spelling is much more indirectly related to phonetic forms, of course, as in pairs like *sign—signify*, where the *i* and the *g* indicate the morphological relationship instead of the phonetic difference. Insofar as a preschool child is able to abstract from phonetic distinctions, he is on his way toward this aspect of standard spelling. In order to help him, we should distinguish between his attempts to represent phonetic facts too narrowly, as in employing a consistent spelling for reduced vowels (see Footnote 7, page 336) and his attempts to abstract, as in pairing [tr] with [č] instead of [t]. In the latter case, we should credit the child with applying the right principle, even though he generalizes in the "wrong" direction.

We cannot make this distinction if we continue to think of learning to read and write as a matter of getting in the "habit" of associating phonemes with graphemes. The preschool orthographers collapse phonemic distinctions where necessary, employing an analysis of articulatory features. As in the case of children's understanding of syntactic structure,[14] this analysis is not made evident in their utterances, so our understanding of it is still quite fragmentary and probably shallow. My intention is not to propose yet another poorly motivated literacy program, but to put forth some empirical hypotheses about one aspect of children's phonology. I suggest that we investigate these judgments as an instance of the intricate knowledge that children construct, going beyond their linguistic experience.

References

Anisfeld, M., Barlow, J., & Frail, C. Distinctive features in the pluralization rules of English speakers. *Language and Speech*, 1968, *11*, 31—37.

Chomsky, C. *The acquisition of syntax in children from 5 to 10.* Cambridge, Mass.: MIT Press, 1969.

Chomsky, C. Reading, writing, and phonology. *Harvard Educational Review*, 1970, *40*, 287—309.

Chomsky, C. Write first, read later. *Childhood Education*, 1971, 47 (No. 6), 296—299.

Chomsky, N. Phonology and reading. In H. Levin & J. P. Williams (Eds.), *Basic studies on reading*. New York: Basic Books, 1970.

Chomsky, N., & Halle, M. *The sound pattern of English.* New York: Harper, 1968.

Gates, A. I., & McKillop, A. S. *Reading diagnostic tests.* New York: Teachers College Press, 1962.

Jakobson, R. *Child language, aphasia, and phonological universals.* The Hague: Mouton, 1968.

Jones, D. *The phoneme: Its nature and use.* Cambridge, Eng.: Heffer, 1962.

Maher, J. P. English-speakers' awareness of the distinctive features. *Language Sciences*, 1969, *5*, 14.

Malécot, A. Vowel nasality as a distinctive feature in American English. *Language*, 1960, *36*, 222—229.

Menyuk, P. The role of distinctive features in children's acquisition of phonology. *Journal of Speech and Hearing Research*, 1968, *11*, 138—146.

Menzel, E. M. Children's phonological judgments of English vowels. Unpublished manuscript, Dep. of Curriculum and Instruction, University of Wisconsin, 1971.

Messer, S. Implicit phonology in children. *Journal of Verbal Learning and Verbal Behavior*, 1967, *6*, 609—613.

---

[14] Carol Chomsky (1969) demonstrates more conclusively a somewhat similar situation in the child's knowledge of syntax at age 5 and beyond. A child may use certain syntactic structures, apparently as an adult does, and yet on examination it turns out that he understands certain relations quite differently.

Montessori, M. 1964. *The Montessori method*. Cambridge, Mass.: Robert Bentley, 1964.

O'Neil, W. The spelling and pronunciation of English. In W. Morris (Ed.), *The American Heritage dictionary of the English language*. Boston: Houghton, 1969.

Pitman, J., & St. John, J. *Alphabets and reading: The initial teaching alphabet*. London: Pitman, 1969.

Read, C. Children's perceptions of the sounds of English. Unpublished doctoral dissertation, Harvard University, 1970.

Read, C. Pre-school children's knowledge of English phonology. *Harvard Educational Review*, 1971, *41*, 1—34.

Read, C. *Children's categorization of speech sounds in English*. NCTE Research Report No. 17. Urbana, Ill.: National Council of Teachers of English, 1975.

Ryder, F. G. Off-rimes and consonantal confusion groups. *Lingua*, 1963, *12*, 190—198.

Scott, C. T. Towards a formal poetics: metrical patterning in "The Windhover." *Language and Style*, 1974, 7, 91—107.

Venezky, R. *The structure of English orthography*. The Hague: Mouton, 1970.

Wilding, J. M. The school child's acknowledgement of the sound pattern of English. Paper presented at the Easter conference of the Linguistic Association of Great Britain, Lancaster, April, 1971.

20. The Relation between Spoken and Written Language

Frank Smith

Spoken language and written language are closely related, but not at the superficial level of spelling—sound correspondence. Contemporary linguistic theory indicates that English orthography is more closely related to underlying aspects of language involving meaning than to the sound pattern of any one dialect. Psycholinguistic evidence supports the view that predictions of meaning are and must be in advance of the eye in reading, the visual function being simply to sample the text in order to confirm or disconfirm cognitive expectations. These linguistic and psycholinguistic views are contrary to conventional assumptions that written language is a visual representation of speech and that reading requires decoding text to sound.

Introduction

It has been widely held—in the English-speaking world at least[1] (Mathews, 1966)—that writing is speech written down, that reading involves the "decoding to sound" of written language to speech, and that reading instruction requires teaching children to blend the sounds of letters. In this chapter, I shall outline some

---

[1] Although the qualification "English" will generally be omitted, such terms as "language" and "language user" in the present chapter should be taken as referring only to English and speakers of English. Because of the varieties of written language in the world, it is not possible to make general statements about the relation of writing to speech (or about reading instruction). However, statements about linguistic and psycholinguistic aspects of the reading process itself are (or should be) universally applicable.

theoretical and empirical challenges to each of the three conventional assumptions. A contemporary linguistic view is that writing is a parallel or alternative form of language to speech, and that reading, like listening, involves a direct "decoding to meaning," or comprehension. There is psycholinguistic evidence that the prior identification of words, or of their sounds, is neither necessary nor feasible in fluent reading, and that children who become fluent readers do not learn to read on a letter-by-letter, word-by-word basis.

The chapter will include some brief observations on dialect, the alphabet, reading instruction, and second-language learning.

The Nature of Written Language

At the most molar level of discourse it is obvious that speech and writing differ—the unedited transcription of a talk or conversation is an inadequate substitute for a specially written paper, and a text written for a reader is rarely suitable for reading to listeners. Speech and writing respect different conventions of style, partly because of the different demands each medium makes upon the receiver (the listener or reader). For example, writing permits the reader to determine his own speed and sequence, but denies him ready access to supplementary information.

At the syntactic and lexical levels the differences between spoken and written language are less clear, except in relative terms. There appear to be no grammatical constructions in written English that are not available in the majority of spoken English dialects (Wardhaugh, 1969), but they are used in different proportions and degrees of complexity in the various registers or styles of writing and speech (Joos, 1962). Similarly there is no evidence that a different lexicon is used for writing than for speech, although words and word classes occur with different relative frequencies in writing and speech (Miller, 1951, Chap. 4).

In short it would appear that differences *between* written and spoken styles of language are not greater than those occurring *within* spoken language. The evidence supports the view that speech and writing are variants or alternative forms of the same language, but not the more superficial proposition that writing is speech written down.

However, the main points of contention concerning the relation of written language to speech usually center on the degree to which the orthography of written English is taken to represent the phonology of the spoken language, and the extent to which writing must be "decoded to sound" in order to be comprehended. The argument is not whether written language *can* be decoded into speech, which is obviously the case, but whether such decoding is necessary for comprehension. It is argued that the converse applies, and that written language can be read aloud only after comprehension of meaning. There is insufficient information in the spelling of English words for their direct decoding into speech (just as there is insufficient information in the sounds of speech for direct transcription into writing). The language user himself must contribute information to bridge the discrepancy between writing and speech from his prior knowledge of language.

GRAPHEME—PHONEME CORRESPONDENCES

The complex nature of the spelling—sound correspondences of English have been examined intensively by Venezky and his coworkers (e.g., Venezky, 1967), and at the Southwest Regional Laboratory for Educational Research and Development (Berdiansky, Cronnell, & Koehler, 1969). The latter examined 6000 common one- and two-syllable words in the spoken language vocabulary of children from 6- to 9-years old and determined that a total of 166 correspondence "rules" would still fail to account for about 10% of the words (Smith, 1971, Chap. 12).[2] Moreover, there are few rules that have no exceptions or alternatives, almost every graph-meme and sound being involved in more than one rule. Some correspondences are more *probable* than others, but common words are usually not instances of the most predictable rules. Brown (1970) has shown that fluent readers tend to spell by memorization rather than rule—they make many more errors on regularly spelled unfamiliar words than on irregularly spelled familiar words.

Prior knowledge of a word's intonation is sometimes required before a decision can be made about the applicability of a correspondence rule (e.g, the initial sound of *acorn, about*), in other cases a knowledge of morphology (for the *sh* in *bishop, mishap*), syntactic function (present or past tense of *read*; noun and verb form of *convict*), and derivation (*cell, cello*). In short, the spelling of individual words provides insufficient information for the prediction of their sound. However, interest in the relation between graphemes and phonemes diminishes with the realization that the representation of the sounds of speech is not a direct function of English orthography and that the "blending" of the sounds of letters in words is neither a necessary nor a preferred way of identifying words (even unfamiliar words) in reading, either by fluent readers or beginners.

LEVELS OF LANGUAGE

The notion that speech and writing are alternative forms of a common language is clarified by consideration of the dual nature of language. Any statement in language (any utterance or sentence) can be analyzed either in terms of its physical properties (roughly speaking the "sounds" of speech or the alphabetic characters of writing) or in terms of its meaning. As Miller (1965) has forcefully demonstrated in the case of speech, there is no simple correspondence between these two aspects of language. Features occur predictably in the physical manifestation of speech that have no significance for meaning, while significant differences in meaning may have no obvious physical correlate. As just one example, the silent intervals

---

[2] Johnson (1969) has calculated that in the 20,000-word analysis made by Venezky (1967), 61 different vowel clusters are associated with 92 sound patterns in a total of over 300 *vowel* spelling—sound correspondences alone. Analysis of the complexity of English spelling as a tool for decoding to sound does not necessarily discourage investigators from asserting that some or all of the correspondences should be taught to children; for example phonic instructional materials are being prepared by the Southwest Regional Laboratory.

that physically occur in speech do not correspond to the segmentation into words that we hear—the utterance /Wes tend/ is heard as "West end." The discrepancies between the physical properties of a message and its meaning must obviously be resolved by a contribution on the part of the receiver similar to the "prior knowledge" required to bridge the information gap between writing and speech.

That there is a difference between the physical and communicative properties of language is far from new (N. Chomsky, 1966). However, a useful conceptual framework has been provided by N. Chomsky's (1965) distinction between "deep" and "surface" structure. Deep structure is defined as the level of language at which meaning is interpreted—the "semantic" level—and surface structure the level at which phonological (or graphic) representations are realized. The bridge between the two levels is "grammar," defined as the abstract set of syntactic rules used by an individual to generate or comprehend sentences in his language. According to this view, it is precisely this implicit knowledge of grammar that the receiver must supply in order to impose meaning upon messages, and to convert between the written and spoken forms of language.

Although recent linguistic hypothesis and controversy has thrown doubt on whether syntax and semantics can be so neatly distinguished, and whether linguistic decisions can in fact be made on the basis of syntactic rules alone (e.g., Bach & Harms, 1968; Fillmore & Langendoen, 1971), for present purposes the simplified distinction between deep and surface levels of language will be adequate.

The argument, then, is that physical aspects of spoken and written language— the phonological and orthographic representation—are alternative surface structure forms of a common underlying language that do not map directly on to each other. Writing from dictation and reading aloud are possible only via a loop through a deeper level of language at which meaning is represented, that is, making use of the reader's (or writer's) knowledge of grammar. By the same token, recourse to spoken language is unnecessary when the purpose of reading is to comprehend the meaning, since the surface structure of writing is more directly related to the deep structure of language than to the surface structure of speech.

As an example, consider the sentences

(1) **The none tolled hymn she had scene bear feat inn hour rheum.**

(2)   *The nun told him she had seen bare feet in our room.*

The fact that the spelling anomalies in (1) are so evident clearly indicates that visual aspects of words distinguish meaning independently of their sound. There would be no way of selecting between (1) and (2) if reading were indeed accomplished by decoding written symbols to sound. The example also demonstrates that in some circumstances it is possible to write a phonetic representation that can be interpreted in the way in which speech is interpreted. But this can scarcely be the prior process, since the anomalies of (1) are invariably identified before the alternative meaning associated with the sound, which is then separated from the meaning associated with the spelling. Furthermore it is difficult to find strings of unconventional spellings that map into meaningful sound so felicitously. Phonetic representations and literary dialects are notoriously difficult to comprehend simply because they eliminate much of the meaning carried by the conventional spelling of words. Sentence (1) was composed to avoid the particularly disruptive syntactic ambiguity that occurs in **Wee mite fined sum read buries inn hear** (*We might find some red berries in here*).

THE RELATION BETWEEN SPELLING AND SOUND

N. Chomsky and Halle (1968)[3] have proposed that there is an underlying "lexical" level of our knowledge of language at which words are represented and related independently of their sound pattern or spelling (the two "surface" characteristics). At such an underlying level, for example, the syntactic (and semantic) relationship between pairs of words like *nation* and *national, nature* and *natural, sane* and *sanity*, are in some abstract sense clustered so that the relation between their various derivations is preserved. Although the actual pronunciation of the vowel in the first syllable varies within each of the above pairs of words, this variation is wholly predictable to a speaker of the language. The variation is also very general, since it appears with other vowels in a large number of words, e.g., *extreme* and *extremity, wide* and *width, phone* and *phonic*. There is a similar predictable variation in the pronunciation of consonants in such word pairs as *medicine* and *medical, sign* and *resign, sage* and *sagacious*.

Speakers of English recognize the lexical similarity within such pairs of words despite their variations in sound, or rather because the variation in sound is completely predictable from the speaker's implicit knowledge of how the same underlying lexical structure is reflected in diverse pronunciations.

According to Chomsky and Halle, it is not the function of the orthography to provide the reader with information that he already possesses. Since speakers of English know the rules relating the underlying lexical structure with the surface structure of their dialect, it is more appropriate for the orthography to represent the underlying lexical structure than to represent any particular phonology.

Put in more familiar terms, the English spelling system indicates how words are related in meaning independently of their sound. It would appear to be a principle of English orthography that words that share meaning should look alike (C. Chomsky, 1970), as in all the above examples. A further principle would appear to be that words differing in meaning should look different, even when they are homophones (such as *none, nun*). In this light, written English may be seen as considerably less ambiguous than speech, since a dictionary compiled by Whitford (1966) lists over 1000 frequent homophones but only 160 frequent homographs. Most proponents of spelling or alphabetic reform would, of course, increase the proportion of homographs.

---

[3] A nontechnical exposition of the Chomsky and Halle view of underlying lexical structure is provided by Carol Chomsky (1970). Similar views on the underlying relation between spelling and spoken language have been widely presented elsewhere (e.g., Reed, 1970; Venezky, 1967; Wardhaugh, 1969).

THE FUNCTION OF THE ALPHABET

The preceding linguistic arguments, together with psycholinguistic evidence to be outlined of the manner in which words are identified, has led to the speculation that alphabetic writing may have developed primarily as a convenience for the writer (or the printer and his proofreader), and that the alphabetic principle has proved relatively disadvantageous for the reader, especially in view of its emphasis in much reading instruction (Smith, 1973, Chap. 10).

Certainly the "blending" of sounds according to phonics principles is not a typical resort for the fluent reader who encounters an unfamiliar word. The preferred strategy is usually to ignore the word altogether, the second alternative being to guess at it from context. English is so redundant in most cases that the occasional omission or misidentification of a word is of little importance. There is interesting evidence that children in the process of becoming fluent readers also tend to prefer the "mature" strategies of ignoring or guessing unfamiliar words (Goodman, 1969), often despite considerable instructional pressure to the contrary. No mystery appears to be attached to the propensity of children to manifest such sophisticated reading strategies independently of classroom instruction, since the limitations of the human visual system and memory and the inadequacies of "phonics" make other methods of reading counterproductive.

DIALECT

Chomsky and Halle's view that English orthography is related to an underlying abstract level of language and not to sound implies that differences in spoken dialect should not be relevant to reading. In fact Chomsky and Halle suggest that the orthography is an optimal system for all dialects—the only feasible alternative to having separate orthographies for the sound patterns of many dialects. The suggestion is based on the assumption that the majority of dialects of English vary only at a superficial level, that is, above the level of the underlying lexical structure. That such an assumption is not unwarranted appears likely from such analyses as those of Labov (1970) and Torrey (1970).

It is an egregious error to assume that written language is somehow a closer representation of a particular prestige or standard dialect than of any other. In part this misconception persists because we tend to "hear" written language in terms of our own dialect, and find it odd when someone reads in a dialect different from our own. But if anything, written language should be regarded as a dialect in its own right, mutually comprehensible with speech, just as dialectical varieties of speech are mutually comprehensible because of underlying consistencies.

Differences in dialect frequently cause difficulties in the classroom, but are usually due more to communication problems than to the reading task itself. Some difficulties can be ascribed simply to intercultural conflict, others to unfamiliar auditory discriminations (not in fact relevant to reading per se), and others to teacher expectations that reading aloud should be in the prestige dialect, or at least "word for word."

The Perception of Written Language

The linguistic argument suggests that speech is comprehended not so much by a detailed analysis of surface structure as by a continuous process of prediction and synthesis at a deep structure level. The listener resorts to surface structure only to the extent that he seeks confirmation or disconfirmation of his underlying hypotheses about meaning. Only in this way can the listener supply the semantic and syntactic information required if language is to be comprehended.

There is extensive psychological support for the notion that underlying hypotheses must precede surface structure analysis because of inherent limitations on the amount of incoming information that sensory systems can accommodate and memory can retain. I shall discuss these limitations in terms of visual information because they are most directly relevant to the question of whether decoding to sound could be involved in reading. It should be borne in mind that the same general limitations apply to speech comprehension, and that explicit or implicit "listening" concurrent with reading would itself require additional processing through limited capacity channels.

LIMITATIONS OF VISUAL INFORMATION PROCESSING[4]

Reading is not primarily a visual process (Kolers, 1969). Two quite different sources of information are in fact critical to reading, one source being the author (and the printer) who provides what may be called *visual information*—the ink marks on the page—and the other source the reader himself, who provides *nonvisual information*. Put in another way, reading involves the mixture or interaction of information that the reader receives through his visual system (surface structure) and information that he already has available in his brain.

Suppose, for example, that a book is written in a language that the reader does not understand; obviously there will be very little reading. Knowledge of language is crucial nonvisual information that the reader himself must supply. Similarly, very little reading will take place if the subject matter of the text is completely removed from the experience of the reader. Everything the author takes for granted must be supplied by the reader in the form of nonvisual information.

The distinction between visual and nonvisual information in reading is important because there is a reciprocal relationship between the two—readers can trade-off one for the other. The more nonvisual information a reader can use, the less visual information he needs. And the less nonvisual information a reader can supply, the more visual information he must get from the page. Some aspects of this reciprocal relationship are immediately apparent—we read faster when the material we read is familiar, we can read smaller type, and in a dimmer light.

---

[4]Much of the remainder of this chapter has been taken from several prior publications by the author. Specific sources for statements about limitations of the visual information processing system and memory are contained in Smith and Holmes (1971).

We recognize familiar names and words over a greater distance than unfamiliar ones. On the other hand we tend to peer more closely and read slower when our own contribution to the understanding of what we are reading is limited. This use of nonvisual information to facilitate the work of the eyes is reflected in the way all readers make use of redundancy. If a passage is redundant because the plot is predictable, or because the sentences are simple and almost everything is said more than once, then less visual information is required, and reading is easier.

The trade-off between visual and nonvisual information in reading is critical because of the limit to the rate at which the brain can handle incoming visual information. This limitation is often overlooked because we tend to think that we see everything that happens before our eyes. We are not usually aware of the fact that the eyes simply pick up and transmit information from the visual world to the brain, and that the brain makes the perceptual decisions about what we see. And there is a limit to how fast and how much visual information can be handled by the brain.

For example, it is impossible from a single glance—from what in reading is called a fixation—to identify more than four or five different items. More visual information may be available to the eyes, but four or five identifications is as much as the brain can accomplish from a single fixation. If a reader is allowed just one glance at a sequence of random letters, for example, he will be able to identify no more than four or five of them. This is one of the oldest findings in experimental psychology. And it will take the reader one second to identify these letters. It is not necessary of course for the reader to be looking at the letters for the entire second, in fact a glimpse lasting no more than 5 msec is usually more than enough for the eye to respond to all of the visual information that the brain will be capable of handling for a second. For this reason, attempting to speed up the rate of fixation from the four or five a second that a child—and any other reader—normally makes is a pointless endeavor, since the informational bottleneck is elsewhere in the visual system than the eye.

Of course, we can all read faster than the rate of four or five letters a second (which would work out to a reading rate of barely 60 words a min if we actually read words letter by letter). And, in fact, if the sequence of letters the reader is allowed to glimpse is made up into recognizable words, rather than being selected at random, then from this single fixation he may identify two words, comprising perhaps a total of 10 letters. In other words, if the letters that he is shown are organized into words, then he can identify twice as many in a single glance and in the same period of time. The eye picks up the same amount of information in each of the two conditions, whether the letters it is inspecting are a random sequence or whether they form words that the reader knows. But in the second condition the reader can make use of nonvisual information, namely his knowledge of the way in which letters are organized into words.

Uncertainty about what a letter might be is reduced by half if that letter is part of a word—and the less the uncertainty about what a letter is, the less visual information is needed to identify it. If the first letter of an English word is *t*, the next is almost certainly going to be *h*, *r* or a vowel, although if letters were occurring at random there could be any one of 26 alternatives. In other words, because of prior knowledge, less new information is required to decide what a letter in a known word might be.

Note that it is the prior knowledge of the reader, his nonvisual information, that is the ultimate determinant of whether a sequence of letters is random or not. Is the sequence *przyjezdzac* random or not? The answer depends on whether the reader knows Polish. If he does, then one glance at the word would suffice for its recognition; if not, the reader would be unlikely to be able to report half of it.

If the words a reader is permitted to glimpse actually constitute a meaningful phrase, he will on the average identify four of them, a total of 20 or more letters. In other words, if the reader can supply nonvisual information of a syntactic and semantic nature (his knowledge of the language and the world in general), he will be able to use the same amount of visual information—one glance—to identify over four times as many letters, 20 or more compared with four or five.

It is helpful to look at the preceding phenomenon—which is sometimes called the "span of apprehension" and in other contexts the "effective field of view"— from the opposite point of view. If a fluent reader is allowed a single glance at a long sentence—if he is in effect allowed one second of visual information processing time—he will be able to identify four or five words. In effect he "sees" four or five words. (When we read faster than four or five words a second, we are making even greater use of nonvisual information and not bothering to identify most of the words.) However, if the reader is not able to make extensive use of nonvisual information, either because he has limited knowledge of the subject matter or of language or reading, or—what to him amounts to the same thing— if the letters are organized randomly, then he will literally be unable to see more than five letters. The less nonvisual information he can supply, the less he is able to see—a common consequence of visual overload known as "tunnel vision." Beginning readers are prime victims of tunnel vision; the width of line they can actually see is tremendously constricted by the limited amount of nonvisual information they can supply, especially if the material they are confronted with is relatively nonsensical (which means low in redundancy or predictability) and when demands upon them for literal accuracy (emphasis on visual information) are high.

Obviously, a student trying to read a book on a topic with which he is not familiar does not have very much nonvisual information at his disposal. He will tend to read slower and more hesitatingly than the teacher who knows the topic well. Reading, for such a student, might be compared with trying to read in the half-light for the teacher. Like the beginning reader, he is reading as if he is looking at the page through the wrong end of a telescope. Even if the student can recognize words on sight, he will still need twice as much visual information to identify them as a reader with more nonvisual information—which in essence means more reading experience—at his command.

To appreciate fully the disruptive effect of the limitations of the visual system in reading, it is necessary to examine another aspect of cognitive function that exercises considerable limitation, that of memory.

LIMITATIONS OF MEMORY

We realize that there is a severe limit to how much can be put into working memory (also called "short-term memory") whenever we try to hold a 7-digit telephone number in our head. Unless we can put some kind of pattern to the number or to a sequence of letters (which is the same thing as making use of information that has already been memorized), there is a limit of some four or five to the number of items that can be retained in this way. (The similarity between the four or five random letters that can be read in a single glance and the four or five items that can be held in short-term memory is coincidental. These are two independent limitations on reading, not one. Rather more than five items can be held in short-term memory if we are not concerned with remembering their order as well.)

The limitation of short-term memory in effect restricts the number of items that can be attended to at any one time. It is of the utmost importance, therefore, to use working memory efficiently. If we try to overload short-term memory, if we attempt to fill it beyond its capacity, then for every additional item we try to put in, something will come out. And there are only two fates for information that overflows from short-term memory. Either it is put into our permanent memory store, which is time consuming, or else it is lost altogether.

However, the size of each of the four or five "items" that can be stored in short-term memory is determined not so much by external considerations as by what the brain can do with the information. We may load up short-term memory with four or five letters *or* four or five words, or even with something that is far more difficult to specify precisely, several larger chunks of meaning. We know this "chunking" is possible because we can hold in short-term memory the meaning—but not the exact words—from utterances of a dozen words or more.

Obviously, to read fluently requires using short-term memory efficiently, which means to fill it with items that carry as much meaning as possible. A reader with tunnel vision, putting into short-term memory only meaningless sequences of letters or fragmented words, has not a hope that he will be able to read with comprehension. Unless he is able to make fluent use of deep-level nonvisual information, sampling the surface structure for confirmation only, he will be defeated from the start by the limitations of short-term memory.

The handicap of the bottleneck in short-term memory becomes even more obvious when one considers the limitations of long-term memory—the permanent memory where, in effect, all knowledge of the world is organized and stored.

Information that goes into long-term memory is not transitory like that in short-term memory, but rather appears to involve a permanent chemical change in the molecular structure of the brain. Similarly, long-term memory appears to be practically infinite in capacity; it suffers from none of the limitations of size and duration of short-term memory. However, having something in long-term memory is no guarantee that it can be retrieved. Generally the question of whether information can be recovered from long-term memory depends on how well it is organized and how efficient are the memory probes employed to find and retrieve it.

However, we are more concerned at the moment with the rate at which new information can be put into long-term memory, which is very slow and limited indeed compared with the more volatile short-term memory. From 3 to 5 sec. is required to put one item of information into long-term memory—whether the one item of information is a letter, a word, or an entire chunk of meaning.

Some of the implications of the limitations of the visual system and of short- and long-term memory are particularly critical for reading and have been spelled out in Smith and Holmes (1971). For example, it is probably impossible to read with comprehension at slower than 200 words a min.—the units we are trying to get into short- and long-term memory will be too small and fragmented to be of use. Similarly, it is impossible to read for meaning if we stop to read every individual word; short-term memory will soon overflow with a meaningless clutter of disconnected words and bits of words, and it would be most impractical to try to cram such "information" into long-term memory.

A student often finds that he is expected to acquire and store far more visual information than he can cope with, or he may have developed the crippling reading habit of trying to get more information from the text than his memory can handle. The classroom practice of "testing" reading by asking numerous "comprehension" questions is basically an imposition upon long-term memory. Pressure upon a reader to put more information through the slow and narrow entry into long-term memory may have the reverse effect; short- and long-term memories become jammed with trivial and incoherent pieces of information, and as a result the reader understands and remembers less. For this reason many books that a student of any age might read of his own volition out of school become unreadable within the educational context.

In any situation where an individual is anxious, or unsure of himself, or has experienced an unhappy succession of "failures," his behavior exhibits an inevitable consequence—he demands far more information before he makes a decision. His very hesitancy aggravates his difficulties, regardless of the material he is reading or his underlying reading ability. The more anxious he is, the less likely he is to rely on nonvisual information. The ironic consequence is that such demanding behavior makes the probability of error and of misunderstanding greater rather than less. Where the relaxed individual sees order, tenseness creates visual confusion. Whether the source of the unrealistic demand lies in the student himself or in the teacher, overdependence on visual information will overload the otherwise competent reader.

Related Issues

READING INSTRUCTION

The view of the reading process that I have outlined, and the general theories of language and language acquisition with which it is most compatible (e.g., McNeill, 1970; Slobin, 1971), contain several important implications for reading instruction. It is clear that a distinction should always be drawn between teaching and learning; that there can be no question of providing children with explicit "rules" for reading, because these rules are at an underlying level of language and not accessible to direct inspection.

Nevertheless many children do learn to read at school, suggesting that they can find the information that they need in reading instruction, even if this information is not what the teacher believes he is providing. This ability of some children to learn to read (and others never to learn) whatever the method of instruction points to a distinction between theories of reading and reading instruction often blurred in the literature. If the linguist or psychologist makes a theoretical advance, it is still not appropriate for him to insist upon a change on the part of the teacher, since anything that worked in the classroom before the theorist's insight will surely continue to work after. By the same token, a successful method of instruction does not "prove" anything for or against a theory of reading, since instructional methods may work (or not work) for reasons completely different from the rationale of the teacher.

The realization that much of our skill in language lies beneath the surface of the phenomenon suggests that the only way to learn reading is by reading (just as the only way in which a child learns spoken language is by talking and listening). (A number of these issues are discussed in Smith [1973], especially Chapters 12–16.)

It must be concluded that expectations about improving the quality of reading instruction are unlikely to be realized through the production of new methods of instruction. Instead, a better understanding is required on the part of educators generally about the nature of the reading process. There can be no "psycholinguistic method" of teaching reading (Smith & Goodman, 1971); rather the nature of the reading process, and of learning to read, must be better comprehended by the teacher himself so that he can respond more directly and appropriately to the specific information needs of children learning to read.

SECOND-LANGUAGE LEARNING

Many of the previous assertions concerning the relationship of writing to speech and the distinction between deep and surface structure are relevant to second-language learning. It is still widely assumed that translation involves a simple "decoding" from the surface structure of one language to the surface structure of another (despite the failure to develop automatic computer translation systems). It is often believed that foreign languages are understood when one "decodes" from them into one's own spoken language. But translation requires the determination of underlying structure just as much as reading (and as the comprehension of one's native tongue). The surface structure of the target language lacks the same information as written text or native speech. The same limitations upon information processing and memory apply to second language comprehension.

Chomsky and Halle's assertion that the orthography of English does not bother to tell the speaker what he already knows about his native language is clearly relevant—it is precisely this "implicit" knowledge that the non-English speaker does not possess. For the non-native speaker, the surface structure of writing is an inadequate representation of both the sound structure of the target language and its meaning. Learning the underlying structure of the target language is as much of a bootstrap operation as the initial process of learning a mother tongue. There is no facile way in which any language learner can be "told" the rules that he needs in order to learn.

FURTHER SOURCES

The journal *Reading Research Quarterly* has published the results of extensive literature searches into (1) language models and reading, (2) learning to read, and (3) the reading process, as part of the United States Right to Read program. The report by Athey (1971), centers particularly upon the type of linguistic theory and psycholinguistic analysis outlined in this chapter.

Several summary chapters by linguists and psychologists whose work is central to much of this chapter appear in Levin and Williams (1970) and in Smith (1973), and there is a more developed and integrated general theory of the relation between comprehension and learning in Smith (1975). The present chapter does not represent the only current view of reading and of the relationship between spoken and written language. For a vigorous defense of the three "conventional" assumptions that this chapter has tried to refute, see Gough (1972).

References

Athey, I. J. Language models and reading. *Reading Research Quarterly*, 1971, 7, 16–110.

Bach, E., & Harms, R. (Eds.) *Universals in linguistic theory.* New York: Holt, 1968.

Berdiansky, B., Cronnell, B., & Koehler, J. Spelling-sound relations and primary form-class descriptions for speech-comprehension vocabularies of 6–9 year olds. Technical Report No. 15, Southwest Regional Laboratory for Educational Research and Development, 1969.

Brown, H. D. Categories of spelling difficulty in speakers of English as a first and second language. *Journal of Verbal Learning and Verbal Behavior*, 1970, 9, 232–236.

Chomsky, C. Reading, writing, and phonology. *Harvard Educational Review*, 1970, 40, 287–309.

Chomsky, N. *Aspects of the theory of syntax.* Cambridge, Mass.: MIT Press, 1965.

Chomsky, N. *Cartesian linguistics.* New York: Harper, 1966.

Chomsky, N., & Halle, M. *The sound pattern of English.* New York: Harper, 1968.

Fillmore, C. J., & Langendoen, D. T. *Studies in linguistic semantics.* New York: Holt, 1971.

Goodman, K. S. Analysis of oral reading miscues: applied psycholinguistics. *Reading Research Quarterly,* 1969, *5,* 9—30.

Gough, P. One second of reading. In J. F. Kavanagh & I. G. Mattingly (Eds.), *Language by ear and by eye: The relationships between speech and reading.* Cambridge, Mass.: MIT Press, 1972.

Johnson, D. D. *Vowel cluster-phoneme correspondences in 20,000 English words.* ERIC Document 039 092. Madison, Wisconsin: University of Wisconsin Research and Development Center, 1969.

Joos, M. The five clocks. *International Journal of American Linguistics, Monographs,* 1962, No. 28.

Kolers, P. A. Reading is only incidentally visual. In K. S. Goodman & J. T. Fleming (Eds.), *Psycholinguistics and the teaching of reading.* Newark, Del.: Int. Reading Ass., 1969.

Labov, W. The logic of nonstandard English. In F. Williams (Ed.), *Language and Poverty.* Chicago: Markham, 1970.

Levin, H., & Williams, J. P. (Eds.) *Basic studies on reading.* New York: Basic Books, 1970.

McNeill, D. *The acquisition of language.* New York: Harper, 1970.

Mathews, M. M. *Teaching to read: Historically considered.* Chicago: Univ. of Chicago Press, 1966.

Miller, G. A. *Language and communication.* New York: McGraw-Hill, 1951.

Miller, G. A. Some preliminaries to psycholinguistics. *American Psychologist,* 1965, *20,* 15—20.

Reed, D. W. A theory of language, speech, and writing. In H. Singer & R. B. Ruddell (Eds.), *Theoretical models and processes of reading.* Newark, Del.: Int. Reading Ass., 1970.

Slobin, D. I. *Psycholinguistics.* Glenview, Ill.: Scott, Foresman, 1971.

Smith, F. *Understanding reading.* New York: Holt, Rinehart and Winston, 1971.

Smith, F. *Psycholinguistics and reading.* New York: Holt, Rinehart and Winston, 1973.

Smith, F. *Comprehension and learning,* New York: Holt, 1975.

Smith, F., & Goodman, K. S. On the psycholinguistic method of teaching reading. *Elementary School Journal,* 71, 177—181.

Smith, F., & Holmes, D. L. The independence of letter, word, and meaning identification in reading. *Reading Research Quarterly,* 1971, *6,* 394—414.

Torrey, J. Illiteracy in the ghetto. *Harvard Educational Review,* 1970, *40,* 253—259.

Venezky, R. L. English orthography: Its graphical structure and its relation to sound. *Reading Research Quarterly,* 1967, *2,* 75—106.

Wardhaugh, R. *Reading: A linguistic perspective.* New York: Harcourt, 1969.

Whitford, H. C. *A dictionary of American homophones and homographs.* New York: Columbia Univ. Teacher's college, 1966.

21. Specific Developmental Dyslexia

Macdonald Critchley

Learning disability is a vogue expression in the contemporary family setting. It covers a diversity of problems, some of them endogenous, others the product of environmental factors. Delay in the acquisition of reading skills looms very large in this context, and here again a variety of etiological circumstances may be discerned leading to a like number of "types" of reading retardation. Set firmly within this complexity, like gold in a nugget, there can be isolated a group of cases where the *dyslexia*—the term currently employed—is *specific*, i.e., it stands alone; and it is developmental, i.e., genetically determined. Unpropitious environmental circumstances may further hinder a particular dyslexic's scholastic progress, but they are definitely not causative. This type of dyslexia is independent of intellectual status, of perceptual defects, and of behavioral aberrations. Brain damage, even of minimal degree, plays no role. This, then, is the setting for a discussion of specific developmental dyslexia.

The condition has been defined by the World Federation of Neurology as follows:

A disorder manifested by difficulty in learning to read despite conventional instruction, adequate intelligence, and sociocultural opportunity. It is dependent from fundamental cognitive disabilities which are frequently of constitutional origin.

It constitutes one of the principal—although not the commonest—causes of delay in learning to read.

The history of our ideas about this entity dates from an analogy with dysphasic loss of the ability to recognize the meaning of graphic symbols. Possibly the first mention of this defect was by Johannes Schmidt in 1676. It received but little attention until the middle of the last century, by which time aphasia or dysphasia had assumed an important role in brain pathology. By 1865 it became pretty firmly established that lesions of the middle two-thirds of the dominant cerebral hemisphere were liable to be followed, not only by a contralateral hemiplegia, but also by a difficulty in communication. The pattern of this speech impairment varied considerably from one patient to another. Roughly speaking, the more forward the situation of the lesion, the more likely it was that the principal linguistic defect would consist in a difficulty in expressing ideas and wishes both by articulate utterance and by way of writing. Rather later it became apparent that more posteriorly sited lesions could be followed by fewer expressive troubles but greater problems in the perception of the meaning of speech. Indeed, it ultimately came to light that some patients, as the result of acquired brain disease, might lose their ability to read, whether silently or aloud, the power of articulate utterance being spared. Moreover, there were cases where the patient could express himself quite adequately on paper, but without afterward being able to read back what he had written.

As a rule, the inability to comprehend graphic symbols was not total. The dysphasic patient might be able to identify a word (or a letter) here and there, and not necessarily a short or commonplace word. That is to say, confronted with a sheet of newsprint he might fail to discern meaning in the brief prepositions or articles, and yet identify a polysyllabic and relatively unfamiliar word. This was not invariable, however, and indeed the dysphasic's performance might fluctuate from day to day. Provided the letters or words were printed in large enough type, the patient could sometimes hit on the meaning by resorting to the device of tracing the outlines with his fingertip, or even by sweeping his gaze slowly and carefully over them.

These receptive disorders attracted the attention of such aphasiologists as Dejerine and Broadbent, and gradually the term *word-blindness* entered the literature. In Stuttgart, however, Professor Berlin preferred to use the Greek equivalent, "dyslexia."

In 1895 a Glasgow oculist, James Hinshelwood, became interested in this subject and published a number of such cases in an article in the *Lancet*.

This communication prompted Dr. Pringle Morgan, a general practitioner in Seaford, where there were, and still are, several preparatory schools, to publish the case of a boy who, though very intelligent, was quite unable to master the art of reading. Had all his instruction been given orally, he said, this boy would have been top of his form. Could it be, Pringle Morgan went on, that one is dealing here with a case of "congenital word-blindness"?

At about the same time, and quite independently, a school medical officer of Bradford also mentioned in his official report in 1896 the existence of a group of children with this same syndrome of congenital word-blindness.

The foregoing story represents the "discovery" of a variety of delayed acquisition of speech, comparable with the cases of children who were late talkers, and also those rare instances of congenital auditory imperception.

The medical profession accepted readily and with considerable interest this conception of an inherent and specific defect in acquiring the ability to recognize meaning within the printed or written characters placed before them. The difficulty was one of transmodal integration, for the task that proved so onerous was to correlate the meaning and the acoustic properties with the visual appearances of words that were quite familiar to the child in their oral usage.

As interest grew, other features emerged. It became obvious that this disability was often familial in its appearance, and, furthermore, that boys were more often affected than girls. As a natural corollary of the difficulties in reading, considerable defects became obvious in the written compositions of those who had painfully acquired some mastery over letters and some simpler words.

The story then temporarily switched away from the neurological scene. It became obvious to teachers and educators that the population of poor readers and spellers within the community was not inconsiderable. Figures ranging from 10—15% of all school children were mentioned as belonging here. Scrutiny of these cases revealed that they were diverse in nature and etiology, and that they did not all conform with the characteristics of the congenital word-blindness (or dyslexia) familiar to the medical profession. Some of the late readers were frankly dullards; others were emotionally disturbed by reason of a variety of circumtances; others were clearly brain-damaged. Others, again, had been deprived in a culturo-educational sense, having had little or no schooling, or else instruction that was faulty as regards technique. The conception grew up of a continuum of poor readers, ranging from those at one end of the scale who were of low intellectual caliber, while at the other extreme were youngsters of adequate or high IQ but who were virtually problems within the province of child psychiatry.

Unfortunately, the neurological type of case, where there is a genetically determined and specific type of learning disability, was only too often passed over through unfamiliarity or, indeed, even regarded as nonexistent.

The scene has changed now, and it is widely accepted, if not universally so, that within this spectrum of poor readers there lies a hard core of cases. These constitute the problem that is today spoken of as "specific developmental dyslexia."

The main hallmarks of such cases are to be found in the definition given at the outset.

1. *Intelligence.* Specific developmental dyslexia is not the product of inadequate mental caliber. Indeed the cases most readily recognized occur in children of high average and often superior IQ.

2. *Perceptual disorders.* The developmental dyslexic shows no visual or ocular defect. True, a recording of the eye movements may be anomalous, but these abnormalities are the product, not the *cause*, of the difficulty in reading. Again, audiometry typically shows no defect. This is not to deny, however, that in some dyslexics an element of dysphonemia may at times be demonstrable.

3. Inadequate teaching is not responsible for specific developmental dyslexia. However, it is only common sense that a dyslexic's halting progress with reading will be still further hindered if the techniques employed are unsatisfactory.

4. Unpropitious sociocultural background is not the cause of developmental dyslexia, and when such a state of affairs exists within a dyslexic's environment, it is coincidental.

5. Specific developmental dyslexia is a cognitive disorder—a defect of transmodal integration—as has already been stated. The etiology is uncertain, but the most convincing hypothesis to date is that of a delayed maturation of this particular aspect of cerebral development within the wider ambit of language acquirement.

The presence of neurotic symptoms or of emotional disturbance must not be regarded as being etiologically significant in cases of specific developmental dyslexia. The temptation to invoke the trauma of domestic disharmony—families disrupted by divorce or bereavement; one or more callous, cruel, or drunken parents—must be resisted. Such environmental circumstances, if they exist, cannot provoke what is actually an endogenous, genetically determined developmental delay, however much they interfere with the dyslexic's struggle to cope with a difficult and perhaps distasteful item within the school curriculum.

As years go by, however, the child with specific developmental dyslexia is all too liable to develop increasing ideas of inferiority and frustration. Several reactive patterns of behavior may result: undue dependence on the mother; projection into athletic prowess and gamesmanship; attention seeking by way of clowning and buffoonery; occasionally the development of psychosomatic troubles, habit spasms, and even school phobia. Most important of all is aggression, which may slip readily into juvenile delinquency.

The foregoing do not necessarily develop, of course. With advancing enlightment within the community, they are likely to become much rarer as recognition of the essential nature of the entity is made more often, more confidently, and at an earlier age. The establishment and acceptance of this diagnosis within the family and the school will act favorably. Early skilled, remedial teaching at the hands of experienced and specially trained staff will both expediate the attainment of reading skill and at the same time avert untoward emotional reactions. Finally, two qualities within the dyslexic himself will materially help his progress and ward off neuroses. *Ceteris paribus*, the higher the dyslexic's IQ, the more likely he is to overcome his initial difficulties. Even more important is the innate factor of ambition, enthusiasm, and sheer determination to master his problems.

The point deserves reemphasis. Emotional disturbances are secondary phenomena and not primary or causative factors.

The suspicion that a very young child is likely to prove to be a case of specific developmental dyslexia usually first arises in the infants' school. The teacher is puzzled because of the discrepancy between the young pupil's good personality and obvious intelligence, and his surprising difficulty in mastering his letters. He steadily falls behind others of his age in acquiring the arts of reading and writing.

The wise teacher will alert the parents, who in their turn would do well to consult their family doctor. This is so because the diagnosis—and more particularly, the differential diagnosis—of cases of reading retardation is a medical issue, often far from easy. After eliminating defects of vision and of hearing, and confirming, psychometrically if need be, that this child is of at least normal intellectual endowment, the doctor next has to distinguish between the various types of reading delay. He will in all likelihood be well acquainted with the family situation. He probably is also fully conversant with the perinatal circumstances and the medical history and rate of development of the putative dyslexic in his infancy.

One of the principal conditions to be eliminated is so-called "minimal brain damage." To exclude this, it is necessary to secure information as to the state of the mother during her pregnancy; factors of prematurity; details of the labor; the immediate neonatal condition of the infant; its rate of motor, mental, and speech development; and the health of the child during its first 3 or 4 years of life.

Finally, a most detailed neurological examination is required, with a search for any of the subtle physical signs that indicate underlying structural brain pathology.

The diagnosis of specific developmental dyslexia can rarely be established with confidence in a child below the age of 7. An exception can be made in the case of a child belonging to a family where a parent or one or more older siblings is a known dyslexic. In such cases, certain phenomena may prove predictive rather than diagnostic.

"Soft neurological signs" is the odd expression sometimes used to describe what an extended physical examination may bring to light. Some of these, at least, are evidences of cerebral immaturity, and might be expected to fade as the young dyslexic grows older. Among these findings one may enumerate:

1. Difficulty in telling the time until a relatively late age. Ordinarily, in Great Britain, a child learns to read a clock at the age of 6 or 7. Delay in acquiring this art may often represent a sort of herald sign of dyslexia.

2. *Infirm cerebral dominance.* By the employment of an extensive battery of tests, it may be found that the dyslexic is a crossed-lateral, or perhaps has an ambiguous type of manual preference. This, again, is perhaps a mark of delayed maturation, and a longitudinal or follow-up study may show that the dyslexic undergoes a steady change and settles down to an ultimate unilateral cerebral dominance, whether left-sided or right.

3. A tendency to confuse lateral dimensions in personal and extrapersonal space. Although this improves as the dyslexic grows older, a mild confusion between right and left, east and west, port and starboard may persist throughout adult life.

Disorders of Writing

As belatedly and hesitatingly the child progresses, despite his initial difficulties with reading, considerable errors show themselves in the written language. The child will learn to copy well enough, and even to transcribe from one style of type to another. The essential difficulties show themselves in writing to dictation and even more so in spontaneous creative writing. As regards the latter, there is an overall reluctance to put pen to paper. Should this task be insisted on, it is found that the dyslexic finds difficulty in expressing himself scriptorially, although he can perhaps do so well in articulate speech. Naturally this contrast shows itself only in the older age group, where a certain competence in reading has been achieved.

It is possible to analyze in great detail the errors typical of the written work of dyslexics. Here it will suffice to enumerate merely some of the principal defects. The child's penmanship is often faulty, being immature and untidy. Individual letters may be poorly constructed so as at times to be scarcely legible. The act of writing is noticeably slow.

Inaccurate spelling is the most conspicuous fault, and in all dyslexics the spelling age lies distinctly below the reading age. It is unnecessary to enumerate every type of error these dyslexics perpetrate. Although some of the mistakes are bizarre in the extreme, it is usually possible to discern some underlying pattern in them. Thus rotations of individual letters (*d* being confused with *b*) are frequent, with a tendency toward the reversal of short-word clusters. With longer words, imperfect serialization is shown in the employment of the right letters but in the wrong order. Other spelling mistakes are essentially phonetic in character, and in an English-speaking dyslexic these are manifold. Letters may be omitted altogether, as well as groups of letters and syllables; this, rather than elongation of the word, is the rule.

The net result is often not wholly comprehensible even to the parents who are accustomed to receiving weekly letters from their dyslexic youngsters away at their preparatory schools. Furthermore, the child himself, confronted with his own written work, may not be able to interpret it with confidence.

Spelling disabilities continue to show themselves long after the dyslexic has "caught up" with his reading and has reached the stage at which he can read for pleasure. These "ex-dyslexics," as they may be termed, belong, of course, to late teenage or adolescent age groups, who have made considerable strides either as the result of special remedial training, or spontaneously by dint of a combination of ambition, sheer doggedness, and superior intellectual caliber. Although now perhaps in the category of avid readers, they may prove on scrutiny to be both slow and inaccurate in their accomplishment. They find it somewhat embarrassing to read aloud, because the simultaneous task of correct pronunciation and exact comprehension is not easy. Foreign languages in their written form are always peculiarly difficult, although they can be picked up by ear well enough.

The eventual mastery of reading is a somewhat fragile achievement and may temporarily deteriorate in circumstances of stress or during intercurrent neurotic illness.

These "ex-dyslexics" usually remain inaccurate spellers throughout life, a circumstance that may handicap them unfairly during written examinations. Thereafter they can often cover up by resort to dictation rather than writing. Often spelling unorthodoxies linger on as an aberration accepted by the family as something of a joke.

22. Literacy as a Mode of Communication on the Warm Spring Indian Reservation[1]

Susan U. Philips

In this chapter, reading and writing are together treated as a mode of communication—the literate mode—one among many modes that may be part of any speech community's communicative repertoire. Specific examples of the social uses of literacy on the Warm Springs Indian Reservation, in central Oregon, are used to demonstrate the ways in which a view of literacy as a mode of communication can contribute to our understanding of cultural variation in patterns of use of different modes of communication, and to the development of workable literacy programs in formal education.

Introduction

In recent years social scientists have devoted increasing attention to the acquisition of communicative competence in children. Much of the sociolinguistic research in this area has focused on the interaction between school and community, as evidenced by the work of Basil Bernstein on elaborated and restricted codes (Bernstein, 1972), of William Labov on the use and non-use of Non-Standard English (NSE) in the classroom (Labov, 1974), of Courtney Cazden and Vera John

[1] I would like to express my appreciation to Rudy Clements, Lloyd Smith, and Dennis Leonard of the Warm Springs Tribal Education Department and to Darryl Wright, Assistant Superintendent of the Jefferson County School District, for increasing my awareness of the educational needs of the people of Warm Springs; to Dell and Virginia Hymes for their general contribution to clarification of thoughts on communication at Warm Springs, to Erving Goffman for a careful reading of the manuscript, and to the National Science Foundation for past research support.

on different styles of learning in North American Indian communities (Cazden & John, 1968), and by recent collections focusing on language usage in the class- room, such as that of Cazden, Hymes, and John (1973).

Perhaps of most general relevance has been the increasing recognition of the diversity of codes and speech styles within any given speech community (Hymes, 1970, p. 308), and the awareness that the acquisition of competence in any range or combination of these depends in part on the particular social contexts in which a child is raised and trained to be a participant. This emphasis on diversity has in turn led to an awareness that school systems can no longer assume that all students come into the schools with a shared background of communicative skills that will be further developed and/or relied upon for the transmission of various sorts of knowledge in the classroom. Rather, they come from diverse speech communities, differing in dialect, in notions of what is socially appropriate speech, and in degrees of familiarity with the dialect and notions of socially appropriate communica- tion that are dominant in the classroom situation.

The major implication of this is a new awareness that children entering schools without having already acquired the communicative competencies that the school assumes will have difficulty learning what is being taught. They will not be able to understand what is going on in the classroom, and they will have difficulty participating in the learning process, because the required modes for participation will be unfamiliar to them.[2]

In light of this orientation, it is surprising that the one aspect of communicative competence on which schools focus considerable attention, namely literacy, or reading and writing, has not received much attention from sociolinguists. There *is* recognition that literacy programs can entail an important practical application of knowledge derived from sociolinguistic research (Fishman, 1972). But until recently (Basso, 1975; Hymes, 1973; Kochman, MS), literacy has not been recog- nized as a mode of communication that may, like the verbal mode, have specialized social functions that vary cross-culturally in ways we should understand, if the goal of literacy through formal education is to be achieved for any given group of people.

In Goody's "Introduction" to *Literacy in Traditional Societies* (Goody, 1968), he considers the significance of writing in human culture:

The importance of writing lies in its creating a new medium of communica- tion between men. Its essential service is to objectify speech, to provide language

---

[2]What follows from this in the way of changes in classroom procedure is subject to debate. On the one hand, schools may consciously attempt to instruct the students formally in the modes of com- municative competence used in the schools with which they are not familiar. Such an approach is exemplified by programs being developed to instruct speakers of Non-Standard English (NSE) in Standard English (SE). On the other hand, schools may attempt to modify teaching methods in such a way as to approximate more closely the modes of communication with which students are already familiar in their community. The hiring of Blacks to teach Blacks and Indians to teach Indians can be interpreted as an effort to move in this direction. However, this approach remains as yet largely unexplored.

*with a material correlative, a set of visible signs. In this material form speech can
be transmitted over space and preserved over time; what people say and think can
be rescued from the transitoriness of oral communication.
The range of human intercourse can now be greatly extended both in time and
in space [pp. 1—2.].*

Given the potential usefulness of literacy, Goody asks why literacy has been
"restricted," or the skills of reading and writing accessible to only a few in
some traditional societies. And he suggests an approach that will answer this
question.

*One way of tackling the problem is to explore the "ethnography" of literacy in
"traditional" or preindustrial societies, to analyse in detail the uses made of writing in a particular social setting to approach the question from the standpoint not so
much of the library scholar but of the field worker with experience of the concrete context of written communication [p. 2].*

Goody then goes on to document cultural situations in which reading and writing
were used only for specific purposes, under the control of persons in highly defined
roles, and he suggests reasons behind these kinds of specificity. For example, the
ritual leader and teacher may orally transmit the contents of sacred texts which
only he can read.

*The GURU tradition is characteristic of situations of restricted literacy, where
the role of the teacher as the mediator of knowledge is given pre-eminent importance. He adds personal charisma to book-learning, in a combination of oral and
literate modes of communication [p. 13].*

Goody, then, sensitizes us to the special inherent features of communication
through writing (i.e., preservation over time and transmission through space), and
to the variation in the social functions of "restricted" literacy in "traditional"
societies. And in these respects, he has developed an orientation very much like
the one advocated here.

However, it is difficult to find reasons for limiting analysis to situations of
restricted literacy in traditional societies. To begin with, one is likely to encounter
diversity in the uses of literacy within any given society where literacy exists,
whether there is only restricted literacy (which we take to mean that only some
people can read) or full literacy (where everyone can read and write to some
degree). In the latter case, one will always find that different people use reading
and writing for different purposes and are "literate" to varying degrees in various
uses of literacy.

It might be possible to argue that in societies where literacy was not traditional,
and has been introduced only through contact with the Western European tradition
of literacy uses, one would encounter merely an unrevealing imitation and

duplication of that tradition. However, as later discussion of literacy on the Warm Springs Reservation should demonstrate, it is more likely that in each of the various cultural situations into which literacy is introduced, there will be culturally varying responses to different uses of literacy and innovation in usage. The overall pattern of usage, then, will be distinctive to the group adopting it.

In addition, to more effectively account for why one encounters the particular patterns of usage that one does, it may be more instructive to view literacy as one of the many modes of communication comprising the communicative repertoire of a community rather than to view the functions of literacy in isolation. Thus, just as sociolinguists have heretofore considered the functions of different linguistics codes within a given community (Blom & Gumpetz, 1972; Gumperz, 1972), one would consider the functions of different modes of communication (verbal, non-verbal, literate) in the same way.

In this regard, it is especially useful to keep in mind what the inherent potentialities and limitations of any given mode of communication are and how these affect the role it may play in communication. Mention has already been made of the potential for preservation of literate communication through time. There are other inherent features of literacy, not all of which would be considered "advantageous." For example, as Goody and Watt point out (1968, pp. 59—60), reading is essentially a solitary activity. The same holds true of writing. And not only does one do these activities alone, but also to the exclusion of other physical activities. Verbal communication, in contrast, is done in the immediate presence of and with other people, and can be maintained while doing other kinds of activities.

From this, one can see that where reading and writing are being introduced into a nonliterate society, they will be replacing other activities, in terms of how people spend their time. How likely reading and writing are to be taken up would depend considerably on how valued are the activities they might replace. This kind of issue would be especially relevant in the development of educational programs in literacy.

It may be useful, then, to consider how the inherent features of one mode of communication differ from those of another mode in ways that affect the uses of literacy in a given community. It may also be useful to consider what the particular functional needs of a community are and through what modes of communication those needs might best be met. If, for example, one lived in a society where everyone whom one knew was within walking distance, one would have no motivation to learn how to read and write for the purpose of writing letters (unless a value was placed on indirect communication), because one would have no need to write letters in order to communicate. This example should also indicate how communicative needs may be closely related to the social structure of a given community.

Finally, it is also important to consider the cultural attitudes toward different modes of communication. In discussions of factors involved in selecting a "national language" for a given country where feelings about cultural or national identity are closely bound up with the language one speaks, it is recognized that a group's attitudes toward a given verbal code or language must be understood and taken into consideration in determining what language is to be selected as the national language (Fishman, 1968). The same sort of orientation is useful in understanding why and when reading and writing, rather than speaking and listening, are used for communication; attitudes toward the literate and spoken modes may often run counter to what would be expected on the basis of the inherent potentialities and limitations of particular modes and the communicative needs of a given group of people.

To summarize this perspective on literacy, I would note the following: 1) Literacy can be viewed as one among many modes of communication used by members of any given society; 2) The use of literacy is related to the use of other modes of communication. How different modes are used relative to one another is determined in part by the inherent limitations and potentialities of different modes of communication. But the use of different modes is also related to the social organization, communicative needs, and language attitudes of different societies; 3) The uses of a literate mode of communication will thus vary within a given society, and also cross-culturally.

The usefulness of this perspective can best be demonstrated through description of the functions of literacy in particular communities. In the discussion to follow, an effort is made to provide both a description of some of the social uses of literacy on the Warm Springs Indian Reservation, and an analysis of the ways such description can contribute to the development of literacy programs.

Literacy on the Warm Springs Indian Reservation: An Introduction

The Warm Springs Indian Reservation is located in the high plateau country of central Oregon. The Indian population of approximately 2000 is descended from three groups who presently call themselves Warm Springs, Wasco, and Paiute. The Warm Springs Indians, who aboriginally spoke a Sahaptin dialect, are the largest group, with the Wasco, formerly speakers of a dialect of Chinookan, next largest in size.

Both groups were moved onto the reservation, when it was established in 1855, from areas to the north as far as the Columbia River 50 miles away. They continued to move back and forth between the reservation and the Columbia River until their fishing sites were destroyed by dam construction in the 1950s. Although the two groups spoke different languages, and differed culturally in some respects, they were neighbors traditionally and shared much in the way of life style.

The Paiutes, numerically the smallest group today, originally lived in southeastern Oregon. They were settled on the reservation in the late 1870s, following a series of raids against both Indians and non-Indians already at Warm Springs.

Today there is considerable intermarriage among the three groups, as there has been in the past, and although they maintain a working awareness of their separate identities, these reservation propulations form an integrated community in many respects, particularly in the extent to which they are set apart from the surrounding white communities.

Published descriptions of the culture of the people in this area are not numerous. General area studies placing the Warm Springs Reservation people in the context of the Plateau cultural area complex would include notably the early work of Ray (1939), and the more recent work of Anastasio (1955). Perhaps the most detailed and recent cultural descriptions of Warm Springs people specifically are available in the works of anthropologists David and Katherine French (D. French, 1961; K. French, 1955), while attention to sociolinguistic description can be found in the work of Hymes (1966, 1972) and Philips (1970).

Formal efforts on the part of the Bureau of Indian Affairs (BIA) to educate the Warm Springs Indians in "white men's ways," which would, of course, include the teaching of English and of reading and writing, began soon after the reservation was created. The first school was established in 1862, and from the 1890s on, a BIA boarding school was in regular operation. In 1961, the public school system took over the operation of the BIA school, and a few years later boarding of students was completely discontinued.

Presently, Warm Springs Indian children attend the first six grades on the reservation, where almost all of the students are Indians. For the last six grades they are bused into the predominantly "white" town of Madras, 15 miles away from the nearest reservation border, where they are outnumbered by white students in a ratio of 5 : 1.

For our present purposes, it would be appropriate to stress that during this period of almost 100 years there has been an effort on the part of the school system to move the Warm Springs people from a completely nonliterate, or oral, cultural tradition to that of a combined oral and literate tradition. Moreover, this literary tradition has been based on English, rather than the Indian languages, and modeled after the tradition of the uses of literacy that derives from Western European culture.

Today, most of the Indians of Warm Springs speak English (although some continue to be bilingual, speaking Sahaptin or Wasco Chinook as well) and can read and write. However, the school administration and the tribal administration are not satisfied with the "degree" of their literacy skills; in this area, the Indian students consistently score lower than their white peers and lower than the national averages in tests designed to measure reading and verbal achievement (Zentner, 1960), from the time they take a reading readiness test in the first grade, on through high school.

Many attempts have been made and are being made to change this situation. A few of these attempts have indicated an awareness that literacy uses are socially patterned, whether or not the awareness was explicitly formulated in this way. For example, about a decade ago, it was recognized (as it apparently was for many minority groups at about that same time) that there are few magazines and books in Indian homes—"few" compared to white middle-class homes, presumably. It was also noted that very few Indian parents read stories to their children. Both the presence of reading materials in the home and the social activity of the story reading were felt to be important factors contributing to children's success in learning how to read and write in school. To introduce their "positive" effects into Indian homes at Warm Springs, VISTA workers were asked to go out into the community armed with books to read to the children.

The project was short-lived, and was not considered a success. The VISTA workers did not feel welcome in the Indian homes, and the Indian parents were in fact apparently not enthusiastic about the project. Many people at Warm Springs are somewhat weary of non-Indians coming to the reservation to tell them how they should run their lives, and such a project would be perceived by some as a case of this common-enough event, in spite of the fact that it was sponsored by the tribal administration. But, more relevant to our interests here, the project also represented an effort to introduce a white middle-class pattern of literacy uses into the Warm Springs culture. White middle-class parents perceive story-reading as a way of giving attention and affection to their children; to them it serves that function. Indian parents, however, have other ways of their own of giving attention and affection to their children and so would not have that motivation for reading to them.

The main flaw in the line of thinking that led to such a project lies in the assumption that children *need* this preschool experience to learn how to read easily. But the main reason they need it is because the design of most primary school reading programs *assumes* it and builds on it. It is "stories," accompanied by drawings depicting events in the stories, that children encounter in their first contact with literacy, regardless of whether the stories deal with white suburban children playing on the grass or black ghetto children playing on the streets. Why stories? The most obvious answer is that they are used because they are the form of literacy most familiar to the children. But this is true only of the white middle-class children.

This account of the story-reading project, then, introduces evidence that non-Indian social uses of literacy differ from those of Warm Springs Indians. It also indicates the relevance such differences can have for formal literacy programs.

A Comparative Analysis of Social Uses of Literacy

With this brief illustration in mind, let us approach the discussion of literacy in a more systematic fashion through further comparison between the reservation town of Warm Springs and the "white" off-reservation town of Madras. Such a comparison can be enlightening in several ways. The towns are similar in size. To the extent that the Indians have been under pressure to assimilate into non-Indian society (and the pressure here has been severe), the Madras population can be taken to represent most closely the culture of non-Indians to which the

Warm Springs Indians have been assimilating; the people in Madras are the type of non-Indians with whom the Indians have the most contact. And it is the Madras model for social uses of literacy (rather than that of urban Portland, Oregon, 100 miles away, for example) that is most available and most likely to be adopted by the originally nonliterate Indians, to the extent that their uses are based on available models.

Comparison of the two towns, then, should make most evident the ways in which the Warm Springs use of literacy continues to be culturally distinctive in spite of the hundred years of exposure to non-Indian patterns of usage. And, it should be most relevant in contributing to our understanding of the difference in "success" in the acquisition of the communicative skills of reading and writing between the Indian children and their non-Indian peers mentioned earlier.

The description of literacy uses is not intended to be comprehensive. Rather, attention will be given to the use of public signs as forms of written communication, and relatedly, to some of the cultural attitudes affecting the socially appropriate uses of literacy. Public signs, as treated here, include: 1) permanently fixed signs on or near public buildings, indicating their function or purpose; 2) street signs that indicate the names of streets; and 3) directional signs indicating how to get to named places.

These forms of written communication serve primarily to guide and direct people to particular places. They are relied upon most heavily by persons who are unfamiliar with the location of particular places in a strange town, but once this means of location has been used initially, it also later becomes relied upon by those familiar with the places for visual cuing in locating them. Types of indicators other than written signs are also used or can be used for such purposes, sometimes in combination with signs. For example, a store front can often be identified by its large plate glass windows and by items on display in them; specific types of gas station chains may always use the same colors and symbols on their buildings; and governmental buildings are often characterized by columned gray façades. Nevertheless, written signs typically play an important role in transmitting directional information in the United States.

The reading of public signs might appear at first to require little "skill," insofar as the vocabulary used in signs is familiar to most, and there is rarely complex sentence syntax to be mastered in the reading of signs. However, like many forms of written communication, signs require their own special types of reading skills. First of all, one must know what *kinds* of public signs are placed in what *types* of locations. For example, street name signs are always on corners, but conventions differ from city to city regarding which way the signs will face, and whether street numbers will be indicated on such signs; commercial buildings often bear neon signs, whereas government buildings rarely do. In addition, one must often be familiar with the rules involved in the abbreviated syntax of signs to comprehend their meaning. For example, a sign that reads *Lot Full*, placed in the appropriate context, must be understood to mean that a particular parking lot has no more spaces free for cars; and, one must be able to distinguish between the optional *Eat Here* and the obligatory *Stop* in the use of the imperative on signs.

Without these kinds of knowledge required for the use of signs, geographical mobility and access to important resources can be considerably restricted, as travelers in foreign countries, where sign conventions differ from the "native" conventions, are aware. The use of signs, then, while a simple skill in some respects, does have its special requirements, and can have very important functions in the day-to-day maintenance of people's lives.

There is considerable difference between the non-Indian town of Madras and the Indian town of Warm Springs in the extent to which public signs are used. While there are numerous signs throughout the town of Madras, of all the sorts mentioned above, there are relatively few of any kind in the town of Warm Springs.

This difference can in part be accounted for by differences in the social make-up of the two communities, and in part by differences in the kinds of public activities and social services that the two towns make available to people. With regard to social make-up, the Warm Springs Reservation is still primarily a kin-based social unit. Most of the Indians who live there were born there, and are descended from the aboriginal inhabitants of this Plateau area. Most of the socializing that is done is done with consanguineal and affinal kinsmen. Residents who were not born there and are not tribal members are usually related by marriage to those who are. For a number of reasons, housing for people who are not tribal members is rarely available, and priority in job hiring is given to tribal members. Of the small number of non-Indians working in the *town* of Warm Springs, most live in the town of Madras, and those who do not can only rent tribally owned homes in a part of the town that is somewhat set apart from the areas where most Indians live.

Of the people who live in Madras, in contrast, most were not born there, and few have kinsmen living in the town. Residence in the town is usually based on job availability, and circles of social contact are determined to a considerable degree by occupational and religious affiliations.

In terms of the public activities and social services available in the two towns, there is again considerable difference. Madras functions as a minor commercial center for the region around it. Its numerous stores draw their clientele from the surrounding rural farming area, including the reservation, and the nearest town with more services is an hour's drive from Madras. Madras also provides facilities for a variety of commercial forms of public entertainment including restaurants, bars, a bowling alley, and a movie theater. And, finally, it is the county seat for Jefferson County.

These facilities are used not only by the town residents and the surrounding rural population, but also by "strangers," mainly tourists, campers, and hunters traveling through the area via one of the two major highways giving access to central Oregon, which passes through both Madras and Warm Springs.

Warm Springs, in contrast, does not function as a commercial center in any of the respects mentioned above, in part, no doubt, because of federal laws regulating reservation commercial ventures. Along the main highway, which does not run through the center of town as it does in Madras, there are simply two gas stations and two restaurants in operation. There is one general store in the town located off the highway.

To the extent that signs serve the function of locating places for people who are unfamiliar with their location, it is possible in light of the above information to see why Warm Springs would have few signs. Because there are almost no people who move to Warm Springs as "strangers," there is little need to have signs indicating what buildings serve what functions or where certain facilities are. In a sense, everyone already knows or has been shown by his or her kinsmen as a child. One would have to infer that in this early learning, nonliterary modes of place location and identification become relied upon. Because the town provides very few services that would be of interest to people who are nonresidents, signs are not required, for the most part, for visitors passing through.

The few signs there are in the town of Warm Springs refer primarily to facilities that are used by both outsiders and local residents. Thus, whereas the facilities on the highway along which strangers travel are loaded with signs, the off-highway general store used by residents bears only a US post office sign. The community center and central BIA and tribal offices, where outsiders often meet with residents for business purposes, bear outside signs. But other buildings, housing facilities such as the day care center and tribal education offices, which are used primarily by residents, do not.

It is possible, then, to see a difference in use of signs in the two communities. In Warm Springs there is a distinction between public areas used for outsiders and strangers, and public areas used by residents. This is reflected in the use of signs. In Madras the distinction between "strangers" and "residents" is blurred, in part because strangers are always in the process of becoming residents, and in part because strangers and nonresidents use these areas in the same way that residents do. Again, this is reflected in the use of signs for all public areas.

In the effort to establish differences in use of signs, I have dealt thus far primarily with what one might term the "productive" use of signs. In other words, where Indians and non-Indians put signs has been discussed, and it has been maintained that Indians do not put them up, or produce them, for the same purposes. However, not enough has been said about the extent to which there is a difference in the "receptive" competence in sign usage, or in other words, in how frequently Indians as opposed to non-Indians read or use signs that already exist, in making their way from place to place.

The suggestion was made that Indian children learn to use non-literary cues in making their way around their own community when they are first taught by kinsmen, and that they continue to do so. There is some evidence that this is true also in their movements outside their own community. While residence in the Warm Springs community is highly stable, many people do a great deal of traveling around, especially during the summer. But the places they go to tend most often to be the same ones year after year and tend also to be places where other

Indians live or come together. Examples would include traditional fishing and berry-picking areas, other reservations, Indian pow-wows, and rodeos. Even in going to a new place, people are most likely to be accompanied by someone who has already been there. Children would then learn directly from the kinsmen with whom they travel now to find places. And this would be less likely to involve learning reliance on public signs than would be the case for the non-Indian children, whose parents are more often strangers in the places they visit. The skills that sign-reading involves, then, probably go largely unused by the Indians, with some few notable exceptions in widely traveled individuals. That these skills are not only not used but also not known by many, also seems likely.

In the preceding discussion, an effort has been made to approach the description of the use of signs in the manner proposed in the introduction. The differences between the two communities' usage of signs was described, and differences in the social structure of the two communities were put forth to account for the usage differences. We can now add to this the suggestion that what we have been considering here also falls in line with the type of analysis proposed, in that it demonstrates a difference in the communicative needs of the two communities and in the extent to which one mode of communication is used rather than another to meet the same needs in the community. More explicitly, because of the Warm Springs community composition and life style, Warm Springs Indians do not need signs to direct strangers to public places: there are few strangers in town; many public places in Warm Springs are not intended for use by strangers; and finally, the people themselves rarely go as strangers to new places. They do not, then, have the communicative need for sign use that the people in Madras do.

However, people in both communities rely upon *some* kind of visual cuing to make their way from place to place, even after they have first been there. In Madras, public signs are used. In Warm Springs, nonliterary cues like topographical features and structural shapes are relied upon more. Thus we see that although in this respect the communicative needs are the same, the non-Indians continue to rely upon written symbolization for information, whereas the Indians rely upon visual input of a nonlinguistic nature. We would say that in this case different modes of communication are being used to meet the same kind of need.

But not all of the differences in patterns of literacy use can best be understood in terms of communicative needs interpreted within the framework of the social structure of a community, even in this limited discussion of the use of public signs. Sometimes modes of communication are used or fail to be used in ways that run counter to what would be considered most "effective" from the point of view of the outsider. Culturally learned notions of what is the most appropriate mode of communication for a given social activity may figure significantly in accounting for patterns of usage.

For example, in Warm Springs, the Christian churches that were established by white missionaries on the reservation, and which presently have Indian congregations, have written signs outside identifying them. The Indian religious centers for the Worship Dance and Shaker Church do not. This difference cannot be accounted for in terms of the preceding lines of reasoning: both the non-Indian and Indian-derived religions are participated in mainly by people from the community, so there is little need to identify them. However, both, under different circumstances, sometimes host groups invited from outside the community. According to the arguments already presented, either both kinds of places should have signs, or neither should, being similar in the relevant respects that have been considered so far.

But there is a sense in which Christian churches by definition and tradition have signs, whereas Indian religious centers do not. There is in Western Christianity a strong tradition of authority being invested in the written word, and of use of written materials in religious services. The most obvious example is the use of the Bible as representing "the word" of God. But there are other, present-day, evidences of use of written materials in the role that hymnals and even "programs" play in religious services.

In the Indian religions mentioned, although they have been strongly influenced by Christian beliefs, there is an equally strong oral tradition. The Indian position articulated by some is that God put "the word" into people's *heads* because they could not read the Bible. It is held that if one has a good heart and a good head, he will remember the songs and teachings. In many respects the Indian religions are "the same" as Christianity, from the Indians' point of view; it is held, however, that different peoples have different religious ways or paths, and the Indian (as opposed to the white) way, as received by them from God, was to be "shown" through dreams and visions, which are then told to others who remember them and pass them on orally.

There is a sense in which to write these Indian teachings down and read them in the Western way would be to do violence to their sacredness. It is difficult to suggest what might be analogous in non-Indian experience, where memorization is rarely valued. But perhaps the non-Indian would be as struck by the inappropriateness of an adult having to read aloud the "Pledge of Allegiance" or the "Star Spangled Banner," as the Indian would be by the reading of sacred songs, even though many more people would be able to join in on the Indian singing. For both Anglo and Indian there would be the sense that to read the words rather than to know them "by heart" indicates less strength of feeling and less true belief in what is being uttered.

Behind this difference in the use of public signs for religious institutions with which we began, then, are two different cultural traditions, and in each the attitudes about the social appropriateness of the use of written communication in the context of religious activities are very different indeed.

The preceding discussion should provide some indication of the relevance of attitudes toward different modes of communication in our understanding of why different modes are used in the ways in which they are in a given cultural context.

The relatively infrequent use of public signs in the Warm Springs community and the absence of use of literacy in Indian religious activities have one very important consequence that deserves mention here. They serve to keep "outsiders" out of the community, and to keep them relatively uninformed about the nature of traditional Indian activities on the reservation. Non-Indians passing through the reservation are sometimes curious about the Indians. They want to see what they look like and how they live. The lack of signs in the community, combined with the unfamiliar and unusual sociospatial arrangement, discourages these tourists from exploring for these purposes, because they cannot tell what is located where, and are uncertain about what they will encounter. Though the tribe often formally sponsors or hosts groups that are interested in learning more about the reservation, many people feel that random exploration by tourists subjects them to examination akin to that given animals in the zoo. So this discouragement is all to the good, although it is probably not done deliberately by the residents of Warm Springs.

The absence of the use of literacy in relgious activities is more deliberate. In addition to the religious justifications for maintaining an oral tradition, there is also the motivation to keep certain kinds of knowledge of the religion within the Indian community, and not have it spread to non-Indians. Although such knowledge can be spread verbally, there is greater control over who has access to the information and the uses to which it is devoted than would be the case if it were written down.

There are probably several reasons why the people want to keep this information to themselves. One important reason is the religious persecution they have experienced at the hands of the non-Indians. For many years Indian doctors, or shamans, were arrested and punished for practicing their medicine. Information that has passed out of the community has consistently been misunderstood, and this misunderstanding has brought ridicule and humiliation to the people. It is easy to understand why they are reluctant to share what they know with non-Indians by allowing it to be written down. One might argue that sharing the information could contribute to the opposite effect—increasing understanding and respect— but there is little precedent in the Warm Springs people's experience to cause them to view this as probable.

From these observations, it is possible to see how certain inherent potentialities of literacy, in this case its potential for being freed of the original communicator or message-sender and reaching a greater number of people, can be perceived as disadvantageous, as well as advantageous. Here the disadvantage from the Warm Springs people's point of view, would be that written communication is less subject to control over who uses it and the uses to which it is put than is verbal communication.

Some Implications for Literacy Programs

In this discussion of some aspects of the social uses of literacy on the Warm Springs Indian Reservation, an attempt has been made to demonstrate (1) some ways in which uses of literacy will vary cross-culturally, even in a situation where there has been and is tremendous pressure for a minority group with an oral tradition to adopt in toto the specific tradition of literacy of the dominant culture; and (2) how our understanding of cultural variation in patterns of social usage of literacy can be increased by attention to variation in communicative needs, the functioning of different modes of communication, *among* them the literate mode, in meeting those needs, and the ways in which differences in social structure and cultural attitudes toward different modes of communication and their inherent potentialities can account for such variability.

There yet remains the task of indicating further the relevance such an analysis may have for programs of formal instruction in reading and writing.

Returning first to the educational situation at Warm Springs, we recall that people in the community are concerned about increasing the ease with which the Indian children acquire the communicative skills of reading and writing and that, among other things, they have tried changing literacy usage patterns by introducing the reading of stories to children into Indian homes.

The role of public sign usage in the acquisition of literacy skills is in some ways similar to that of stories; whereas non-Indian children are likely to be motivated to learn how to read signs by observing their parents' reliance upon them, and would become familiar with written symbolization by having their attention drawn to signs, Indian children would be less inclined to do so. In addition, just as the non-Indian Children are motivated to imitate their parents and test their literacy skills by reading stories to their parents, they are often eager to try to make out the meaning of signs when they are first learning how to read. The use of signs differs from that of stories for non-Indian children, in that it is not made use of in the classroom, but the experience they gain in reading signs is a kind of outside "practice" that feeds back into their classroom learning. These things would not be true to the same degree for the Indian children.

However, there is *more* of a precedent for Indian children reading signs and coming into contact with them than would be true of stories. There are *some* signs in the community, and everyone must use them on occasion (e.g. "stop" signs). In addition, the potential usefulness of signs may be more readily demonstrable to the Indian children than that of stories. Thus classroom use of public signs and encouragement by teachers in learning how to read them in the early stages of teaching reading could be of greater interest to the children than the focus on stories.

This does not necessarily mean that classroom work with signs is optimally desirable in working with Warm Springs children. The main point here is that educators need more of the kind of information reported here than they typically have before they can determine what kind of literacy learning material would be most effective in the classroom. What kinds of written materials *do* Indian children see their kinsmen using, in what contexts, and for what purposes? It could be the labels on cans, the comic books of older siblings, western adventure or true romance magazines, or mail-order catalogues. What kinds of literacy skills do the children's parents want them to have? What do they see as useful skills that they themselves lack? Probably the Warm Springs tribal member who has been repeatedly fined by the police for driving without a license, because the unreadability of the test he would have to pass to get the license makes him avoid the test completely, does not want his children to have to experience the same thing. In a situation like that of Warm Springs, then, efforts can be made to design programs that build on current local uses of literacy, and on current needs—not on presupposed uses that are in fact nonexistant.

To speak in terms that are more generally applicable to a wide range of circumstances, I maintain that there is a strong need to acquire the kind of information presented here before efforts are made to design literacy programs. It is necessary to know the communicative needs of a community and the people's attitudes toward appropriate uses of various modes of communication for various purposes, if reading and writing are to find their place in a community's—or a nation's—communicative repertoire. Above all, it is necessary for the outsider who is asked to share his special literacy skills to determine to the best of his ability what the people's goals with regard to literacy are and to carry out those goals he learns to respect, rather than to maintain an outsider's notions of what those goals should be and imposing them on the people.

References

Anastasio, A. Intergroup relations in the southern plateau. Unpublished doctoral dissertation, University of Chicago, 1955.

Basso, K. The ethnography of writing. In J. Sherzer and R. Bauman (Eds.), *Towards an ethnography of speaking.* Cambridge: Cambridge University Press, 1975.

Bernstein, B. A sociolinguistic approach to socialization; with some reference to educability. In J. Gumperz & D. Hymes (Eds.), *Directions in sociolinguistics.* New York: Holt, 1972, Pp. 465—497.

Blom, J-P., Gumperz, J. Social meaning in linguistic structures: Code-switching in Norway. In J. Gumperz & D. Hymes (Eds.), *Directions in sociolinguistics.* New York: Holt, 1972. Pp. 407—434.

Cazden, C. B., Hymes, D., & John, V. P. (Eds.) *The functions of language in the classroom.* New York: Teachers College Press, 1973.

Cazden, C. B., & John, V. P. (Editors). Learning in American Indian children, In *Styles of learning among American Indians: An outline for research.* Washington, D.C.: Center for Applied Linguistics, 1968.

Fishman, J. A. Sociolinguistics and the language problems of developing countries. In J. A. Fishman, C. A. Ferguson, & J. Das Gupta (Eds.), *Language problems of developing nations.* New York: Wiley, 1968.

Fishman, J. *Language in sociocultural change.* Stanford: Standord University Press, 1972.

French, D. H. Wasco-Wishram. In E. Spicer (Ed.), *Perspectives in American Indian culture change.* Chicago: Univ. of Chicago Press, 1961.

French, K. Culture segments and variation in contemporary social ceremonialism on the Warm Springs Reservation, Oregon. Unpublished doctoral dissertation, Columbia University, 1955.

Goody, J. Introduction. In J. Goody (Ed.), *Literacy in traditional societies.* London & New York: Cambridge Univ. Press. 1968.

Goody, J., & Watt, I. The consequences of literacy. In J. Goody (Ed.), *Literacy in traditional societies.* London & New York: Cambridge Univ. Press, 1968.

Gumperz, J. Introduction. In J. Gumperz & D. Hymes (Eds.), *Directions in sociolinguistics.* New York: Holt, 1972. Pp. 1—25.

Hymes, D. Two types of linguistic relativity: Some examples from Amerindian ethnography. In W. Bright (Ed.), *Sociolinguistics.* The Hague: Mouton, 1966.

Hymes, D. Linguistic method in ethnography. In P. L. Garvin (Ed.), *Method and theory in linguistics*. The Hague: Mouton, 1970.

Hymes, D. Breakthrough into performance. In K. S. Goldstein (Ed.), *Folklore as communication. Semiotica*, 1972, Spec. Issue.

Hymes, D. On the origins and foundations of inequality among speakers, *Daedalus* 1973, *102*, (3), 59—86.

Kochman, T. Orality and literacy as factors of "black" and "white" communicative behavior. University of Illinois, Unpublished manuscript.

Ladov, W. *Language in the inner city*. Philadelphia: University of Pennsylvania Press, 1974.

Philips, S. Acquisition of rules for appropriate speech usage. In *Monograph series on languages and linguistics* Georgetown University, 1970, No. 23, 77—96.

Ray, V. *Cultural relations in the plateau of northwestern America*. Publications of the F. W. Hodge Anniversary Publication Fund, Vol. III. Los Angeles: Southwest Museum, 1939.

Zentner, H. *Warm Springs research project. Vol. II. Education*. Corvallis: Oregon State College, 1960.

23. On Written Language: Its Acquisition and Its Alexic-Agraphic Disturbances

E. Weigl

The focus of this chapter is on the basic rules that relate written language to oral language, discussed particularly by Bierwisch (1972). Of particular interest are their acquisition during childhood, the mastery of reading and writing during maturity, and the preservation of these basic rules even in cases of severe alexia and agraphia. The brain correlates of written language are discussed and are related to the theory of functional cerebral systems proposed by Vygotsky and his students, in conjunction with Lenneberg's conceptualization of language acquisition and brain maturation.

Introduction

The acquisition and the mastery of written language, in both receptive and expressive reading, as well as the different forms of writing (spontaneous, to dictation, copying), is an extraordinarily complex process. The study of the neuropsychological and psycholinguistic preconditions of this sort of human transfer of information is still in its infancy, in comparison with the study of spoken language. Important preliminary work has been done in this direction through psychological research into normal reading and writing[1] and into alexia and agraphia (Hécaen, Angelergues, & Douzenis, 1963; Leischner, 1957; Luria, 1950, 1970); recently contributions have also been made from the side of linguistics and psycholinguistics

---

[1] For a general survey, see Kainz (1956); see also in Hiebsch, Klix & Vorwerg (1957), particularly articles by Galperin, Kostjuk, and Luria.

(Bierwisch, 1972, Fries, 1964; Gibson, Pick, Osser, & Hammond, 1969; Schlesinger, 1968). Another source of insight into the processes underlying the acquisition of written language is our centuries-old experience with teaching reading and writing. In this chapter we shall discuss a number of basic psycholinguistic and neuropsychological aspects of the acquisition and mastery of written language, as well as the relevant sequelae to brain damage.

Psycholinguistic Aspects

Our form of writing, with its many letters and combinations of letters, as well as its various type faces, constitutes a signal system complete in itself and, with respect to its structure, entirely distinct from spoken language. The individual characters may be analyzed in terms of a limited number of basic elements (stroke, arch, loop, etc.; Eden, 1961), whose combination makes it possible to produce any character of the alphabet. The combination of these basic elements does not occur randomly, but is governed by rules (Bierwisch, 1972). Both visual perception and writing depend on the efficiency of these basic rules.

These structural rules of written language are not related in any way to factors of spoken language. Their acquisition is truly independent, and is by no means facilitated by the earlier acquisition of spoken language. It would, however, be impossible to acquire written language merely by learning letters and their combinations. Written language can be learned only as a consequence of the rule-governed correspondence between graphic and acoustic structures.

We are indebted to recent psycholinguistic investigations for important contributions to our understanding of the functional relationships between graphic and sound structures. Gibson (*et al.*, 1969), investigating psychological problems, and Bierwisch (1972), making a linguistic analysis, were both able to show that the relationships between written and spoken language may be characterized, for any letter-writing system whatever, in terms of grapheme—phoneme correspondence rules. However, owing to the lack of an isomorphism between sound and written structures, there is no one-to-one correspondence between phonemes and graphemes. The graphic unit for reading and writing processes is not the individual letter, but letter clusters; each graphic unit stands in a specific, invariant, context-dependent relationship to a phonological unit, either phonemic or phonetic.

The exceptions to the rules are determined by lexical entries that indicate graphemic idiosyncracies (Bierwisch, 1972). Information of this sort in the lexicon is necessary in all those cases where the grapheme—phoneme correspondence rules fail to specify the graphemic structure. This is particularly true for the many graphemic ambiguities (word pairs such as *raze—raise, beach—beech, altar—alter, sign—sine*). In contrast to those graphemic structures that are assignable to phonemic structures according to specifiable rules and that therefore need no lexical entries, such graphemic irregularities must be specifically noted in the lexicon (and therefore marked accordingly in long-term memory). Although phonemically ambiguous words are rarer, those that occur also require specific entries—for example, pairs such as *read* (present) and *read* (past); *permit* (noun) and *permit* (verb); *concrete* (noun) and *concrete* (adjective).[2]

A graphemic ambiguity such as *raise—raze* must be taken into account by the hearer, the writer, and the receptive reader. On the other hand, when reading aloud, one must disregard these ambiguities as the graphemic input is recorded into the corresponding articulatory pattern.

It is impossible to attribute to written language a syntax and lexicon that is independent of spoken language. Written language assumes mastery of the phonology, morphology, syntax, and lexicon of its respective natural language. (A similar point of view has been expressed by Vygotsky, 1964.) This means that knowledge of the grammar of a given language (Chomsky's (1965) *competence*) is also at the basis of the written performance—competence in oral language is an integral part of written language. Nevertheless, written language includes, in addition, the grapheme—phoneme correspondence rules; it therefore seems reasonable to regard competence in written language as *augmented* competence.

Neuropsychological Aspects

An important part of developmental neuropsychology is the study of the biological prerequisites, particularly those of a morphological and neurophysiological nature, for the acquisition of higher psychic functions. Important beginnings of such research have been discussed by Lenneberg (1967), especially in connection with the ontogenesis of the capacity for language acquisition. As a preliminary for the eventual discovery of neuroanatomical and neurophysiological correlates of language acquisition, Lenneberg proposes the study of all of those changes that take place in man's brain during and after the "critical period" for language acquisition. (At the same time, he is correct in cautioning us not to deduce causal relationships between the observed biological data and language acquisition.) "It is not so much one or the other specific aspect of the brain that must be held responsible for the capacity of language acquisition but the way the many parts of the brain interact. Thus it is mode of function rather than specific structures that must be regarded as the proper neurological correlate of language [Lenneberg, 1967, p. 170]."

In this respect, Lenneberg approaches, in my opinion, the point of view expressed by Vygotsky and his disciples, Leontiev, Luria, Galperin, Shinkin, and others, who maintain that one must understand the development of the higher psychic functions in general, and language in particular, as the result of integration of functional cerebral systems. According to this view, the specific and differentiated cortical zones begin to interact and form cerebral systems during the course of ontogenesis, a process based on the child's communication with his environment

---

[2]For these examples I am indebted to M. Bierwisch. Examples in German are: *malen—mahlen; Stil—Stiel; Seite—Saite; Weise—Waise; Hexe—Kleckse;* etc.

and facilitated by the interaction of sensory and motor functions. The Russian neuropsychologists refer to this as the system-specific character of higher cortical functions and their dynamic localization.[3]

In the course of oral or written language performances, many processes come together, particularly cognitive processes such as acoustic and optic perception, language comprehension, memory, inner speech, and also motor processes for speech production and reproduction. The complexity of the linguistic task, in which all of these become integrated, gives us an idea of the close and complex network of intracerebral connections. Since oral language comes prior to written language, we must assume that the execution of the latter requires further cerebral zones that must become integrated with those already engaged in oral language. Thus processes of the temporal lobe play a certain role in writing to dictation because of the verboauditory components of the latter. The premotor and sensory-motor segments of the cortex also enter into the task of reading aloud. Spontaneous, voluntary speech and writing are related to prefrontal cortical areas (Luria, 1970), etc.[4] Thus the cortical areas involved in reading and writing are larger than those involved in oral language.

Once established, the higher psychic processes function differently from the way they functioned during the formative period. Whereas during acquisition various functional cerebral systems interacted, there is a gradual reduction in this functional complexity once a certain degree of mastery has been attained. Certain intracerebral connections are no longer needed once the function is perfected; however, such connections continue to be potentially available and may be reactivated in case of need. Vygotsky regards this type of modification in the interfunctional relationships as the most important aspect of psychological development (Vygotsky, 1964, p. 148). This notion of reduction in functions is of particular importance in understanding the transition from the learning phase to the mature stage of mastery of written language. This can be illustrated by consideration of the processes of acquisition and automatization of comprehension, reproduction, and production of graphemic structures.

In the course of the acquisition of reading and writing, several aspects of oral language are involved, including the auditory perception of phonemic structures (the teacher pronounces the written word) and their reproduction (the pupil articulates the word that he has heard and seen). At a later phase, the pupil himself must produce the sound pattern of the words he has learned to write, either by saying them to himself (inner speech) or by reading them aloud. Phonemic structures

[3] For hypothetical formulations of code learning see Bruner (1967), who demonstrated relationships between perception, motor coordination, and linguistic rules in the human infant. Bruner regards the active cognitive integration of experience as most important for development. Experiments on problem solving in which subjects must discover certain rules are only indirectly relevant to our topic. The same is true of concept-formation experiments. However, some of the theoretical models proposed in connection with problem-solving and concept-formation experiments might be profitably related also to the interrelation of distinctive features and categorization and generalization processes (see Duncker, 1963; Klix, 1971; other references may be found in Smith & Miller, 1966).

[4] For further details and bibliography, see Luria (1970, Chapter I).

are paired with graphemic structures (as soon as the student has learned these correspondences, he will "know" the meaning of the words).[5] A similar process is at work during the acquisition of writing.[6]

In short, acquisition of written language requires the construction of a chain of interacting functions; a number of recoding processes are required between the various sensory modalities and the processes of inner speech and of the grapho-motoric stereotypes. The latter may become complicated through feedback systems of an auditory and optic nature.[7] During the transition from reading or writing single words to reading or writing whole sentences, syntactic processes also begin to play a role.

In school, certain paradoxes may occur; a word that is well-known to the student may not be read correctly because he is fixed on individual letters, and thus the word or sentence may lose its identity. This happens when reading comprehension is preceded and overtaken by the recoding of grapheme to morpheme, which leads to reading without understanding, to wrong accentuation and intonation, and so forth.

Later, reading becomes more automated, and the various recoding processes become reduced. The role of phonology is reduced to a minimum; it is no longer necessary to hear the words as internal speech or by manifest articulation in order to understand what is being read. Experiments (Sokolov, 1967; Weigl, 1964; Weigl, Böttcher, Lander, & Metze, 1971; and others) have shown that reading comprehension is not impaired by suppression of articulatory movements. This means that the semantic decoding of graphemic structures may take place immediately after optic perception and without a deviation via oral language. However, when difficulties in meaning arise, one falls back on phonological aids (Sokolov, 1968). The same is true of writing.

It is sufficient to understand a word in order to reproduce it graphically. Normally in this process there is no strict copying, no direct transcription, but an immediate recoding according to the sense and content. Ordinarily, we are unconscious of motoric control when writing. However, this reduction of consciousness may vary with the difficulty of the material to be written (for instance, the beginnings and ends of sentences, new paragraphs, punctuation, etc.). The free flow of writing processes requires the programming of a particular graphic picture and the evocation of a correlated pattern of innervation that will control the movements of the writing hand. In view of the little need for concentration during automatic writing, and the rather high speed at which it is done, the following questions

---

[5] During primary education in reading, the phonological relations are further supplemented by pictorial material.

[6] In this connection, Nasarova's (1955) investigations on coarticulation during the learning of writing are of importance. The author showed that a child's writing task becomes more difficult if he is forced to write with wide-open mouth and protruding tongue. Under these circumstances the incidence of writing mistakes increases appreciably. Thus written reproduction is facilitated by simultaneous speech movements; inhibition of these movements produces encoding difficulties.

[7] See Weigl et al. (1971) for the distinctions between inner and outer speech, prearticulation and latent and manifest articulation.

arise. Is there a new programming for every writing act and a new synthesis of graphomotoric impulses, or does the writing act proceed by means of the realization of stored motor stereotypes (cf. Luria, 1970, p. 140, who speaks of kinesthetic engrams). If the latter, are these stereotypes limited to graphemes or words, or do they comprise structural sequences (syntagmata)? What is the relationship of the grapheme—phoneme correspondence rules to the graphomotoric stereotypes? Only future research can answer these questions.

Reduction in the area of psychic functions is important in the case of oral and written language because it implies a substantial reduction of the original tasks necessary for such activities. This results in a noticeable liberation of certain cerebral functional systems. The greater the independence of receptive reading from oral manifestations, the faster and the more immediately may the processes of semantic decoding act. Reduction of the dependence on oral language does not imply an abandonment of the relations that were built up in the course of learning. As the difficulty of the material increases, the subject may return to their use. That they are not abandoned is particularly well illustrated by the normal person's ability to read nonsense words aloud—words he pronounces correctly, but for which there are no meanings. Similarly, a normal person can write nonsense words correctly from dictation.

As a consequence of the completed development of the higher psychic functions, relatively autonomous partial systems take shape, which, despite their integration into the whole system, may operate quite independently from one another (Weigl, 1969, 1972). Such an autonomy is also evident in the various forms of oral and written language, where comprehension and speaking, receptive and expressive reading, copying, writing to dictation, and so forth, become quite independent. We shall return to this independence when discussing pathological conditions, which illustrate the point dramatically.

The field of alexia and agraphia can serve as a proving ground for the validation of various hypotheses on the nature of graphemes and syntactic-semantic relationships and their respective psychological realities. On the other hand, the neuropsychological analysis of reading and writing disturbances raises a number of basic problems that require a new set of psycholinguistic hypotheses (Weigl & Bierwisch, 1970). In this connection, language competence is a central problem in cases of alexia and agraphia. We have postulated (Weigl & Bierwisch, 1970) that competence is not "lost" even in severe cases of aphasic disturbances. We have furnished a number of arguments in support of this view based on aphasiological investigations. Of special importance were the following facts: even total aphasia may be completely or partially reversed; further, losses are usually confined to specific performances, such as comprehension or production; and finally, it is possible to "de-block" aphasic interferences, and so forth (Weigl, 1961, 1968). Such facts make it unlikely that language disturbances are due to interference with the basic rules that govern verbal behavior.

A discussion of the problem of competence is of particular practical and theoretical importance when it comes to understanding cerebral language disorders.

As shown by Lenneberg (1967), there are temporal limitations imposed upon the effortless acquisition of language during childhood, which are conditioned by maturational processes of the brain and cerebral lateralization. During the "critical period" of language acquisition, the immature brain has the capacity, to acquire the competence, that is the knowledge of the basic rules, and to store them, processes that occur spontaneously and are based on generalization and classification procedures. We agree with Lenneberg that at the close of the critical period, the human brain is no longer able to accomplish this.

If language competence were lost in the case of aphasia, the patient would be faced with the task of forming de novo the respective basic rules, despite his damaged cortex. This would imply that language could, in fact, be reacquired from the start, which is precisely what is frequently attempted in the course of rehabilitation training. In view of the limited period of brain maturation, such an assumption is neuropsychologically untenable. We are in agreement with a number of authors (e.g., Lenneberg, 1967; Wepman, 1951; and to a certain degree also Luria, Vinarskaya, Naydin, & Tsvetkova, 1969; and others) that the objective of aphasia therapy should not be a fresh start in primary language acquisition but, in contrast, should aim at reactualization of disturbed forms of language. We have been confirmed in this view by the results of our own research on de-blocking, which we cannot discuss here (Weigl, 1961, 1968, 1969). Suffice it to say that it is possible to couple successively the use of specific intact modalities and thus reactualize language usage that had been blocked. Our success implies that competence remains basically intact despite the partial disturbance of certain modalities, and this confirms the psychological reality of our assumptions. Our most recent experience with de-blocking has shown that severely disturbed language functions may be rehabilitated and that the patient may regain the capacity for making syntactic transformations (as demonstrated by Irina Weigl (see E. Weigl & Bierwisch, 1970; Böttcher, Metze, & I. Weigl, 1969); these accomplishments do not signify de novo acquisition but are reactualizations of stored basic grammatical rules.

However, there are some additional problems of competence in the area of written language that are not easily solved. As already mentioned, competence underlying written language is augmented relative to the competence underlying oral language. It is conceivable that in the case of alexia and agraphia, precisely this augmentation is affected and the storage of the graphemic—phonemic correspondences is thus compromised. There is no question that one must treat the problem of competence for writing separately from that of competence for speaking. In this connection, it is particularly important that reading and writing can be learned after cerebral maturation is complete; therefore, perhaps, the rules governing these later acquisitions are more labile and more subject to pathological interference than are the basic rules of language.

The main evidence that would support such a view would be the existence of patients who have lost all aspects of written language—that is, a combination of alexia and agraphia—but whose oral language has been completely spared.

However, such patients are extremely rare. Insofar as they do exist, one could argue that only the superstructure of additional rules for reading and writing has been affected. Such an hypothesis would never do for any of the other cases of alexia and agraphia, since in these cases—the vast majority—only one or the other form suffers. When losses are selective, we may not attribute them to interference with "augmented competence."[8] Moreover, alexic and agraphic disturbances may fluctuate considerably, and they are invariably amenable to de-blocking.

From the foregoing, it is evident that the majority of the aphasic, alexic, and agraphic disturbances must be regarded as a limitation of one or more aspects of performance. But how can this happen? What is the meaning in this case of selective aspects of performance? The short-sighted explanations in terms of cerebral localization can hardly be considered appropriate. Most aphasiologists are unanimous in believing that specific, localized cerebral lesions are not sufficient cause for selected losses in the presence of otherwise intact language functions. No doubt concepts such as "disturbance of a fundamental nature" (Goldstein) or "disturbances in the mode of action of given factors" (Luria—for instance, simultaneity or sequence; Lenneberg speaks of timing factors) are more suggestive. Nevertheless, it seems to us that the assumption of autonomous partial systems gets us still a step closer to a solution of the problem.

If it is correct that during the automation of certain functions there is a reduction in the interaction of various partial systems which had to interact during acquisition, then it is possible that these systems might become "protected" as they become independent one from another; this then may clarify the nature of selected losses. In other words, the more autonomous a given partial system, the less likely would an interference of that system implicate other, even related systems, provided, naturally, that the common competence remains intact. Thus it becomes understandable that limitations of comprehension in oral language need not affect comprehension in written language (acoustic sensory aphasia with receptive alexia) or that a patient with a motor aphasia may be able to read out loud correctly, etc.

In view of the problem of localized lesions, the following hypothesis may not be unreasonable. Circumscribed disturbances of partial systems due to circumscribed cerebral lesions can occur only after reduction and automatization have taken place. In contrast to this are the results of lesions during childhood, at which time functions are in the process of acquisition and establishment, requiring the interaction of all of the partial systems at the same time, together with their respective cerebral structures and cerebral interconnections.[9] During this period, there should be a very low probability that focal cortical lesions would produce selective dis-

---

[8] Among 50 aphasic patients of various types examined by us, there was only one in whom every function of spoken language (on the level of words) was intact, whereas receptive and expressive reading and copying were practically abolished. But even in this case, there was one graphic capacity that was almost completely spared—writing to dictation.

[9] See Vygotsky (1965) and Luria (1970, p. 55) on the different consequences of cerebral lesions upon psychological functions at various developmental stages.

turbances. Of course, this hypothesis must be further verified on appropriate clinical material.

We propose a further hypothesis: disorders of written language due to cerebral lesions (alexia and agraphia) should have different symptomatology depending on whether the skills were acquired during infancy or adulthood; the augmented competence should be less susceptible to interference in the former case than in the latter.

I should like to conclude this discussion of the neuropsychological problems of central disturbances of written language by reporting on some results of research on 50 aphasic patients of different types, undertaken in collaboration with my Romanian colleagues A. Fradis, L. Mihăilescu, and N. Gheorghiţă (for the methodology of this work see Weigl, 1966)—and by interpreting these results in the light of the problem of the grapheme–phoneme correspondence rules.

To determine whether our alexic patients still had the necessary optical and cognitive prerequisites for the tasks of reading and writing, we asked them to select identical written letters from a long series of letters. Of the thirteen patients with partial or total receptive alexia, eleven were able to select these correctly. This means that despite their alexia, they had no disturbance in form perception.

In another experiment, we tried to determine whether the grapheme–phoneme correspondence rules were still effective among the alexic patients when semantics was excluded. We asked the patients to select equivalent words that were written in different type faces. In five cases of total or severe receptive alexia, the patients were able to perform the task correctly, even though they were unable to understand any of the meanings. Also, my collaborators, R. Böttcher and Irina Weigl, were able to demonstrate the same thing on other patients with definite receptive alexia.

Unquestionably, the significance of these results is less obvious than may at first appear. A certain invariance must exist, which enables correct identification of the written structures in the absence of semantic correspondences. The only common denominator in these different type faces is their relationship to their phonological values. The proper performance of this identification task by our patients serves as proof of the psychological reality of the grapheme–phoneme relationships and their respective transformational rules.

In another set of experiments, we examined patients who were alexic and suffered from acoustic-sensory aphasia. There were 11 patients who presented with both receptive alexia and word deafness. Different words were spoken to these patients, who then had to identify one of these words from a series of written words in front of them. Although they were unable to understand the words in either their auditory or their optic form, six patients were able to make correct identifications in about 75—100% of the cases (there were 20 words for each (see Weigl, 1974). In this case, the correct matching in the absence of semantic understanding in either the acoustic or the graphic form could have been due only to the effective operation of the grapheme–phoneme correspondence rules, which, according to these findings, were apparently not affected.

Our method of de-blocking offers a further opportunity for the study of the relationship between written and oral language. It is possible to de-block disturbed reading comprehension (receptive alexia) by first having the patient repeat orally given words and sentences or by having him copy the material or write it from dictation; the naming of the objects also helps; finally, a coupling of the remaining spared functions is brought about (Weigl, 1968, 1969). In these tasks, one deals not only with the graphemic-phonemic aspects, but also with semantic ones. At first, we believed that the results of these de-blocking procedures were due only to the channeling of intact semantic models through different avenues. We must now add to this assumption; the semantic accomplishments have as prerequisites the intact operation of the grapheme—phoneme correspondence rules.

A final remark. In this article, I have tried to bring some neuropsycholinguistic views to bear upon written language. I was most anxious to demonstrate the close relationships that exist between psychology, linguistics, and medical brain research (see also Weigl, 1972; Weigl & Bierwisch, 1970). I trust I will be excused for the shortcomings of this chapter, which are due to lack of space; in particular, the discussion on the level of sentences has been shortchanged (for amplification, see Weigl, 1972).[10]

References

Bierwisch, M. Schriftstruktur und Phonologie. *Probleme und Ergebnisse der Psychologie*, 1972, *43*, 21–44.

Böttcher, R., Metze, E., & Weigl, I. Untersuchungen der Beziehungen zwischen intakten und hirnpathologisch beeinträchtigten psychischen Funktionen im Dienste der Erforschung und Rehabilitierung aphasischer Störungen. *Probleme und Ergebnisse der Psychologie*, 1969, *28/29*, 103–113.

Bruner, J. S. *Toward a theory of instruction*. Cambridge, Mass.: Harvard Univ. Press, 1967.

Chomsky, N. *Aspects of the theory of syntax*. Cambridge, Mass.: MIT Press, 1965.

Duncker, K. *Zur Psychologie des produktiven Denkens*. Berlin & New York: Springer-Verlag, 1963.

Eden, M. On the formalization of handwriting. In R. Jakobson (Ed.), *Structure of language in its mathematical aspect*. Providence, R.I.: Amer, Math. Soc., 1961.

Fries, C. C. *Linguistics and reading*. New York, Holt, 1964.

Gibson, E. J., Pick, A., Osser, H., & Hammond, M. The role of grapheme-phoneme-correspondence in the perception of words. In J. P. De Cecco (Ed.), *The psychology of language, thought, and instruction*. New York: Holt, 1969.

Hécaen, H., Angelergues, R., & Douzenis, J. A. Les agraphies. *Neuropsychologia* 1963, *1*, 179.

Hiebsch, H., Klix, F. & Vorwerg, M. (Eds.). *Ergebnisse der sowjetischen Psychologie*. Berlin: Akademie-Verlag, 1967.

Kainz, F. *Psychologie der Sprache*. Vol. 4. Stuttgart: Enke, 1956.

Klix, F. *Information und Verhalten*. Berlin: VEB Deutscher Verlag der Wissenschaften, 1971.

Leischner, A. *Die Störungen der Schriftsprache (Aphasie und Alexie)*. Stuttgart: Thieme, 1957.

Lenneberg, E. H. *Biological foundations of language*. New York: Wiley, 1967.

[10] *Editor's note*: Parts of Professor Weigl's original article had to be omitted by the editors because of overlap with other chapters in this volume. The interested reader should consult the expanded German version, published in 1972.

Luria, A. R. *Zur Psychologie des Schreibens*. Moscow: APW Verlag, 1950. [In Russian.]

Luria, A. R. *Die höheren kortikalen Funktionen des Menschen und ihre Störungen bei örtlichen Hirnschädigungen*. Berlin: VEB Deutscher Verlag der Wissenschaften, 1970.

Luria, A. R., Vinarskaya, E. N., Naydin, V. L. & Tsvetkova, L. S. Restoration of higher cortical functions. In P. Vinken & G. de Bruyn (Eds.), *Handbook of clinical neurology*. Vol. 3. Amsterdam, 1969.

Nasarova, L. K. Die Rolle der kinästhetischen Sprechweise beim Schreiben. [In Russian.] In *Beiträge zur Anwendung der Lehre Pawlows auf Fragen des Unterrichts*. Berlin: Volk und Wissen Volkseigener Verlag, 1955.

Schlesinger, I. M. *Sentence structure and the reading process*. The Hague: Mouton, 1968.

Smith, F. S., & Miller, G. A. (Eds.) *The genesis of language; A psycholinguistic approach*. Cambridge, Mass.: MIT Press, 1966.

Sokolov, A. N. Untersuchungen zum Problem der sprachlichen Mechanismen des Denkens. In *Ergebnisse der sowjetischen Psychologie* Hiebsch, H., Klix, F. & Vorwerg, M. (Eds.). Berlin: Akademie-Verlag, 1967.

Sokolov, A. N. *Inner speech and thought*. Moscow: Verlag für Pädagogik, 1968. [In Russian.]

Vygotsky, L. S. *Sprache und Denken*. Berlin: Akademie-Verlag, 1964.

Vygotsky, L. S. Psychology and localisation of functions. *Neuropsychologia*, 1965, *3*, 381—386.

Weigl, E. The phenomenon of temporary deblocking in aphasia. *Zeitschrift für Phonetik, Sprachwissenschaft und Kommunikationsforschung*, 1961, *14*, 337—364.

Weigl, E. Die Bedeutung der afferenten, verbo-kinästhetischen Erregungen des Sprachapparates für die expressiven und rezeptiven Sprachvorgänge bei Normalen und Sprachgestörten. *Cortex*, 1964, *1*, 77—90.

Weigl, E. On the construction of standard psychological tests in cases of brain damage. *Journal of Neurological Sciences*, 1966, *3*, 123—127.

Weigl, E. On the problem of cortical syndromes. In M. L. Simmel (Ed.), *The reach of mind: Essays in the memory of Kurt Goldstein*. New York: Springer, 1968.

Weigl, E. Beiträge zur neuropsychologischen Grundlagenforschung. *Probleme und Ergebnisse der Psychologie*, 1969, *28/29*, 87—102.

Weigl, E. Zur Schriftsprache und ihrem Erwerb; Neuropsychologische und psycholinguistische Betrachtungen. *Probleme und Ergebnisse der Psychologie*, 1972, *43*, 45—105.

Weigl, E. Neuropsychological experiments on transcoding between spoken and written language structures. *Brain and Language*, 1974, *1*, 227—240.

Weigl, E., & Bierwisch, M. Neuropsychology and linguistics: Topics and common research. *Foundations of Language*, 1970, *6*, 1—18.

Weigl, E., Böttcher, R., Lander, H.-J., & Metze, E. Neuropsychologische Methoden zur Analyse der Funktionen und Komponenten sprachfunktionaler Teilsysteme, Ein Beitrag zum Problem der inneren und äusseren Sprache. *Zeitschrift für Psychologie*, 1971, *179*, 444—494.

Wepman, J. *Recovery from aphasia*. New York: Ronald Press, 1951.

Subject Index

sensory, 22—26, 60, 198
spatial orientation in, 99—100
speech areas in, 21—29
speech and thought in, 102—103
subclassification in, 5
types of, 22
verbal transformation in, 87
Aphasic language, versus normal language, 76
Aphasic neologisms, 85
Aphasic speech, amobarbital and, 109—110,
   see also Aphasic language; Aphasic transformations
Aphasic transformations, 75—93
   articulation level in, 78
   basic operations in, 82—83
   computer analysis of, 90—91
   dyssyntactic, 88
   examples of, 81—82
   phonemic paraphasias and, 84—85
Aphasiology, 1
   brain in, 4—6
   electrophysiological data in, 11—13
   as science, 3—9
   symptomatology in, 7—9
Apraxia, 117—119
   aphasia and, 119—125
   constructional, 117, 119, 122
   defined, 97, 117
   hemispheric dominance in, 119—120
   ideational, 117—118, 121
   ideomotor, 118, 122
   "programming," 117
Apraxia for dressing, 119
Articulation defects, 209
Articulation tests, 201—205
Articulation, three levels of, 78
Association cortex, 14
Asymmetrical space, in brain lesions, 69—70
Athetosis, language processing in, 265
Atresia, choanal, 231
Attitude, defined, 298
Autism, symptoms and speech defects in,
   241—242

B

Babbling
   by deaf baby, 150—151
   speech development through, 149
Behavior, neurophysiology of,
Bilingualism, 358—359
Blind child

compared with sighted child, 188—192
   I/Me usage in, 178—180, 191
   observations of, 177—192
   self-image of, 179—192
Blindness, 135ff.
Brain, *see also* Left hemisphere; Right hemisphere
   cerebral hemisphere maturation in, 107—114
   dominance in, 21, 112—113
   electrophysiological data on, 11—13
   hemispheric involvement and, 107—109,
      112—113
   information storage in, 138
   lateralization in, 13—14, 247—248
   networks in, 12—13
   "plasticity" of, 14
   speech and, 4, 12, 21—29, 126, 139
   "splitting" of, 108—109
   tissue destruction in, 10—11
   in written language acquisition, 385—386
Brain damage, *see also* Brain lesions
   aphasia and, 23
   bilateral, 23
   thinking and, 170
Brain function
   nature of, 4
Brain lesions
   amnesic aphasia and, 32—33
   apraxia and, 120
   asymmetric space and, 69—70
   grammatical structure and, 67—68
   language and, 11, 14
   literal paraphasia and, 60
   music and, 97—98
   pantomime impairment and, 95
   pathological changes in, 59
   plasticity and, 14, 17
   right hemisphere and, 107—108
   speech and, 5, 65, 70, 95, 112
   vocabulary changes and, 59
Brain tissue
   destruction of, 10—11
   electrical stimulation of, 12
Broca's area, 4, 12
   speech stabilization and, 21—29
Bureau of Indian Affairs, 372

C

Central deafness, 252
Cerebral cortex, *see also* Left hemisphere;
      Right hemisphere
   language and, 15—18